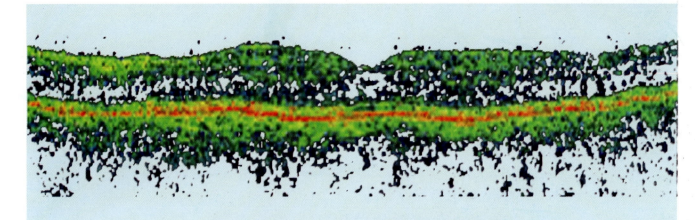

Optical Coherence Tomography

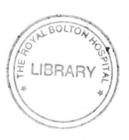

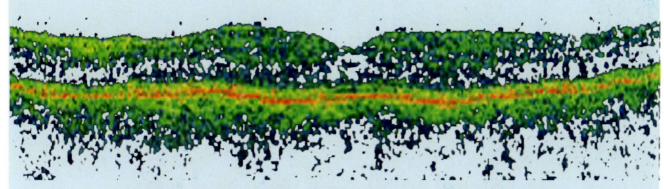

Optical Coherence Tomography

Editors

Sandeep Saxena

Fellow, Barnes Retina Institute and Anheuser Busch Eye Institute, St. Louis, USA
Fellow, New York-Presbyterian Hospital, New York, USA
Visiting Professor, University of North Carolina at Chapel Hill, Chapel Hill, USA

Associate Professor, Department of Ophthalmology
King George's Medical University, Lucknow, India

Travis A Meredith

Sterling A Barrett Distinguished Professor
Chairman, Department of Ophthalmology
University of North Carolina at Chapel Hill, Chapel Hill, USA

Foreword
Stanley Chang

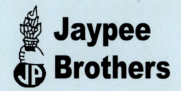

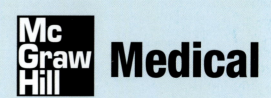

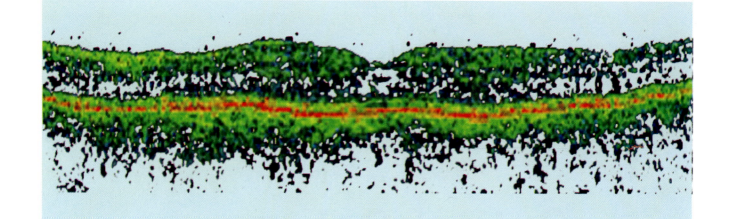

First published in India in 2008 by

Corporate Office
4838/24 Ansari Road, Daryaganj, **New Delhi** - 110002, India, +91-11-43574357

Registered Office
B-3 EMCA House, 23/23B Ansari Road, Daryaganj, **New Delhi** 110 002, India
Phones: +91-11-23272143, +91-11-23272703, +91-11-23282021,
+91-11-23245672, Rel: +91-11-32558559 Fax: +91-11-23276490, +91-11-23245683
e-mail: jaypee@jaypeebrothers.com, Visit our website: www.jaypeebrothers.com

First published in USA by The McGraw-Hill Companies, 2 Penn Plaza, New York, NY 10121.
Exclusively worldwide distributor except South Asia (India, Nepal, Sri Lanka, Bhutan, Pakistan,
Bangladesh, Malaysia).

ISBN-13: 978-0-07-160187-0
ISBN-10: 0-07-160187-2

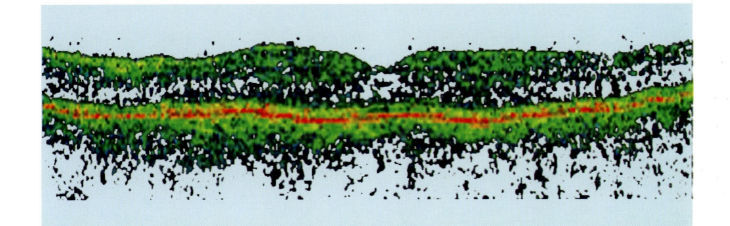

To
Our Family Members

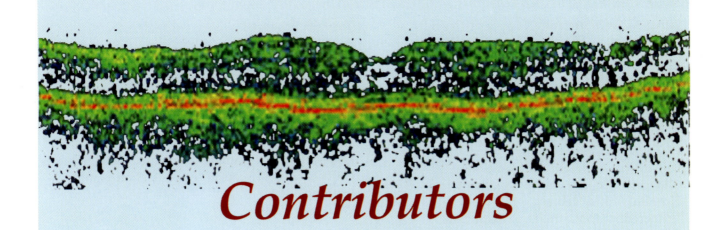

Contributors

Takayuki Baba MD
Department of Ophthalmology and Visual Science
Tokyo Medical and Dental University
Tokyo, Japan

Muna Bhende MS
Consultant, Vitreoretinal Service
Medical Research Foundation
Sankara Nethralaya, Chennai, India

Jyotirmay Biswas MS
Director, Uvea Department
Medical Research Foundation
Sankara Nethralaya, Chennai, India

A Boixadera MD
Vitreoretinal Department of Institut de
Microcirugia Ocular (IMO)
Barcelona, Spain

Borja F Corcostegui MD
Professor of Ophthalmology
Universitat Autonoma de Barcelona
Director of Institut de Microcirugia Ocular (IMO)
Barcelona, Spain

Gabriel Coscas MD, FEBO
Professor of Ophthalmology, University Paris XII
Creteil, France

Arno Doelemeyer PhD
Novartis Institutes for Biomedical Research
Basel, Switzerland

Kimberly A Drenser MD, PhD
Associated Retinal Consultants, PC
Royal Oak, USA

Wolfgang Drexler PhD
Associate Professor
Director, Christian Doppler Laboratory
Center for Biomedical Engineering and Physics
Medical University, Vienna, Austria

Ali Erginay MD
Hopital Lariboisiere
Paris, France

Erdem Ergun MD
Department of Ophthalmology
General Hospital of Vienna Medical University
Vienna, Austria

Marni Grage Feldmann MD
Department of Ophthalmology and Visual Sciences
University of Wisconsin, Wisconsin, USA

Sharon Fekrat MD, FACS
Associate Professor, Vitreoretinal Surgery
Albert Eye Research Institute
Duke University Eye Center, Duke University
Durham, USA

Adolf F Fercher PhD
Center for Biomedical Engineering and Physics
Christian Doppler Laboratory
Medical University Vienna, Vienna, Austria

James G Fujimoto PhD
Department of Electrical Engineering and
Computer Science and Research Laboratory of
Electronics
Massachusetts Institute of Technology
Cambridge, USA

Jose Garcia-Arumi MD
Professor of Ophthalmology
Universitat Autonoma de Barcelona
Chairman, Department of Ophthalmology
Hospital Vall d'Hebron
Vitreoretinal Department of Institut de
Microcirurgia Ocular (IMO)
Barcelona, Spain

Satpal Garg MD
Professor
Dr. Rajendra Prasad Centre for Ophthalmic
Sciences
All India Institute of Medical Sciences
New Delhi, India

Alain Gaudric MD
Professor of Ophthalmology, Universite Paris 7
Head of the Department of Ophthalmology,
Hopital Lariboisiere
Paris, France

Richard Hamilton MD
The Eye Institute
Medical College of Wisconsin
Milwaukee, USA

Andrea Hassenstein MD
Department of Ophthalmology
University Medical Center Hamburg-Eppendorf
Hamburg, Germany

Boris Hermann PhD
Center for Biomedical Engineering and Physics
Christian Doppler Laboratory
Medical University Vienna
Vienna, Austria

Tomohiro Iida MD
Professor and Chairman
Fukushima Medical University
Fukushima, Japan

Yasushi Ikuno MD
Assistant Professor
Department of Ophthalmology
Osaka University Medical School
Osaka, Japan

Michael S Ip MD
Associate Professor
Department of Ophthalmology and Visual Sciences
University of Wisconsin, Fundus Photograph
Reading Center
Wisconsin, USA

Yasuki Ito MD, PhD
Assistant Professor
Department of Ophthalmology
Nagoya University School of Medicine
Nagoya, Japan

Motohiro Kamei MD
Department of Ophthalmology
Osaka University Medical School
Osaka, Japan

Judy E Kim MD
Associate Professor
The Eye Institute
Medical College of Wisconsin
Milwaukee, USA

Tony H Ko PhD
Department of Electrical Engineering and
Computer Science and Research Laboratory of
Electronics
Massachusetts Institute of Technology
Cambridge, USA

Peter Kroll MD
Professor and Chairman
Department of Ophthalmology
Philipps-University Marburg
Marburg, Germany

Maurice B Landers III MD
Professor of Ophthalmology
Department of Ophthalmology
University of North Carolina at Chapel Hill
Chapel Hill, USA

Pascale Massin MD
Professor of Ophthalmology, Universite Paris 7
Hopital Lariboisiere
Paris, France

Carlos Mateo MD
Associate Professor of Ophthalmology
Universitat Autonoma de Barcelona
Vitreoretinal Department of Institut de
Microcirurgia Ocular (IMO)
Barcelona, Spain

Miguel A Materin MD
Oncology Service, Wills Eye Hospital
Thomas Jefferson University
Philadelphia, USA

Travis A Meredith MD
Professor and Chairman
Department of Ophthalmology
University of North Carolina at Chapel Hill
Chapel Hill, USA

Carsten H Meyer MD
Department of Ophthalmology
Philipps-University Marburg
Marburg, Germany

Keisuke Mori MD, PhD
Associate Professor of Ophthalmology
Department of Ophthalmology
Saitama Medical School
Saitama, Japan

Max Motta MD
Vitreoretinal Surgeon
Hospital de la Santa Creu i de Sant Pau
Universitat Autonoma de Barcelona
Barcelona, Spain

Bijoy K Nair MS
Vitreoretinal Service
Medical Research Foundation
Sankara Nethralaya
Chennai, India

Masahito Ohji MD
Professor and Chairman
Department of Ophthalmology
Shiga University of Medical Sciences
Seta Tsukinowa-cho, Otsu, Japan

Elzbieta Polska PhD
Novartis Institutes for Biomedical Research
Basel, Switzerland

Giuseppe Querques MD
Fellow
Creteil University Eye Clinic, University Paris XII
Creteil, France

Gisbert Richard MD
Professor and Head
Department of Ophthalmology
University Medical Center Hamburg-Eppendorf
Hamburg, Germany

Hirokazu Sakaguchi MD
Department of Ophthalmology
Osaka University Medical School
Osaka, Japan

Harald Sattmann PhD
Center for Biomedical Engineering and Physics
Christian Doppler Laboratory
Medical University Vienna
Vienna, Austria

Sandeep Saxena MS
Associate Professor
Department of Ophthalmology
King George's Medical University
Lucknow, India

Ulrich Schaudig MD
Department of Ophthalmology
University Medical Center Hamburg-Eppendorf
Hamburg, Germany

Christoph Scholda MD
Department of Ophthalmology
General Hospital of Vienna
Medical University Vienna
Vienna, Austria

Robert F See MD
Fellow, Vitreoretinal Surgery
Albert Eye Research Institute
Duke University Eye Center, Duke University
Durham, USA

Carol L Shields MD
Professor of Ophthalmology
Thomas Jefferson University
Co-Director/Attending Surgeon
Oncology Service, Wills Eye Hospital
Philadelphia, USA

Jerry A Shields MD
Professor of Ophthalmology
Thomas Jefferson University
Director, Oncology Service, Wills Eye Hospital
Philadelphia, USA

Gisèle Soubrane MD, PhD, FEBO
Professor of Ophthalmology
University Paris XII
Creteil, France

Eric H Souied MD, PhD
Assistant Professor
Creteil University Eye Clinic, University Paris XII
Creteil, France

Parul Sony MD
Dr. Rajendra Prasad Centre for Ophthalmic Sciences
All India Institute of Medical Sciences
New Delhi, India

Richard F Spaide MD
The Vitreous-Retina-Macula Consultants of
New York
New York, USA

Michael Stur MD
Department of Ophthalmology
General Hospital of Vienna
Medical University Vienna
Vienna, Austria

S Sudharshan DO
Uvea Department
Medical Research Foundation
Sankara Nethralaya
Chennai, India

Yasuo Tano MD
Professor and Chairman
Department of Ophthalmology
Osaka University Medical School
Osaka, Japan

Hiroko Terasaki MD, PhD
Professor and Chairperson
Department of Ophthalmology
Nagoya University School of Medicine
Nagoya, Japan

Michael T Trese MD
President, Associated Retinal Consultants, PC
Chief, Pediatric and Adult Vitreoretinal Surgery,
Beaumont Eye Institute
William Beaumont Hospital-Royal Oak
Clinical Professor of Biomedical Sciences, Eye
Research Institute,
Oakland University, Rochester, USA

Angelika Unterhuber PhD
Center for Biomedical Engineering and Physics
Christian Doppler Laboratory
Medical University Vienna
Vienna, Austria

Pradeep Venkatesh MD
Associate Professor
Dr. Rajendra Prasad Centre for Ophthalmic Sciences
All India Institute of Medical Sciences
New Delhi, India

Mathias Wirtitsch MD
Department of Ophthalmology
General Hospital of Vienna
Medical University Vienna
Vienna, Austria

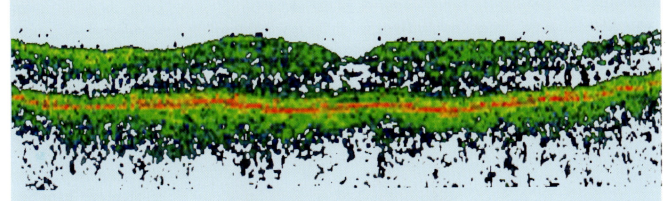

Foreword

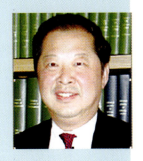

In less than a decade, Optical Coherence Tomography (OCT) has revolutionized the diagnosis of retinal and macular diseases. This technology is indispensable in providing quality patient care by expanding the clinical observations with a view of the retina with higher resolution than is appreciated by the human eye. Saxena and Meredith have edited a book that demonstrates both the qualitative and quantitative advantages of OCT as applied to the patterns of various retinal disorders. These disorders range from vitreoretinal interface disorders, such as epiretinal membranes and macular holes, to intrinsic disorders within the retina (macular edema), and choroidal processes. The authors are selected respected international authorities from both medical and surgical subdivisions of the retinal domain.

Optical coherence tomography has shown us the role of the vitreous in the evolution of macular holes and the masquerading processes that can sometimes be difficult to differentiate clinically. The postoperative confirmation of a successful anatomic outcome is often comforting to the patients who has maintained the prone position for prolonged periods of time, and would like to see the results of their diligence. In cystoid macular edema resulting from retinal vascular diseases, OCT is the best method for quantitatively assessing the outcome of any medical or intervention. It is a reliable, accurate and cost-effective in following patients who are being treated with systemic or local treatments for macular disease. In entities such as myopic foveoschisis, and macular anatomy after retinal detachment, OCT has added new information to the understanding of visual loss by revealing anatomical changes that were not visible by slit lamp biomicroscopy previously. Understanding the anatomic relationships at the vitreoretinal juncture allows development of a more effective surgical rationale.

It is encouraging that improvements in OCT technology continue to develop. Currently the axial resolution of 10 microns, and lateral resolution of 20 microns still make it difficult to separate layers within the retina. Higher resolutions shown by Dr. Drexler in this book, promise axial resolutions of 3 microns that demonstrate the different cellular layers within the retina. This will be a useful tool of studying *in vivo* the effects of vitreoretinal interface changes on the layers of cells within the retina, and final outcomes of surgical intervention on the retinal structure.

It is apparent that OCT has become the most useful non-invasive diagnostic modality. Expansion of this technology to glaucoma and the anterior segment is undoubtedly not far behind. This book summarizes the state of the art in practical and clinical aspects of OCT for retinal disorders. I congratulate Dr Saxena and Dr Meredith for compiling a most useful reference.

Stanley Chang MD
Edward S Harkness Professor and Chair
Department of Ophthalmology, New York-Presbyterian Hospital
Director
Edward S Harkness Eye Institute
Columbia University College of Physicians and Surgeons
New York, USA

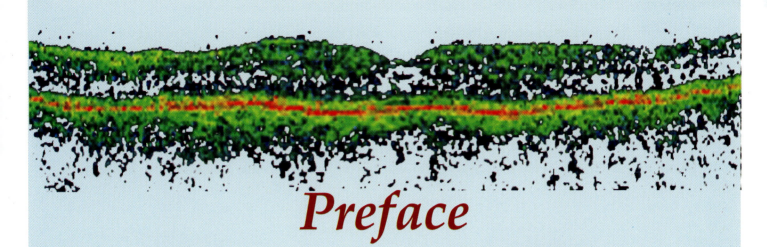

Preface

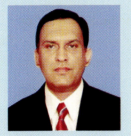

Sandeep Saxena

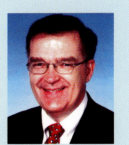

Travis A Meredith

Novel imaging technologies can improve not only the diagnosis and clinical management of retinal diseases but also the understanding of its pathogenesis. Therefore, they promise to have a significant impact in clinical practice and research. A need has existed in medicine for a technology capable of *optical biopsy*, imaging at or near the resolution of histopathology without excisional biopsy. In the past decade, advances in optics, fiber optics, and laser technology have led to the development of a noncontact, high-resolution optical biomedical imaging technology, called Optical Coherence Tomography. Optical coherence tomography achieves cross-sectional imaging of tissue by measuring the echo delay and intensity of back-reflected infrared light from internal tissue structures. Using a classic optical measurement technique known as low-coherence interferometry in combination with special broad-bandwidth light, optical coherence tomography achieves high-resolution cross-sectional visualization of tissue morphologic characteristics.

Optical coherence tomography is the best way of determining the anatomic effect of a treatment. It can be used to identify and quantify macular edema, and to measure retinal thickness changes in response to therapy. It helps in making clinical decisions and also in patient education and medical record documentation.

This book summarizes the present knowledge of optical coherence tomography in various medical and surgical management of diseases of retina. The value of this book lies in the clinical experience and expertise of the contributing authors.

Optical coherence tomography is the beginning of a new imaging revolution. New technology including ultrahigh resolution optical coherence tomography or combined optical coherence tomography and scanning laser ophthalmoscope technology or fusion technology of optical coherence tomography and ultrasonography will increase our insight into the pathophysiology of retinal disease, better define indications for surgery, help plan the operative procedure and assess the outcome.

This book would not have been possible without the untiring efforts of Ms Kay Walker of M/s Jaypee Brothers Medical Publishers, New Delhi also deserve special mention for an excellent publication effort.

Sandeep Saxena
Travis A Meredith

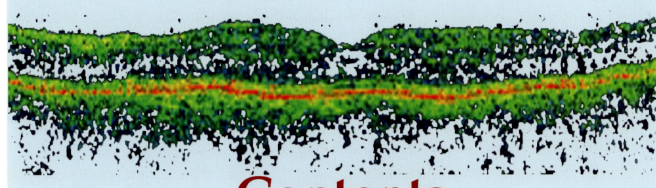

Contents

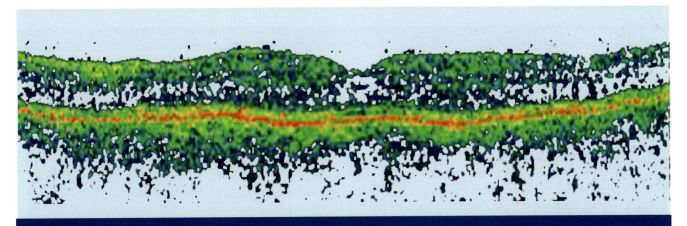

CHAPTER

1

Optical Coherence Tomography

Sandeep Saxena, Travis A Meredith

INTRODUCTION

A retina specialist uses a variety of imaging techniques to evaluate retinal pathology. Fundus photography, fluorescein and indocyanine green angiography, and ultrasonography, are among the frequently used methods. However, these techniques do not give detailed information regarding cross-sectional retinal anatomy, and do not provide quantitative retinal thickness measurements.

New emerging medical imaging technologies can improve not only the diagnosis and clinical management but also the understanding of pathogenesis of disease. Therefore, they promise to have a significant impact in clinical practice and research. Imaging instruments, including optical coherence tomography (OCT; Carl Zeiss Meditec Inc., Dublin, California, USA), the Retinal Thickness Analyzer (RTA; Talia Technology Inc., Tampa, Florida, USA), and the Heidelberg Retinal Tomograph (HRT; Heidelberg Engineering, Heidelberg, Germany) have been used to produce cross-sectional and surface topographic retinal images, and quantitative retinal thickness data.

A need has existed in medicine for a technology capable of 'optical biopsy,' imaging at or near the resolution of histopathology without excisional biopsy.[1] Advances in optics, fiberoptics, and laser technology have led to the development of a noncontact, high-resolution optical biomedical imaging technology, called optical coherence tomography (OCT).[2-5] In 1990, OCT was invented at the Massachusetts Institute of Technology in Boston. In 1993, the first *in vivo* human retina images were obtained. In 1995, the first clinical retinal images were obtained.

Optical coherence tomography is a new technique for high-resolution cross-sectional visualisation of retinal structure.[6] Optical coherence tomography achieves 2- or 3-dimensional cross-sectional imaging of retina by measuring the echo delay and intensity of back-reflected infrared light from internal tissue structures. Using a classic optical measurement technique known as low-coherence interferometry[7-13] in combination with special broad-bandwidth light, OCT achieves high-resolution, cross-sectional visualisation of tissue morphologic characteristics at depths significantly greater than the penetration depth offered by conventional bright-field and confocal microscopy.

A- and B-scan ultrasonography require physical contact with the eye and are routinely used in ophthalmic diagnosis, with a typical longitudinal resolution of 150 μm.[14,15] Imaging with OCT is analogous to ultrasound B-scan in that distance information is extracted from the time delays of reflected signals. However, the use of optical rather than acoustic waves in OCT provides a much higher (≤ 10 micron) longitudinal resolution in the retina versus the 100-micron scale for ultrasound. This is due to the fact that that the speed of light is nearly a million times faster than the speed of sound. Use of optical waves also allows a non-contact and noninvasive measurement. This technique is presently being used increasingly to evaluate and manage a variety of retinal diseases. Optical coherence tomography has been used to identify epiretinal membranes and macular holes, to differentiate macular holes from simulating lesions, to identify lamellar macular holes, macular cysts, vitreomacular traction, subretinal fluid, pigment epithelial detachment, and choroidal neovascularisation. It can be used to identify and quantify macular edema, and to measure retinal thickness changes in response to therapy.[16] The ability to non-excisionally evaluate tissue can have a significant impact on the diagnosis and management of a wide range of diseases.[17]

BASIC PRINCIPLE

Optical coherence tomography is based on the principle of Michelson interferometry.[7-13] Low-coherence infrared light coupled to a fiber-optic travels to a beam-splitter and is directed through the ocular media to the retina and to a reference mirror, respectively. Light passing through the eye is reflected by structures in different retinal tissue layers. The distance between the beam-splitter and reference mirror is continuously varied. When the distance between the light source and retinal tissue is equal to the distance between the light source and reference mirror, the reflected light from the retinal tissue and reference mirror interacts to produce an interference pattern. The interference pattern is detected and then processed into a signal. The signal is analogous to that obtained by A-scan ultrasonography using light as a source rather than sound. A two-dimensional image is built as the light source is moved across the retina. The image is in the form of a series of stacked and aligned A-scans, which produces a two-dimensional cross-sectional retinal image that resembles that of a histology section. This imaging method thus can be considered as a form of *in vivo histology*. Digital processing aligns the A-scans to correct for eye motion. Digital smoothing techniques are used to further improve the signal-to-noise ratio.[18]

Image Display

Stratus OCT (OCT-3; Carl Zeiss Meditec Inc., Dublin, California, USA) is an advanced imaging device. It can be used in the absence of dilation in many individuals, and usually requires a 3-mm pupil for adequate visualisation. The imaging lens is positioned 1 cm from the eye to be examined and adjusted independently until the retina is in focus. An infrared-sensitive charge-coupled device video camera documents the position of the scanning beam on the retina.

The OCT image can be displayed on a gray scale where more highly reflected light is brighter than less highly reflected light. Alternatively, it can be displayed in color whereby different colors correspond to different degrees of reflectivity. On the currently commercially available OCT scanners, highly reflective structures are shown with bright colors (red and white), whereas those with low reflectivity are represented by darker colors (black and blue). Those with intermediate reflectivity appear green.

Image Resolution

Optical coherence tomographic image resolution depends on several factors. Resolution can be considered in the axial (z axis) or transverse (x-y) planes.

Axial resolution depends on the wavelength and bandwidth of the incident light. Shorter wavelength light, in the 800 nm range, is not absorbed as much as longer wavelength light by high water content structures such as the cornea and vitreous. This property allows adequate light penetration to the retina, and excellent axial resolution. Hence, light with a broader spectral bandwidth enhances axial resolution by producing a shorter coherence light beam. Current commercial scanners employ a low coherence super-luminescent diode source (820 nm). The presently available model Stratus OCT (OCT-3) has a theoretical axial resolution ≤ 10 micron.

Transverse resolution is essentially wavelength-independent. It is limited to a theoretical maximum of approximately 10 microns. Depending on the scan mode, OCT-3 can produce 512 scan points in the x-axis. Furthermore, the reference mirror in the OCT, scans four times more rapidly than that of the older generation

OCTs. The light detector has been improved too. Together, these modifications produce images with significantly greater transverse resolution at a higher scan speed.

VOLUMETRIC OPTICAL COHERENCE TOMOGRAPHY

Jaffe and Caprioli[18] have coined the term "volumetric optical coherence tomography (VOCT)" to quantify retinal thickness throughout the macula. To obtain such tomogram using commercially available software on the Stratus OCT, the retinal thickness map (RTM) scan mode and analysis function, or the fast retinal thickness map (FRTM) scan mode and analysis function, is used. With these scan modes, six radial scans are obtained.

In the RTM mode, each of the six individual scans is manually acquired sequentially by the operator; while, in the FRTM mode, each of the sequential scans is obtained automatically by the OCT software. Each of the six scans is oriented radially, 30 degrees from one another, and intersect at the foveal center. Each radial scan (typically obtained at a scan length of approximately 6 mm) produces a cross-sectional image. [19] The OCT software locates the inner retina at the vitreoretinal interface and the outer retina at the retinal pigment epithelial-photoreceptor outer segment interface, based on differences in the image reflectance patterns. The software then places a line on the inner retina and another on the retinal pigment epithelium. A retinal thickness measurement is determined as the distance between these lines at each measurement point along the scan's x-axis. From these scans, a surface map reconstruction is created. The surface map is displayed as a false color image whereby retinal thickness at each point is represented by a different color. Bright colors (for example, red and white) represent thick regions, and dark colors (for example, blue and black) represent thin areas. Intermediate thickness regions are displayed as green and yellow. Because the data point density is greater centrally than peripherally, interpolated thickness measurements of regions further from the fovea are determined from fewer measurements, and may be less accurate, than those in central regions.[18]

Typical RTM or FRTM scan and analysis OCT printout yields a lot of data. These include:
1. Cross-sectional images for each of the six radial scans,
2. Measurement of central foveal thickness (calculated as the mean and standard deviation of the retinal thickness at the intersection of the six radial scans),
3. Measurement of retinal thickness in nine separate regions in the macula,
4. Surface map reconstruction display,
5. Measurement of retinal volume contained under the area represented by the surface reconstruction.

The central foveal thickness measurement is particularly useful, as it includes the thickness measurement variability among the six radial scans. Typically, this variability is less than 5%. Volumetric scanning is especially useful to quantify changes in retinal thickness. Thickness measurements determined by this technique are reproducible.[19]

STRATUS OPTICAL COHERENCE TOMOGRAPHY

Instrument

Stratus OCT is an interferometer that resolves retinal structures by measuring the echo delay time of light (broad bandwidth near-infrared light beam; 820 nm) that is reflected and backscattered from different microstructural features in the retina. The instrument electronically detects, collects, processes and stores the echo delay patterns from the retina. With each scan pass, the instrument captures from 128 to 768 longitudinal (axial) range samples, i.e. A-scans. Each A-scan consists of 1,024 data points over 2 mm of depth. Thus, the instrument integrates from 131,072 to 786,432 data points to construct a cross-sectional image (tomogram) of retinal anatomy. It displays the tomograms in real time using a false color scale that represents the degree of light backscattering from tissues at different depths in the retina. The system stores the scans, which can be selected for later analysis.

The instrument delineates intraretinal, cross-sectional anatomy with axial resolution of ≤10 microns and transverse resolution of 20 microns. Its software package includes 19 scan acquisition protocols and 18 analysis protocols. The video camera enables to view the patient's fundus and to store video and scan images together. The data management system enables storage of patient histories, for monitoring patients over time. Images and data can be archived on rewritable DVD-RAM discs. The inkjet printer generates color hard copy.

Patient's Experience

The patient's experience with the Stratus OCT is normally brief and comfortable. An experienced operator can acquire several scans from each eye in the space of 5-7 minutes. An exam usually requires the patient to look inside the ocular lens of the Patient Module for 1-3 minutes at a time for each eye, depending on the number of scans desired. The instrument acquires most scans in about 1 second. The additional time is required to position the 'Patient Module' before scanning and to optimize scan quality. The patient need not remain in the head mount throughout an examination, since the operator can reposition the 'Patient Module' as needed. Internal or external fixation may be selected. During positioning, what the patient sees with the study eye is a rectangular field of red punctuated with a green target light. Normally, the patient can look at this field for several minutes at a time without discomfort or tiredness. During scan alignment, the patient sees the scan pattern in motion on the red field. It is traced rapidly at first, while in scan alignment mode, then more slowly in scan acquisition mode. Finally, during scan acquisition, the patient sees a bright greenish-white flash, like a camera flash. This is the video camera acquiring a red-free fundus image for storage with the scan image. The operator has the option of acquiring scans without the flash and, therefore, without a high contrast image.

ADVANTAGES OF OPTICAL COHERENCE TOMOGRAPHY

There are several advantages of OCT as a diagnostic imaging technique:
1. It is noncontact unlike ultrasound and noninvasive, unlike fluorescein angiography.
2. Patients, especially children, easily tolerate it.
3. It is extremely helpful in providing quantitative information regarding macular thickness changes over time.
4. It is a valuable teaching tool for the physicians as well as patients.

DISADVANTAGES OF OPTICAL COHERENCE TOMOGRAPHY

Although OCT is an extremely valuable technique, there are limitations and potential pitfalls to its use:

1. Optical coherence tomographic images are degraded in the presence of media opacity, for example dense cataract.
2. Scan quality is dependent on the skill of OCT operator.
3. Optical coherence tomographic scanning may not be possible with uncooperative patients.
4. Measurements of foveal thickness may be inaccurate if the scan is not centered over the fovea.

COMPARISON OF OPTICAL COHERENCE TOMOGRAPHY WITH STANDARD TECHNIQUES

Stereo-fundus photographs and fluorescein angiography are the other methods of evaluating macular thickness. Retinal thickening determined by stereo-fundus photography correlates well with that measured by OCT. Macular hyperfluorescence seen on fluorescein angiography correlates well with increased retinal thickness measured by OCT. However, occasionally, eyes with macular hyperfluorescence do not appear thickened by OCT, and, conversely, some eyes without macular hyperfluorescence look thickened by OCT. Fundus photography, fluorescein angiography, and OCT, together, provide complementary information regarding macular disorders.

Fundus photography, unlike OCT, does not yield objective quantitative measurements of retinal thickening, and neither fundus photography nor fluorescein angiography gives information about cross-sectional retinal morphology or high-magnification surface topographic images. However, fluorescein angiography can provide information about the origin of macular fluid leakage, and retinal vascular abnormalities, while fundus photography may demonstrate subtle macular lesions not seen by OCT or clinical examination.[18]

COMPARISON OF OPTICAL COHERENCE TOMOGRAPHY WITH COMMERCIALLY AVAILABLE INSTRUMENTS

HRT and RTA are the other commercially available instruments, in addition to OCT, to measure retinal thickness and to evaluate retinal morphology. All can effectively measure retinal thickness in normal eyes, and in eyes with macular edema. There is a high degree of correlation between retinal thickness determined by OCT and that measured by RTA.[20-23] For patients with very early diabetic retinopathy without clinically significant macular edema, RTA may be more sensitive than OCT to detect macular thickening. However, RTA may produce a larger number of falsely elevated retinal thickness measurements, and produces retinal images less effectively than OCT in eyes with media opacity.[21,22,24] The HRT may be more effective than OCT and RTA to image the outer retina in the presence of retinal hemorrhage and hard exudates.[25] The HRT can also demonstrate surface topology. However, images are acquired relatively slowly.

ULTRAHIGH RESOLUTION OPTICAL COHERENCE TOMOGRAPHY

Standard ophthalmic OCT provides more detailed structural information than any other ophthalmic diagnostic technique. Despite the promising and clinically valuable results of these OCT studies, the axial resolution and performance of standard clinical ophthalmic OCT technology can be significantly improved. Many of the early pathologic changes associated with disease are still below the resolution limit of standard OCT. Intraretinal structures, such as the ganglion cell layer, the photoreceptor layer, and the retinal pigment epithelium, are often involved in early stages of ocular diseases but cannot be resolved with standard OCT. One of the most powerful approaches for obtaining ultrahigh resolution is the use of femtosecond laser light sources for OCT imaging.

Drexler and Fujimoto developed a clinically viable ultrahigh-resolution ophthalmic OCT system based on a commercially available titanium-sapphire laser. This system can be used in a clinical setting, enabling *in vivo* cross-sectional imaging of macular pathologies with unprecedented axial resolution of approximately 3 μm. Ultrahigh-resolution imaging studies were performed which demonstrated that ultrahigh-resolution OCT permits visualisation of all principal intraretinal layers, including the ganglion cell layer, inner and outer plexiform and nuclear layers, external limiting membrane, and the inner and outer segments of the photoreceptor layer in selected macular pathologies. Ultrahigh-resolution OCT imaging using a laboratory prototype femtosecond titanium-sapphire laser light source has recently been demonstrated to achieve an axial resolution of 1 to 3 μm in nontransparent and transparent tissue, enabling unprecedented *in vivo* subcellular[26] as well as intraretinal [27,28] visualisation. Ultrahigh-resolution OCT enables all of the major intraretinal layers to be visualised noninvasively *in vivo*, and images have excellent correlation with known retinal morphologic features. [29]

Comparison of Zeiss Meditec OCT-3 and Ultrahigh-resolution OCT is shown in Table 1.1.

Table 1.1: Comparison of Zeiss Meditec OCT-3 and Ultrahigh Resolution-OCT	
Zeiss Meditec OCT-3	Ultrahigh Resolution-OCT
Prototype superluminescent diode	Low-cost Ti:Sapphire laser
~ 30 nm bandwidth	~ 12.5 nm bandwidth
~ 10 micron axial resolution	~ 3 micron axial resolution
512 cross section A-scans	600 cross section A-scans
1,024 points per line	3,000 points per line

OPTICAL COHERENCE TOMOGRAPHY AND SCANNING LASER OPHTHALMOSCOPE TECHNOLOGY

Optical coherence tomography imaging requires a series of image processing programs. Two specific limitations are recognised with the current device:

a. *Errors in A-scan image correlation and interpolation*: Cross-correlation and interpolation errors of A-scan increase as the scan lengths increase from 3 to 10 mm, making image quality less reliable.

b. *Precise anatomic localisation of the OCT image from the red-free image*: The anatomic localisation is compromised because the red-free image depicting the position of the OCT trace is not pixel linked. The red-free images are derived from live video images by a frame grabber during the examination and serve as a rough estimate of the OCT B-scan anatomic position.

A new device is being developed to create OCT B-scan images (without the use of A-scans) and use simultaneous red-free Scanning Laser Ophthalmoscope (SLO) pixel-linked images for precise OCT image localisation. The OCT B-scan images are created by horizontal scanning (x-y) in the ophthalmoscopic plane, at increasing depths. This technology also permits accumulation of information from entire planes of tissue at varying depths, creating a new image format called C-scan. Numerous C-scan images can be computer processed into 3-D OCT images that permit volumetric and linear measurements. The new technology utilises a beam splitter at the light source to create two channels. One channel uses conventional SLO to create red-free images, while the other channel is used to create simultaneous OCT images. Since the images are pixel linked, precise anatomic localisation of OCT image is possible.

FUSION TECHNOLOGY OF OPTICAL COHERENCE TOMOGRAPHY AND ULTRASONOGRAPHY

Fusion technology of optical coherence tomography and ultrasonography is being developed that produces pixel-wise combination of images of differing modalities to obtain added diagnostic value. It produces a single image from a set of input images. The fused image provides more complete information for interpretation of ocular tissues and layers. This produces improved anatomic delineation. Imaging and identification of tissue boundaries is possible. High resolution of layers increases the accuracy of measuring the thickness of nevi and small melanomas. Accurate choroidal thickness measurement is also possible.

Optical coherence tomography will be used increasingly to diagnose and manage retinal diseases. Improvements in scanning hardware and software will facilitate its use in the future. It is likely that commercial scanners will incorporate ultra-broad spectral bandwidth light sources as they become less costly, a modification that will greatly enhance axial resolution. In addition, more studies are needed to identify the range of retinal diseases for which OCT is useful, and to determine the relative usefulness of OCT to diagnose and follow patients compared with alternative imaging techniques. In many cases, OCT provides information complementary to that available by alternative methods. However, more information is needed to determine when OCT testing alone would suffice. In addition, care is needed to avoid artifacts and image misinterpretation.[18]

Optical coherence tomography has become an established method for imaging retinal diseases. It is now an accepted method for making quantitative measurements in studies on the cause and course of macular holes, vitreoretinal traction, pigment epithelial detachment, macular edema, and diabetic retinopathy. Its potential benefit in the evaluation of age-related macular degeneration and a variety of other diseases is currently under investigation. In clinical practice, optical coherence tomography images add information to the biomicroscopic findings and results of other imaging techniques or functional testing and can significantly help in making critical decisions. Its future role in routine clinical practice will depend on further technical development and the results of long-term studies.[30] This sequential imaging technique will aid in our understanding of the rapid evolution of retinal pathology and response to treatment in the research and clinical setting.[31]

REFERENCES

1. Brezinski ME, Tearney GJ, Bouma B, et al. Optical biopsy with optical coherence tomography. Ann N Y Acad Sci. 1998;9:838:68-74.
2. Huang D, Swanson EA, Lin CP, et al. Optical coherence tomography. Science. 1991;254:1178-1181.
3. Fujimoto JG, Brezinski ME, Tearney GJ, et al. Optical biopsy and imaging using optical coherence tomography. Nat Med. 1995;1:970-972.
4. Fercher AF, Roth E. Ophthalmic laser interferometry. In. Müller GJ, (Ed): Optical Instrumentation for Biomedical Laser Applications. Vol 658. Bellingham, Wash: SPIE; 1986:48-51.
5. Fercher AF. Optical coherence tomography. J Biomed Opt. 1996;1:157-173.
6. Hee MR, Izatt JA, Swanson EA, et al. Optical coherence tomography of human retina. Arch Ophthalmol. 1995;113:325-332.
7. Youngquist RC, Carr S, Davies DEN. Optical coherence domain reflectometry: a new optical evaluation technique. Opt Lett. 1987;12:158-160.
8. Takada K, Yokohama I, Chida K, Noda J. New measurement system for fault location in optic waveguide devices based on an interferometric technique. Appl Opt. 1987;26:1603-1610.
9. Huang D, Wang J, Lin CP, Puliafito CA, Fujimoto JG. Micron-resolution ranging of cornea and anterior chamber by optical reflectometry. Lasers Surg Med. 1991;11:419-425.

10. Swanson EA, Izatt JA, Hee MR, et al. *In vivo* retinal imaging by optical coherence tomography. Opt Lett. 1993;18:1864-1866.
11. Huang D, Swanson EA, Hee MR, et al. Optical coherence tomography. Science. 1991;254:1178-1181.
12. Swanson EA, Huang D, Hee MR, et al. High-speed optical coherence domain reflectometry. Opt Lett. 1992;17:151-153.
13. Hee MR, Huang D, Swanson EA, Fujimoto JG. Polarisation-sensitive low coherence reflectometer for birefringence characterisation and ranging. J Opt Soc Am B. 1992;9:903-908.
14. Olsen T. The accuracy of ultrasonic determination of axial length in pseudophakic eyes. Acta Ophthalmol (Copenh). 1989;67:141-144.
15. Bamber JC, Trstam M. Diagnostic ultrasound. In. Webb S, (Ed): The Physics of Medical Imaging. Philadelphia: Adam Hilger. 1988:319-388.
16. Puliafito CA, Hee MR, Lin CP, et al. Imaging of macular diseases with optical coherence tomography. Ophthalmology. 1995;102:217-229.
17. Fujimoto JG, Brezinski ME, Tearney GJ, et al. Optical biopsy and imaging using optical coherence tomography. Nat Med. 1995;9:970-972.
18. Jaffe GJ, Caprioli J. Optical coherence tomography to detect and manage retinal disease and glaucoma. Am J Ophthalmol. 2004;137:156-169.
19. Hee MR, Puliafito CA, J.S. Duker, et al., Topography of diabetic macular edema with optical coherence tomography. Ophthalmology. 1998;105:360-370.
20. Pires I, Bernardes RC, Lobo CL, Soares MA, Cunha-Vaz JG. Retinal thickness in eyes with mild nonproliferative retinopathy in patients with type 2 diabetes mellitus: comparison of measurements obtained by retinal thickness analysis and optical coherence tomography. Arch Ophthalmol. 2002;120:1301–1306.
21. Polito A, Shah SM, Haller JA, et al. Comparison between retinal thickness analyzer and optical coherence tomography for assessment of foveal thickness in eyes with macular disease. Am J Ophthalmol. 2002;134:240-251.
22. Neubauer AS, Priglinger S, S. Ullrich S, et al. Comparison of foveal thickness measured with the retinal thickness analyzer and optical coherence tomography. Retina. 2001;21:596-601.
23. Konno S, Akiba J, Yoshida A. Retinal thickness measurements with optical coherence tomography and the scanning retinal thickness analyzer. Retina. 2001;21:57-61.
24. H. Sanchez-Tocino H, Alvarez-Vidal A, Maldonado MJ, et al. Retinal thickness study with optical coherence tomography in patients with diabetes. Invest Ophthalmol Vis Sci. 2002;43;1588-1594.
25. Antcliff RJ, Stanford R, Chauhan DS, et al. Comparison between optical coherence tomography and fundus fluorescein angiography for the detection of cystoid macular edema in patients with uveitis. Ophthalmology. 2000;107:593-599.
26. Drexler W, Morgner U, Kärtner FX, et al. *In vivo* ultrahigh resolution optical coherence tomography. Opt Lett. 1999;24:1221-1223.
27. Drexler W, Morgner U, Ghanta RK, et al. New technology for ultrahigh resolution optical coherence tomography of the retina. In. Lemij H, Schuman JS (Eds): The Shape of Glaucoma: Quantitative Neural Imaging Techniques. The Hague: Kugler Publications; 2000:75-104.
28. Drexler W, Morgner U, Ghanta RK, et al. Ultrahigh resolution ophthalmologic optical coherence tomography. Nat Med. 2001;7:502-507.
29. Drexler W, Sattman H, Hermann B, et al. Enhanced visualisation of macular pathology with the use of ultra-high resolution optical coherence tomography. Arch Ophthalmol. 2003;121:695-706.
30. Schaudig U. Optical coherence tomography. Ophthalmologe. 2001;98:26-34.
31. Toth CA, Narayan DG, Boppart SA, et al. A comparison of retinal morphology viewed by optical coherence tomography and by light microscopy. Arch Ophthalmol. 1997;115:1425-1428.

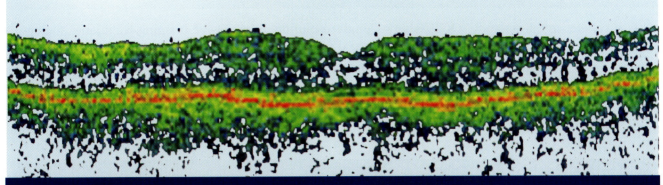

CHAPTER

2

Optical Coherence Tomography: Normal Macula and Interpretation of Images

Sandeep Saxena, Travis A Meredith, Maurice B Landers III, Tomohiro Iida

INTRODUCTION

Optical coherence tomography (OCT) is a new high-resolution, noninvasive imaging technique, analogous to ultrasound B-scan, that can provide cross-sectional images of the retina with micrometer-scale resolution.[1] Optical coherence tomography scans can discriminate the cross-sectional morphologic features of the fovea and optic disc, the layered structure of the retina, and normal anatomic variations in retinal and retinal nerve fiber layer thicknesses with 10-microns depth resolution. Optical coherence tomography is a potentially useful technique for high-depth resolution, cross-sectional examination of the fundus.

NORMAL OCT SCAN

On a normal 10 mm horizontal scan passing through the fovea, one can clearly demarcate two major landmarks, namely, the optic disc and fovea (Fig. 2.1).

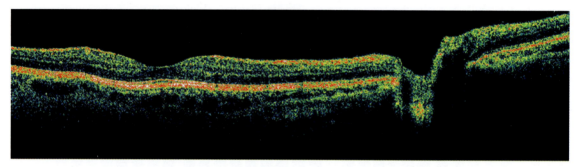

Fig. 2.1: Collage of the OCT scans showing optic nerve and macula

The optic disc is seen towards the right of the tomogram and can be easily identified by its contour. The central depression represents the optic head cup and the stalk continuing behind is the anterior part of optic nerve. The fovea is seen towards the left of the tomogram and can be easily identified by characteristic thinning of the retinal layers. The vitreous anterior to the retina is non-reflective and is seen as a dark space. The interface between the non-reflective vitreous and backscattering retinal layers is the vitreoretinal interface.[1]

Retinal morphology and macular OCT imaging correlate well, with alignment of areas of high and low reflectivity to specific retinal and choroidal elements (Fig. 2.2). Resolution of retinal structures by OCT depends on the contrast in relative reflectivity of adjacent structures.[2]

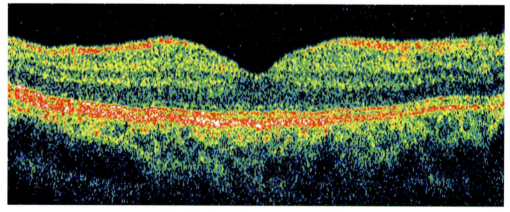

Fig. 2.2: Normal macula on an OCT scan

The nerve fiber layer and ganglion cell layers are reflective, and are seen as bright colors on the false color map. The nuclear layers appear hyporeflective, while interconnecting plexiform layers and axonal layers are relatively hyper-reflective.[2,3] Typically, the photoreceptor outer segments appear slightly hyporeflective compared with the other retinal layers. The retinal pigment epithelium/choriocapillaris complex is seen as a hyper-reflective band. The retinal blood vessels within the neurosensory retina show backscatter and also cast a shadow behind. The choroid is also highly reflective, although it is frequently not well resolved because of light reflection by the overlying retinal pigment epithelium.

OPTICAL COHERENCE TOMOGRAPHY INTERPRETATION

An OCT image can have two modes of interpretation: objective and subjective. For an accurate interpretation, one needs to combine both these modalities.[4]

The purpose of OCT is to detect abnormalities in the retina, in terms of thickness, morphology, and reflectivity. Optical coherence tomography reading must be done in two stages:
1. Qualitative and quantitative analysis
2. Deduction and synthesis
   The analysis stage can be further divided into:

Qualitative Analysis

1. Morphological study:
   a. Morphological variations: overall retinal structural changes, changes in retinal outline, intraretinal structural changes and morphological changes in the posterior layers
   b. Anomalous structures: Preretinal, epiretinal, intraretinal and subretinal
2. Reflectivity study: hyper-reflectivity, hypo-reflectivity, and shadow areas

Quantitative Analysis

Thickness, volumetry and surface mapping

Deductive and synthetic study is performed comparing all the analytical data, the results of the clinical examination and all the other available data.

The OCT software offers the protocols for both qualitative as well as quantitative estimation.

Qualitative Analysis

Various image modification protocols can be used for qualitative analysis.
  i. *Normalize:* This protocol is used to eliminate background noise and to use the whole color scale in the processed scan image. This function normalizes scan images with respect to noise and signal strength. In other words, when one applies this function to scan images made with different noise or signal strength, the resulting images appear equally "bright," i.e. have the same range of color.
     The scan image uses the entire color scale to express the relative reflectivity of the retinal structures between the noise and saturation signal levels
 ii. *Align:* This protocol is used to correct the data for effects due to patient motion in the axial direction. Slight movements of the head toward and away from the instrument cause the scan image to shift

vertically, resulting in low-frequency "wiggles." (This also happens if the scan beam is not perpendicular to the retina over the whole scan. To correct for this movement, this algorithm compares each of the longitudinal samples (A-scans) in the data set with its neighbor in a process called correlation. In effect, it slides A-scan 2 in relation to A-scan 1 until the data align. Then it slides A-scan 3 in relation to the now-aligned A-scan 2, and so on until all A-scans are aligned.

iii. *Gaussian and median smoothing:* The two smoothing functions average out noise and blend the colors of the scan image. Smoothing may be useful to appreciate more fully the large-scale features in the data. However, some small details may be lost.

Gaussian smoothing works by calculating a moving average of signal values in a 3 × 3 region. It weights the signal values according to a Gaussian function, such that the outer points in the region are weighted less than the center point.

Median smoothing is similar to Gaussian smoothing, except that it uses the median value of the 3 × 3 region (i.e. the middle value when ordered by size) instead of the moving average value weighted by location. The advantage of median smoothing is that it removes noise while preserving small details in the data.

Morphological Study

Deformation of Retina
a. *Concavity:* In cases of high myopia and posterior staphyloma in myopia, OCT reveals the presence of pronounced concavity, which can become less evident if the scan is processed using the alignment function.
b. *Convexity:* Convexity is often observed in cup-shaped detachment of the retinal pigment epithelium and subretinal cysts.

Deformation of Retinal Profile
a. *Disappearance of the foveal depression:* This is a sign of clinically significant macular edema (Fig. 2.3)
b. *Epiretinal membrane:* It may be separate form the retina, in contact with it, or adhered to it and may cause folds of retinal surface (Figs 2.4A and B)
c. *Macular pseudo-holes and lamellar holes*
d. *Macular Hole:* The OCT helps in identifying and classifying macular holes, as well as determining their diameter and the extent of detachment (Figs 2.5AtoD).

Intraretinal Structural Changes
a. *Pseudoholes*
b. *Cysts* due to cystoid macular edema (Figs 2.6A to C).
c. *Cotton wool spots* consist of superficial hyper-reflective retinal nodules, which are in contact with superficial retinal layers in the nerve fiber layer. They are located at the margins of ischemic lesions of the nerve fibers.
d. *Hard exudates* occur at the margin of an edematous area and normal retina. They are hyper-reflective in an OCT scan (Fig. 2.7).

Posterior Morphological Changes
a. *Retinal pigment epithelial detachments* deform the posterior limit of retina on OCT scan, forming a steep angle with the choriocapillaris (Fig. 2.8).

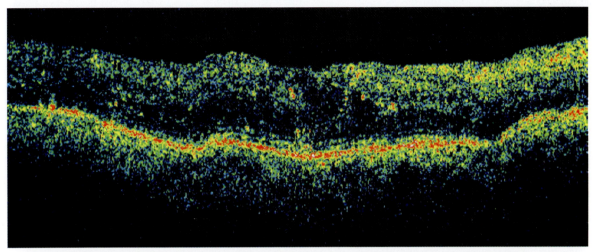

Fig. 2.3: Disappearance of the foveal depression in clinically significant macular edema

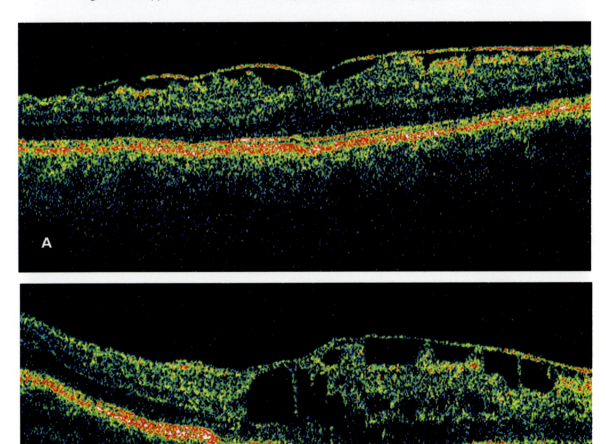

Figs 2.4A and B: Epiretinal membrane

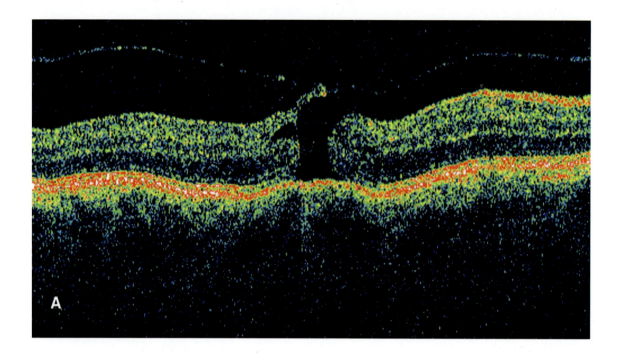

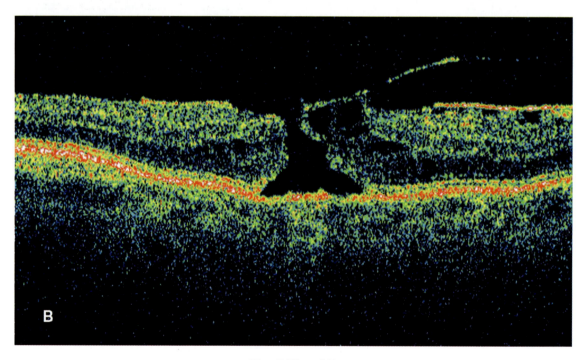

Figs 2.5A and B

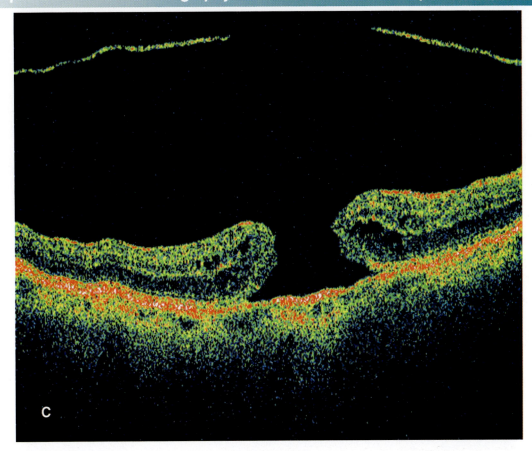

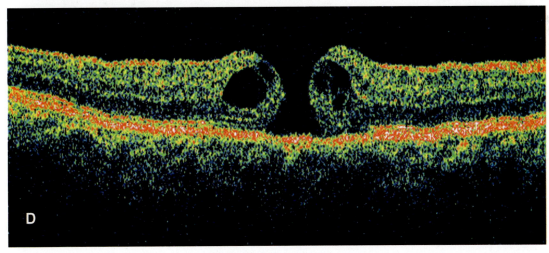

Figs 2.5A to D: Macular hole

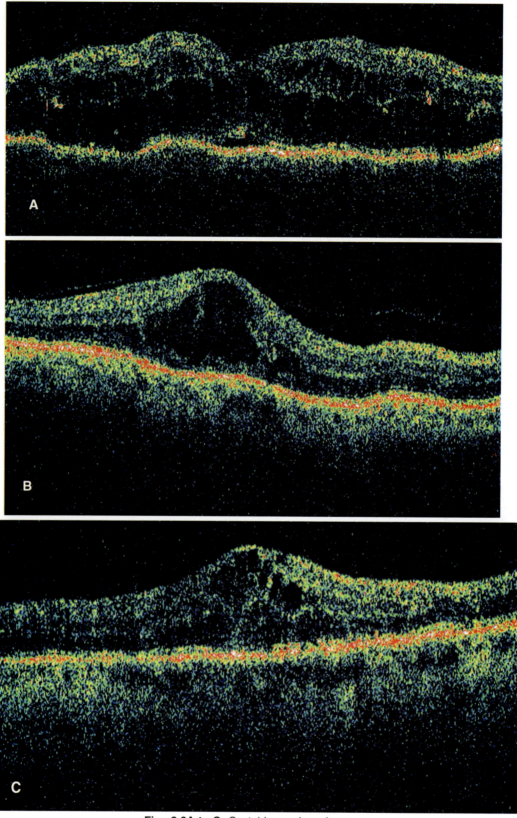

Figs 2.6A to C: Cystoid macular edema

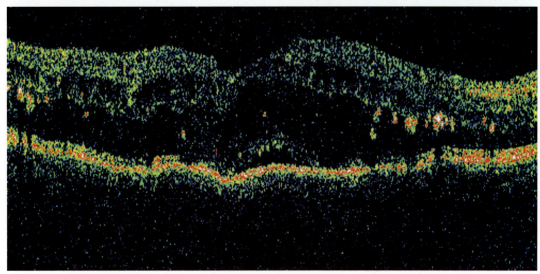

Fig. 2.7: Hard exudates

b. *Serous retinal detachment* of the retina protrude less, and form shallow angles with the retinal pigment epithelium (Figs 2.9A and B).
c. *Drusens* produce irregularities and wavy undulations of the pigment epithelium and choriocapillaris.
d. *Choroidal neovascular membrane* in young or myopic patients are usually visualized as nodular, rounded fusiform structure located in front of the retinal pigment epithelium. This is also true in cases of early neovascular age-related macular degeneration. They may be associated with edema or serous retinal detachment. When choroidal neovascular membranes have had several weeks or months to develop they are much more difficult to detect and may appear as thickening of the retinal pigment epithelium (Figs 2.10A and B). Occult choroidal neovascular membranes are difficult to identify.

Reflectivity Study

When pathology is present, reflectivity may be increased or decreased, or a shadow zone may be observed on an OCT scan. Vertical structures, such as photoreceptors, are less reflective than horizontal structures, such as nerve fibers (Table 2.1).

Shadow Areas

An area of dense, hyper-reflective tissue produces a screen that may be complete or incomplete, thereby creating a shadow area on OCT scan that conceals the elements lying behind it (Fig. 2.11).

Anterior shadow and screen effects
- Hemorrhage
- Exudates
- Retinal vessel (normal)

Posterior shadow and screen effects
- Retinal scars
- Pigment epithelial hypertrophy/hyperplasia

Table 2.1: Reflectivity study of OCT interpretation

High reflectivity
- Pigment accumulation
- Hypertrophy of retinal pigment epithelium
- Nevus
- Scar
- Neovascularisation
- Hard exudates
- Nerve fiber (normal)
- Retinal pigment epithelium-choriocapillaris complex (normal)

Medium Reflectivity
- Plexiform layer (normal)

Low Reflectivity
- Retinal edema
- Cystoid edema
- Nuclear layer (normal)
- Photoreceptors (normal)
- Cavities/cysts
- Pigment epithelial detachment
- Serous retinal detachment

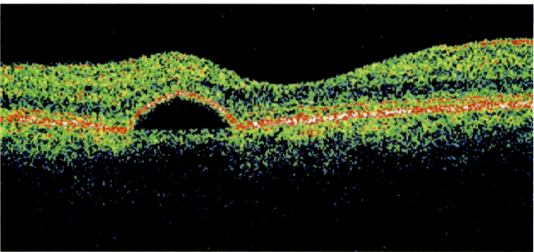

Fig. 2.8: Retinal pigment epithelial detachment

- Pigment accumulation
- Choroidal nevi

Quantitative Analysis

i. *Retinal thickness/volume:* This analysis protocol obtains two circular maps for each eye that depict thickness and volume of retina. It can be displayed either as retinal thickness or retinal volume. The output display includes all the elements of the retinal thickness/volume analysis (Figs 2.12A and B), with a slightly different arrangement to accommodate the table. The output display has the same layout for both thickness

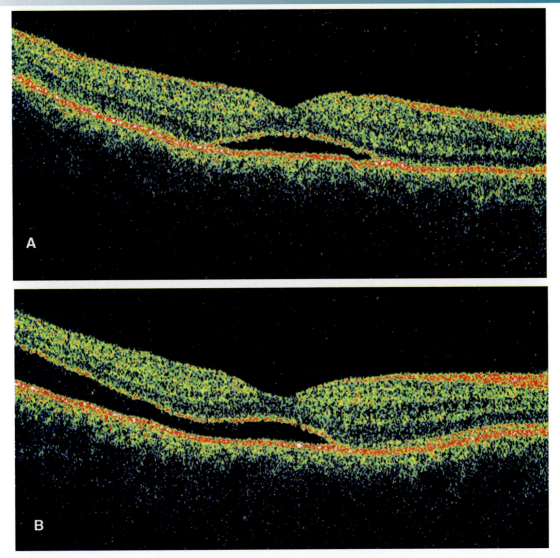

Figs 2.9A and B: Serous retinal detachment

and volume analysis. The upper map always presents retinal thickness using a color code. The color scale appears to the right. The lower map shows either average retinal thickness (in microns) or average volume (in mm^3) in each area. A key of the map circle diameters appears at right below the color scale. The default diameters are 1, 3 and 6 mm. On the lower right, numeric information for each eye includes: Foveal thickness which represents the calculation of average thickness in microns +/− the standard deviation for the center point, where all the scans intersect; and total macular volume of the retinal map area in mm^3.

Mean foveal thickness refers to the average of retinal thickness values in the central 1000 microns central disc, and central foveal thickness refers to the average of 6 values of retinal thickness at the intersection of the six radial scans.

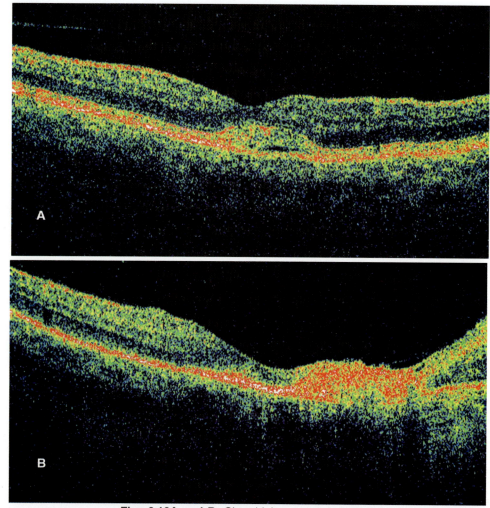

Figs 2.10A and B: Choroidal neovascularisation

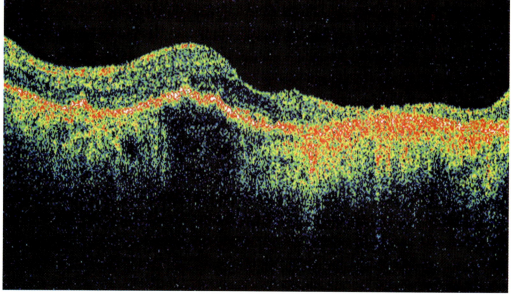

Fig. 2.11: Shadow areas

ii. *Retinal thickness/volume tabular:* This analysis protocol gives the same information as above. It obtains not only all the output of the retinal thickness/volume analysis, but also a data table that includes thickness and volume quadrant averages, ratios and differences among the quadrants and between the eyes.

iii. *Retinal thickness/volume change:* This analysis protocol helps to assess changes in retinal thickness or volume between examinations. The default output displays thickness change between exams.

The output has the same layout for both thickness and volume change analysis. The upper map always presents retinal thickness change using a color code. The color scale appears to the right. The lower map shows the change in either average retinal thickness (in microns) or average volume (in mm^3).

OCT SCAN PROTOCOLS FOR MACULA

The Stratus OCT-3 offers various scan acquisition protocols for examination. To get the most accurate and meaningful information, one needs to apply the appropriate protocol. Scan protocols suitable for macula are:

a. *Line Scan:* This scan protocol gives an option of acquiring multiple line scans without returning to the main window. The default angle is 0° and the nasal position is defined as zero degree. By default, the length of the line scan is 5 mm. However, the length of the line scan and the angle can be altered. As the length scan increases, the resolution decreases. Multiple scans of different parameters can be acquired using this protocol.

b. *Radial Lines:* This scan protocol consists of 6 to 24 equally spaced line scans that can be varied in size and parameters. All the lines pass through a central common axis. The default setting has 6 lines of 6 mm length. Adjusting the size of aiming circle can change the length of these lines. The radial lines are useful in acquiring macular scan and retinal thickness/volume analysis.

c. *Macular Thickness Map:* This scan protocol is similar to radial lines except that the aiming circle has a fixed diameter of 6 mm. This acquisition protocol helps in measuring the macular thickness.

d. *Fast Macular Thickness Map:* This scan protocol is designed for use with retinal thickness analysis. When performed in both eyes, it can be used for comparative retinal thickness/volume analysis. It is a quick protocol that takes only 1.92 seconds to acquire six scans of 6 mm length each. The size and number of scan is fixed and cannot be altered.

e. *Raster Lines:* This scan protocol provides an option of acquiring a series of line scans that are parallel, equally spaced and are 6-24 in number. These multiple line scans are placed over a rectangular region, the area of which can be adjusted to cover the entire area of pathology. This protocol is especially useful in disease conditions like choroidal neovascular membranes, where scans at multiple levels are required. The default setting has 3 mm square with 6 lines.

f. *Repeat:* Repeat protocol enables one to repeat any of the previously saved protocols using the same set of parameters that include scan size, angle, placement of fixation light emitting diode and landmark. This protocol is especially helpful when one is monitoring retinal changes. No parameter except placement can be changed. The landmark can be placed on the point of reference. This helps in reproducibility during repeat scan. The previous image can be displayed for accurate placement of landmark.

STRATUS OCT
Retinal Thickness Analysis Report - Ver. 3.0

ZEISS

DOB: 04/13/1949, ID: 1456890-1, Male

ScanType:	Macular Thickness Map
ScanDate:	03/28/2003
ScanLength:	6.0

OD   OS

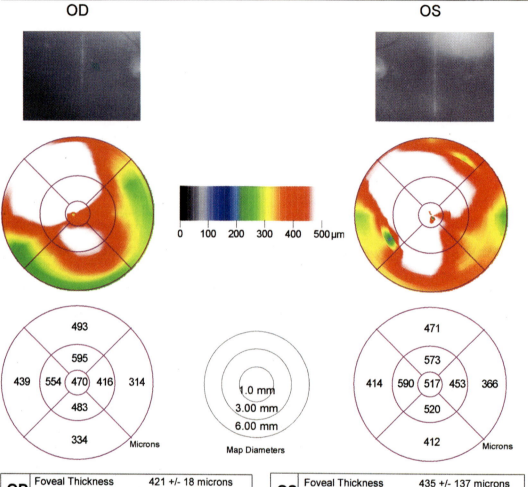

OD	Foveal Thickness	421 +/- 18 microns
	Total Macular Volume	11.96 mm³

OS	Foveal Thickness	435 +/- 137 microns
	Total Macular Volume	12.58 mm³

Signature: _____

A   _____

Physician: _____

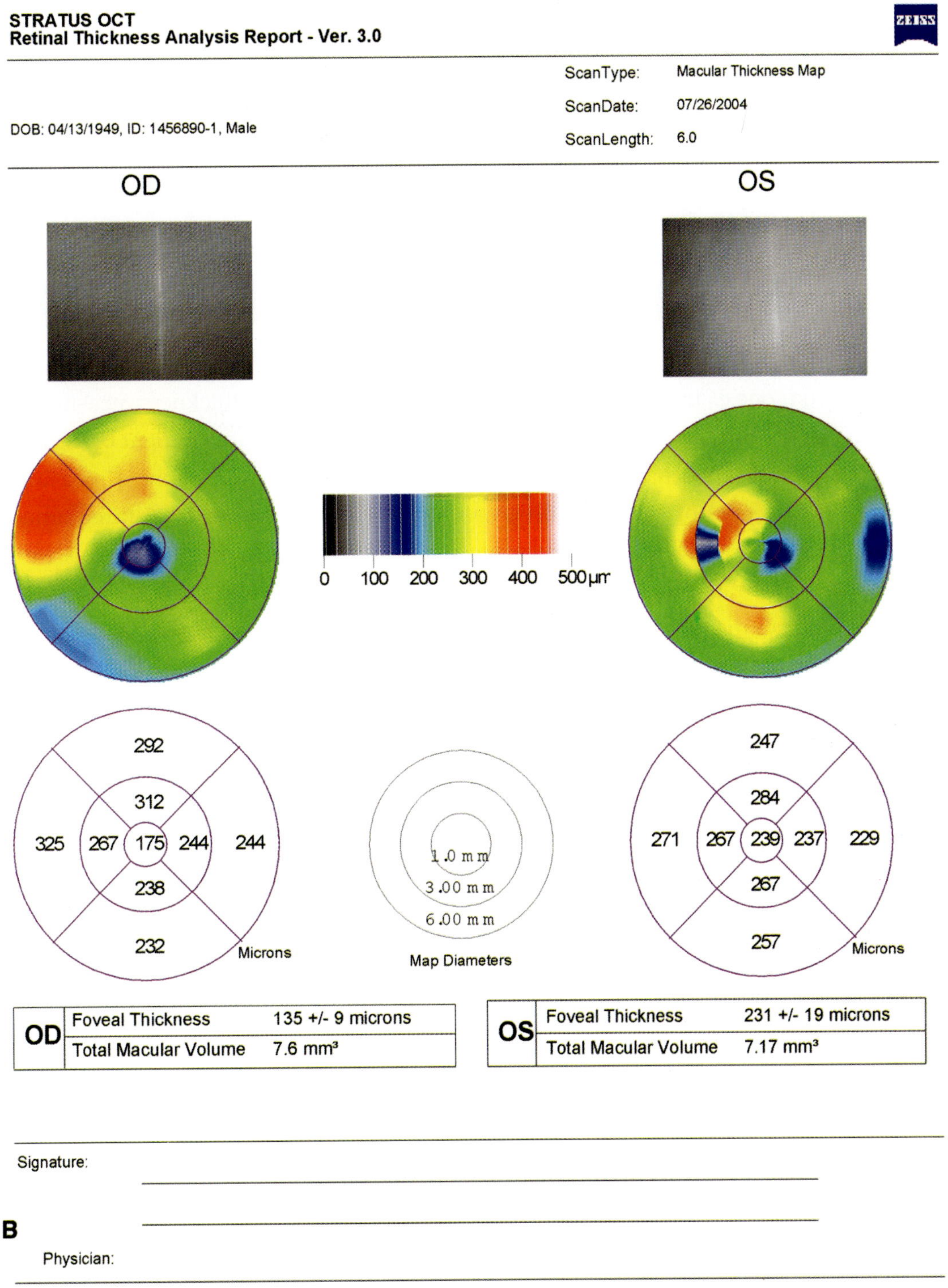

STRATUS OCT
Retinal Thickness Analysis Report - Ver. 3.0

ZEISS

DOB: 04/13/1949, ID: 1456890-1, Male

ScanType:	Macular Thickness Map
ScanDate:	07/26/2004
ScanLength:	6.0

OD   OS

0   100   200   300   400   500 μm

	292	
	312	
325	267 175 244	244
	238	
	232	Microns

1.0 mm
3.00 mm
6.00 mm
Map Diameters

	247	
	284	
271	267 239 237	229
	267	
	257	Microns

OD	Foveal Thickness	135 +/- 9 microns
	Total Macular Volume	7.6 mm³

OS	Foveal Thickness	231 +/- 19 microns
	Total Macular Volume	7.17 mm³

Signature: _____

B

Physician: _____

Figs 2.12A and B: Quantitative analysis

MACULAR THICKNESS DATABASE SOFTWARE UPGRADE

The new version 4.0 software applications for the optical coherence tomography technology include a normative database for macular thickness analysis. This new software compares a patient's macular thickness measurements with a normative database. The results are demonstrated on screen and print outs with color-coded graphs, maps, and tabular data. The software package features a screen display of colored bands that demonstrate the normal distribution of macular thickness measurements in micrometers. The patient's measurements are compared with a normal distribution percentile chart.

REPRODUCIBILITY

Optical coherence tomography measures retinal thickness with a high degree of accuracy and reproducibility for a given patient, from one examination to the next. Furthermore, retinal thickness measurements obtained on a patient by one technician are very similar to those obtained on that same patient by another technician.

Gurses-Ozden and associated assessed the reproducibility of macular thickness measurements using OCT-3. Randomly chosen eyes of healthy individuals were scanned using OCT-3 three times on separate days within a one-month period. Fast and regular macula (128 A-scans) scanning protocols were performed. Intra- and interoperator measurement reproducibility was evaluated. Intraoperator reproducibility was high for macular thickness measurements. There was no difference in mean foveal thickness measurements performed on different days. Interoperator reproducibility was high. Macular thickness measurements are reproducible in normal eyes.

Massin and associates[6] defined the normal retinal thickness in healthy subjects using optical coherence tomography mapping software and assessed the ability of OCT to detect early macular thickening in diabetic patients. Thickening was diagnosed if mean retinal thickness of an area was greater than the mean thickness $\pm/-2$ SD in the corresponding area in healthy subjects; or if the difference between right and left eye exceeded the mean difference $\pm/-2$ SD in a given area in healthy subjects. In healthy subjects, mean retinal thickness in the central macular area 1000 microns in diameter was $170\pm/-18$ microns. There was no significant difference according to age, or left or right eye, but central macular thickness was significantly greater in men than women. No difference was observed between the eyes of healthy subjects and diabetic patients without macular edema on biomicroscopy, but OCT detected early macular thickening in diabetic eyes. In this study average retinal thickness and mean local variations in a normal population was defined using commercially available mapping software. Optical coherence tomography seems to be a sensitive tool for detecting early retinal thickening.

Sanchez-Tocino and associates[7] quantitatively assessed retinal thickness by OCT in normal subjects and patients with diabetes. They noted that foveal thickening over 180 microns measured by OCT may be useful for the early detection of macular thickening and may be an indicator for a closer follow-up of the patient with diabetes.

Muscat and associates[8] assessed the accuracy, precision, repeatability, and reproducibility of measurements made by the OCT. Measurements made from OCT scans were found to be accurate and precise. Retinal

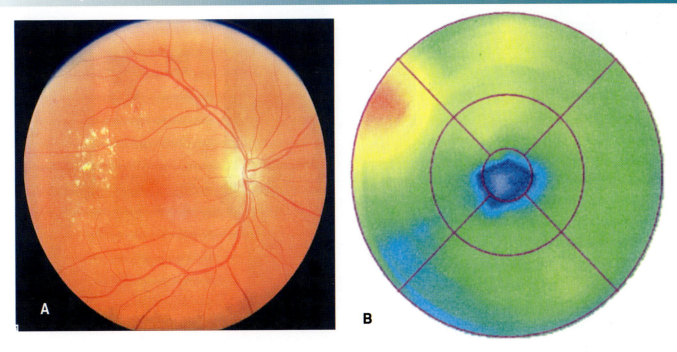

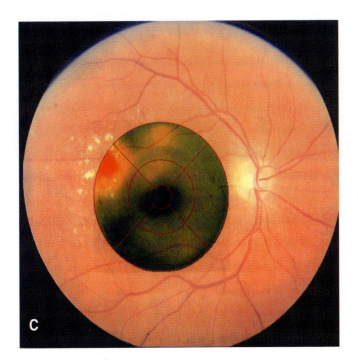

Figs 2.13A to C: Macular map thickness of the OCT scan, depicting macular thickness, can be overlaid on a color fundus photograph to correlate topographically, the macular thickness corresponding to that underlying area

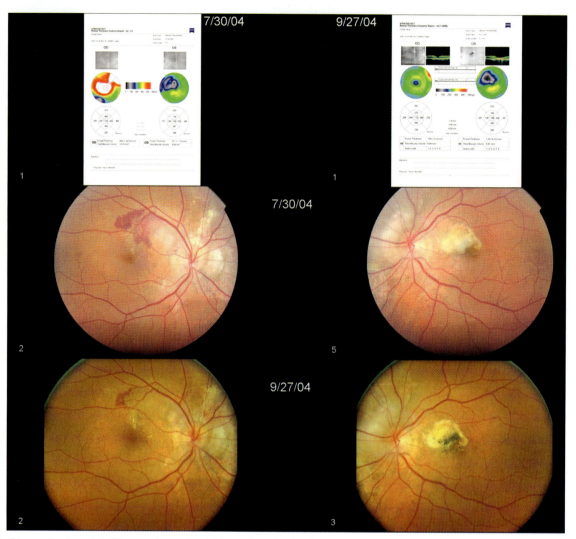

Fig. 2.14: Six-up display of OCT scan (macular thickness) and color fundus photographs of the last visit and the present visit helps in assessment of the current status of the macula

thickness measurements in the macular area were repeatable and reproducible. This demonstrates that OCT is a useful tool in the monitoring of patients with conditions that affect macular thickness, even when there is considerable degradation of the OCT signal.

Baumann and associates[9] determined the reproducibility of retinal thickness measurements in normal eyes and reported that OCT is capable of reproducible measurement of retinal thickness in normal eyes. They noted that computer-driven, automated measurement of retinal thickness within 500 microns of fixation needs to be refined and its reproducibility reassessed in this region.

Massin and associates[10] assessed the reproducibility of retinal thickness measurement. Six radial scans, 6 mm long and centered on the fixation point, were performed Measurement reproducibility was tested by means of 3 series of scans performed by 2 different observers on 2 different days. In healthy subjects, intraobserver, interobserver, and intervisit reproducibility of retinal thickness measurements were excellent. Retinal mapping software of OCT allows reproducible measurement of retinal thickness in both healthy subjects and diabetic patients with macular edema.

OPTICAL COHERENCE TOMOGRAPHY-ASSISTED PATIENT EVALUATION

Fundus Photograph-OCT Overlay

Macular thickness map of the OCT scan, depicting macular thickness, can be overlaid on a color fundus photograph. This helps to correlate topographically, the macular thickness corresponding to that underlying area (Fig. 2.13A to C).

Six-up Photograph Display

In the office, 6-up display of OCT scan (macular thickness) and color fundus photographs of the last visit and the present visit helps in assessment of the current status of the macula (Fig. 2.14). It is a non-invasive, quick and useful method of patient evaluation.

REFERENCES

1. Hee MR, Izatt JA, Swanson EA, et al. Optical coherence tomography of the human retina. Arch Ophthalmol. 1995;113:325-332.
2. Toth CA, D.G. Narayan DG, Boppart SA, et al. A comparison of retinal morphology viewed by optical coherence tomography and by light microscopy. Arch Ophthalmol. 1997;115:1425-1428.
3. Drexler W, Morgner U, Ghanta RK, et al. Ultrahigh-resolution ophthalmic optical coherence tomography. Nat Med. 2001;7:502-507.
4. Puliafito CA, Hee MR, Schuman JS, Fujimoto JG. Optical coherence tomography of ocular diseases. New York: Slack Inc 1996.
5. Gurses-Ozden R, Teng C, Vessani R, et al. Macular and retinal nerve fiber layer thickness measurement reproducibility using optical coherence tomography (OCT-3). J Glaucoma. 2004;13:238-244.
6. Massin P, Erginay A, Haouchine B, et al. Retinal thickness in healthy and diabetic subjects measured using optical coherence tomography mapping software. Eur J Ophthalmol. 2002;12:102-108.
7. Sanchez-Tocino H, Alvarez-Vidal A, Maldonado MJ, et al. Retinal thickness study with optical coherence tomography in patients with diabetes. Invest Ophthalmol Vis Sci. 2002;43:1588-1594.
8. Muscat S, Parks S, Kemp E, Keating D. Repeatability and reproducibility of macular thickness measurements with the Humphrey OCT system. Invest Ophthalmol Vis Sci. 2002;43:490-495.
9. Baumann M, Gentile RC, Liebmann JM, Ritch R. Reproducibility of retinal thickness measurements in normal eyes using optical coherence tomography. Ophthalmic Surg Lasers. 1998;29:280-285.
10. Massin P, Vicaut E, Haouchine B, et al. Reproducibility of retinal mapping using optical coherence tomography. Arch Ophthalmol. 2001;119:1135-1142.

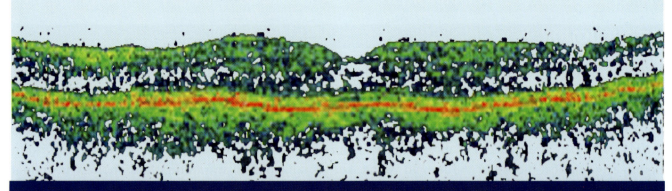

Ultrahigh Resolution Optical Coherence Tomography in Macular Diseases

Wolfgang Drexler, Boris Hermann, Angelika Unterhuber, Harald Sattmann, Mathias Wirtitsch, Michael Stur, Christoph Scholda, Erdem Ergun, Elzbieta Polska, Arno Doelemeyer, Tony H Ko, James G Fujimoto, Adolf F Fercher

INTRODUCTION

Ultrahigh resolution optical coherence tomography (UHR OCT)[1-5] is a recently developed improvement of the well established optical coherence tomography (OCT) technology[6-8] enabling unprecedented *in vivo* sub-cellular[1] as well as intraretinal visualization.[2-5] Ophthalmic UHR OCT exceeds standard resolution OCT by obtaining superior axial image resolution of 3 μm as compared to 10-15 μm achieved so far for retinal imaging and therefore enables enhanced visualization of intraretinal layers and has the potential to perform noninvasive optical biopsy of the human retina, i.e. visualization of intraretinal morphology in retinal pathologies approaching the level of that achieved with histopathology. This quantum leap in imaging and visualization performance is achieved by employing state of the art ultrabroad bandwidth light source instead of super luminescent diodes. The ultimate availability of this UHR OCT technology strongly depends on the availability of such ultrabroad bandwidth light sources, which are suitable for OCT applications. Recently reported, cost effective approaches for broad bandwidth light sources mainly take advantage of the lower power demand with ultrahigh resolution OCT imaging.[9-12] Limiting factors of these systems are relative small bandwidths for ultra low-pump-threshold KLM titanium: sapphire lasers and strongly modulated spectra of Cr^{3+}-ion lasers, thus not perfectly suitable for OCT applications.

For the results presented in this chapter, ultrahigh resolution OCT imaging has been performed employing a laboratory prototype as well as commercially available (INTEGRAL, Femtolasers Produktions GmbH) femtosecond titanium-sapphire laser light source, that are capable of generating up to 176 nm bandwidth at 800 nm center wavelength[13] enabling 3 μm axial resolution in the retina, in combination with a commercially available ophthalmic OCT system (OCT-1) that was provided by Carl Zeiss Meditec Inc. (Dublin, CA, USA). Optical coherence imaging was performed with axial scan rates up to 250 Hz using up to 800 μW incident power in the scanning OCT beam, well below the ANSI exposure limits. Up to date, several hundreds of patients with different macular diseases including macular hole, macular edema, age-related macular degeneration, central serous chorioretinopathy, epiretinal membranes, detachment of pigment epithelium and sensory retina, glaucoma, and different hereditary retinal diseases were included.

IN VIVO OPTICAL BIOPSY OF THE HUMAN RETINA

In order to evaluate the potential of UHR OCT for enhanced visualization of intraretinal structures and to provide an improved basis for correct interpretation of *in vivo* ophthalmic UHR OCT tomograms of high clinical relevance, studies have been conducted to compare and correlate UHR OCT cross-sectional images of *ex vivo* pig[14] and monkey[15] (*Macaca fascicularis*) retinal specimens with histology. The results of these studies allow the extraction of structural retinal information of high clinical relevance *in vivo* ultrahigh resolution ophthalmic OCT tomograms and have reduced major ambiguities allowing correlation of more than 10 intraretinal layers to corresponding signals in UHR OCT tomograms.

Figure 3.1 depicts a typical horizontal *in vivo* cross-sectional UHR OCT image of a normal human macula (bottom) and a two times magnification of the foveal region (top), demonstrating the potential for *in vivo* visualization of all major intraretinal layers. These layers were subjectively correlated to the well know foveal anatomy using the results of the studies comparing UHR OCT with histology of pig and monkey retinal specimens.[14,15] Layers which consist of nerve fibers or plexiform layers are optically backscattering,

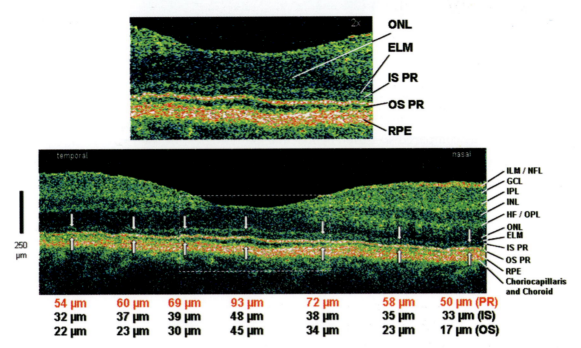

Fig. 3.1: Horizontal UHR OCT image of a normal human macula (bottom) with twofold magnification (top). ILM: internal limiting membrane; NFL: nerve fiber layer; GCL: ganglion cell layer; IPL, OPL: inner and outer plexiform layer; INL, ONL: inner and outer nuclear layer; HF: Henle's fiber layer; ELM: external limiting membrane; IS, OS PR: inner and outer segment of photoreceptor layer; RPE: retinal pigment epithelium. Arrows indicate location of total PR (red PR), IS PR (black IS) and OS PR (black OS) layer thickness measurement

while nuclear layers are less backscattering. The internal limiting membrane (ILM) has previously only been visible with electron microscopy and is not resolved with OCT. The obliquely running photoreceptor axons are sometimes considered as a separate layer in the outer plexiform layer (OPL), known as Henle's fiber layer (HF), and are highly backscattering. It is interesting to note, that the external limiting membrane (ELM) as well as the junction between the inner and outer segment of the photoreceptors (IS PR, OS PR) could be visualized. This structure is not a physical membrane, but an alignment of junctional complexes between Müller cells and photoreceptor cells. The retinal pigment epithelium (RPE), which contains melanin, is a very strongly backscattering layer. Due to the unprecedented performance of the UHR OCT technology, the thickness of the inner and outer segment of the PR layer can therefore be quantified. The distance between the RPE and the ELM indicates the thickness of the photoreceptors and is about 50-54 µm in the parafoveal region, with about 17-22 µm distributed to the outer (Figure 3.1: OS) and about 33 µm to the inner (Figure 3.1: IS) photoreceptor segment. The thickness of the PR layer significantly increases in the central foveal region, consistent with the well-known increase in length of the outer cone segments in this region to about 93 µm, approximately equally distributed to the inner (IS: 48 µm) and the outer (OS: 45 µm) photoreceptor segment. These values have been confirmed in other normal subjects, between 20 and 40 years of age. Visualization and quantification of the major intraretinal layers—especially the photoreceptor inner and outer segment—using ultrahigh resolution OCT has the potential to improve early ophthalmic diagnosis, contributes to a better understanding of pathogenesis of retinal diseases as well as might have impact in the development and monitoring of novel therapy approaches.

EARLY CLINICAL DIAGNOSIS

Recently, this novel OCT technology has been used in a clinical setting for the first time enabling *in vivo* cross-sectional imaging of macular pathologies with unprecedented axial resolution of ~3 μm to evaluate its clinical feasibility.[4,16-18]

Figure 3.2 compares ultrahigh resolution of intraretinal morphology—especially the appearance of the photoreceptor (PR) and outer nuclear layer (ONL) as well as external limiting membrane (ELM) - in a normal human retina as compared to different macular pathologies. In the extreme case of Stargardt's dystrophy the PR, the ONL, and the ELM appears completely degenerated, whereas in different stages of macular hole the PR layer as well as the ELM seem to be less affected in early stages (macular hole # 1 as compared to later stages, macular hole # 2, 3). A displacement of the PR layer as well as the ELM can be seen in acute central serous chorioretinopathy (CSC) and partially in chronic CSC, whereas in age-related macular degeneration (AMD) with minimal CNV the PR layer and the ELM are affected by CNV in the center as well as the retinal and RPE detachment. In patients with AMD and vitelliform lesion, despite retinal detachment, the PR layer, the ELM and the ONL appear quite normal, which explains the preservation of visual acuity in these patients.

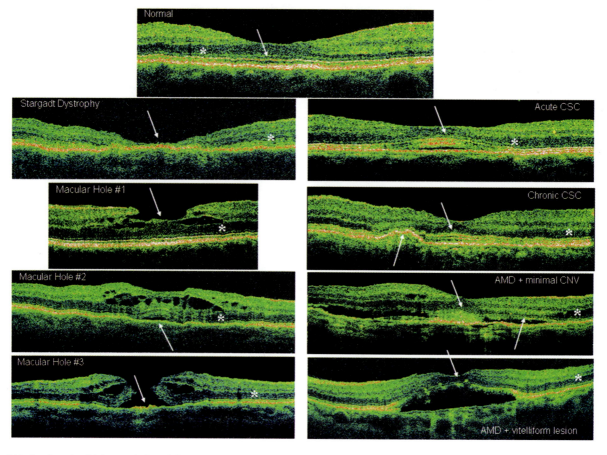

Fig. 3.2: *In vivo* ultrahigh resolution OCT images of the foveal region of a normal human retina as compared to different macular pathologies. Arrows indicate different appearance of the photoreceptor and out nuclear layer; asterisks indicate impairment of the external limiting membrane.

Especially in patients with macular hole, detailed visualization and objective quantification of the photoreceptor layer is an important factor for the therapeutic decision. Figure 3.3 shows the visualization and quantification of the IS and OS PR layer thickness in three patients with different stages of macular holes. Figure 3.3 (top) depicts the right eye of a 59-year-old woman with a visual acuity of 0.9. UHR OCT examination shows a beginning dehiscence of the inner retinal layers at the margin of the fovea, forming flat intraretinal spaces at the inner border of the outer nuclear layer. Although the temporal space seems to be only intraretinal, the nasal spaces seem to communicate with the vitreous cavity. The outer retinal layers, especially the ELM, the IS PR, the highly reflective interface between inner and outer segment of the photoreceptor layer, the OS PR and the RPE can clearly be visualized and appear unchanged. Higher magnification allows for better identification of small intraretinal spaces as well as the quantification of the PR layer, which is about 98 µm in the central and about 70-77 µm in the parafoveal region, indicating quite normal thickness despite the retinal pathology. The findings lead to the diagnosis of an early stage of an inner lamellar macular hole. Figure 3.3 (middle) shows the left eye a 63-year-old woman who suffered from a loss of visual acuity from 1.0 to 0.4. UHR OCT revealed a total interruption of the outer retinal layers, especially the ELM, IS PR, the highly reflective interface between the IS and OS PR and the OS PR. The outer retinal layers seem to be pulled up towards the center of the lesion with about 100-117 µm PR layer thickness. This is probably due to the retinal detachment in this area and therefore the stretched appearance of the PR OS. In the parafoveal region the PR layer thickness is about 76-77 µm, again like in the latter case in a normal thickness range. These findings are consistent with a macular hole stage 1-A to 1-B according to Gass.[19] In Figure 3.3 (bottom) UHR OCT was performed on a patient a full thickness macular hole with adherent vitreous, corresponding to a stage 3 hole as classified by Gass.[19] UHR OCT reveals a marked thickening of the hole wall, small cystoid spaces in the INL and large spaces in the ONL. The PR layers, however, seem to be intact (yellow arrows) almost to the edges of the full thickness tissue defect at the center of the hole (red arrows). The highly reflective layer can be followed almost to the edge of the hole. The RPE – Bruch´s membrane complex shows an increased reflectivity at the center of the hole. Outside the macular hole the PR layer thickness is between 68-73 µm, indicating normal appearance and condition.

Figure 3.4 (top) depicts an UHR OCT scan through the fovea of a 30-year-old female patient with Stargardt's disease (left), central microperimetry measurement (middle), as well as the corresponding location of the UHR OCT scan on the fluorescein angiogram (right). Due to a significant atrophy of the entire intraretinal layer, but especially of the outer nuclear, IS PR and OS PR, reduction of the retinal thickness to only 65 µm is revealed by UHR OCT. In the parafoveal region, small remnants of the IS PR and OS PR with a thickness of about 30-33 µm—significantly thinner than in normal subjects (Figures 3.1 and 3.2)—can be visualized by UHR OCT. Microperimetry measurements revealed the existence of a clear absolute scotoma indicated in Figure 3.4 (top – middle). This absolute scotoma corresponds with the area of transverse PR loss visualized by UHR OCT (red arrows in Figure 3.4 top-left). In a separate study 22 eyes of 14 patients with Stargardt's disease and fundus flavimaculatus were investigated using UHR OCT to compare it with central functional tests[17] employing microperimetry. Statistically, a correlation was seen between visual acuity and photoreceptor loss ($R^2= -0.53$, $p = 0.016$) as well as with scotoma size ($R^2=0.53$, $p=0.024$). There was, however, no correlation between PR loss and scotoma size ($R^2=0.17$, $p=0.51$). A linear regression model for visual acuity and photoreceptor loss showed a highly significant result ($R^2=0.60$, $p=0.006$, Figure 3.4 bottom). This was not seen when scotoma size was related to photoreceptor loss ($r=0.06$, $p=0.81$). The mean

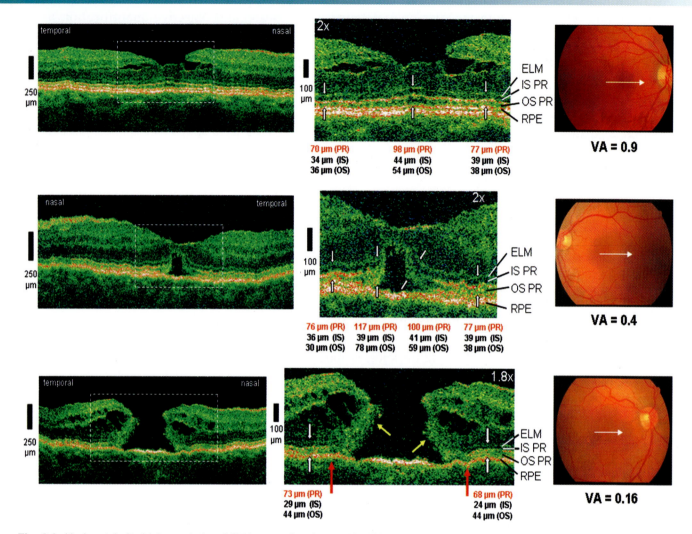

Fig. 3.3: Horizontal ultrahigh resolution OCT image of patients with different stages of macular holes (left), magnification of the central foveal region with quantification of the PR layer thickness (middle) and fundus photo with arrow indicating scan location; ELM, external limiting membrane; IS PR, inner segments of photoreceptors; OS PR, = outer segments of photoreceptors; RPE, retinal pigment epithelium.

foveal thickness was markedly reduced (85 μm ± 39). This did not correlate with PR loss (R^2=0.15, p=0.5) or VA (R^2= –0.32, p=0.16), but there was a significant correlation with scotoma size (R^2= –0.6, p=0.008).

For early glaucoma diagnosis, UHR OCT might enable significantly improved visualization of the retinal nerve fiber layer, especially of its posterior surface, quantification of its circumpapillary thickness distribution as well as topographic information of the optical nerve head.[18] Hence UHR OCT might be a powerful technique to track subtle intraretinal morphology changes associated in early stages of this disease. Figures 3.5A to D demonstrate a possible alternative strategy for early glaucoma detection, by visualizing and quantifying foveal ganglion cell layer thickness. An UHR OCT image of a healthy subject (A) as well as of the same foveal region of a 74-year-old patient with end stage glaucoma (B) documented by visual field (C) and HRT (Heidelberg Retinal Tomogram) (D) are depicted. Due to increased intraocular pressure the foveal depression is less pronounced in the end stage glaucoma patient (B). Nasally no nerve fiber layer thickness

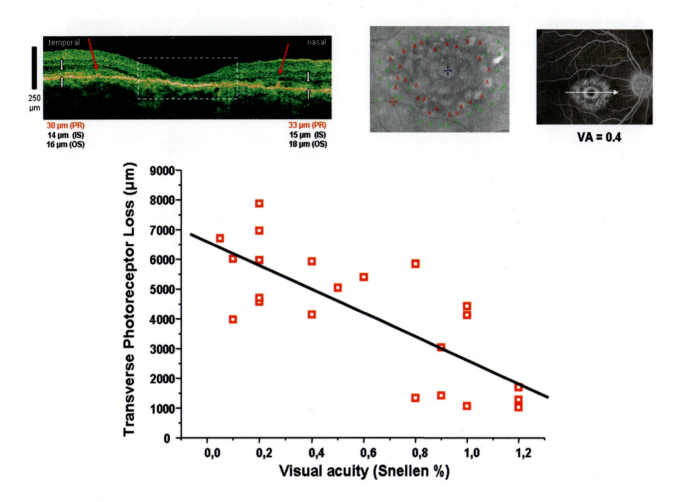

Fig. 3.4: Horizontal UHR OCT image of patients with Stargardt's dystrophy (top, left), microperimetry measurement (top, middle) and fluorescein angiography photo (top, right) with arrow indicating scan location; ELM, external limiting membrane; IS PR, inner segments of photoreceptors; OS PR, = outer segments of photoreceptors; RPE, retinal pigment epithelium. Transverse photoreceptor loss in micrometers as a function of best corrected visual acuity in Snellen percentage (bottom). Black line indicates linear regression graph ($R^2 = 0.6$; $p < 0.01$).

exists anymore in the end stage glaucoma patient (white arrows). Finally the ganglion cell layer is atrophied in case of the end stage glaucoma (circles) and has a mean thickness of about 40 µm (together with the inner plexiform layer) in the parafoveal region as compared to about 120 µm in the case of the normal subject. In addition to the nerve fiber layer thickness distribution around the optic disc, atrophy of the foveal ganglion cell layer might enable a novel approach for a more sensitive and specific early glaucoma diagnosis.

MONITORING OF DISEASE PROGRESSION

Figures 3.6A to F depict *in vivo* horizontal UHR OCT tomograms of the optic nerve head in a non-human primate glaucoma model (*cynomolgous monkey*). Cross-sections are depicted at baseline (A), 20 days (B) as well as 34 days (C) after induction of unilateral ocular hypertension at approximately the same retinal

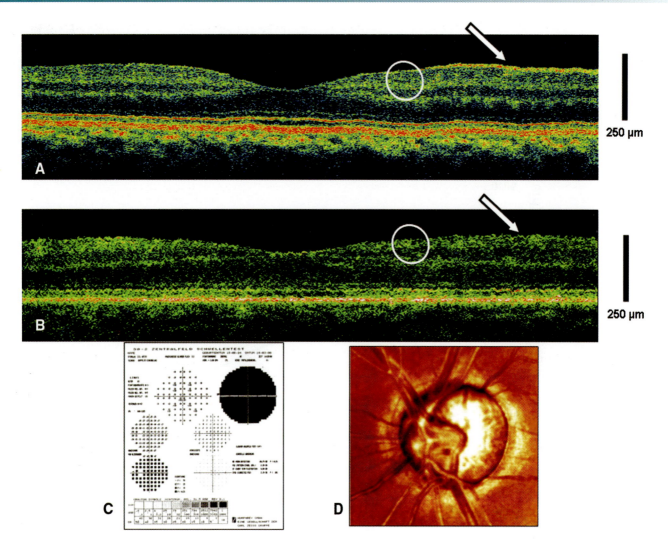

Figs 3.5A to D: *In vivo* ultrahigh resolution OCT detecting and quantifying subtle changes in an end stage glaucoma patient (B) documented by visual field test (C) and Heidelberg Retinal Tomogram (HRT) image (D)) as compared to a normal subject (A): Foveal pit contour changes, lost nerve fiber layer (arrows) as well as atrophy of the ganglion cell and inner plexiform layer (circles) are detected.

location. The retinal nerve fiber layer in the circumpapillary region is clearly visualized despite its atrophy due to increased ocular pressure in twofold magnifications (arrows in D-F). Furthermore the lamina cribrosa is clearly visualized at baseline (A), which might also be used for detecting early glaucomatous changes. In the advanced stages, the lamina cribrosa is severely thinned or even absent (B and C) and vessels appear prominent caused by significant cupping of the optic nerve head due to increased intraocular pressure. These preliminary results demonstrate that UHR OCT enables unprecedented visualization of intraretinal morphology, which had previously only been possible with histopathology and therefore provides a powerful tool for longitudinal monitoring of micro structural changes related to the development of glaucoma and in general retinal diseases. In glaucoma, it provides a tool to investigate the impairment of the foveal ganglion cell layer in early stages of glaucomatous damage and might therefore significantly contribute to a better

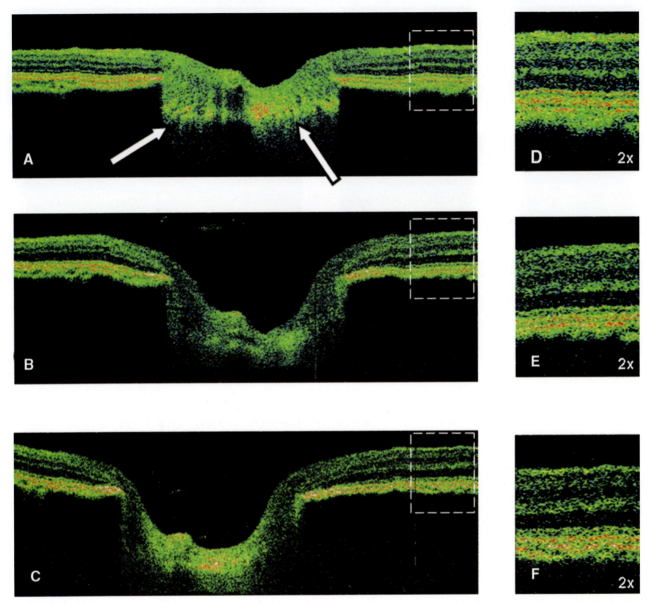

Figs 3.6A to F: *In vivo* ultrahigh resolution OCT of a non-human primate glaucoma model (cynomolgous monkey). Clear topographic (A-C) as well as morphological progression (D-E) is detected by ultrahigh resolution OCT. In addition to clear visualization of the lamina cribrosa (A, arrows), circumpapillary nerve fiber layer thickness despite significant atrophy is clearly visualized (D-E, arrows).

understanding of the pathogenesis of this disease.

MONITORING OF THERAPY

Figure 3.7 demonstrates the potential of ophthalmic ultrahigh resolution OCT to monitor and therefore contribute to a better understanding of novel therapy approaches. In this case the effect of an anti-VEGF drug is investigated. This case describes a 60-year-old woman having regressing drusen with placoid occult

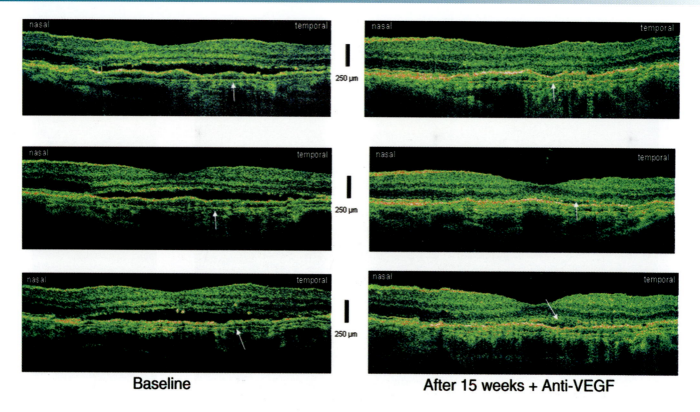

Fig. 3.7: Monitoring of new therapy approaches using *in vivo* ultrahigh resolution OCT: patient with regressing drusen with placoid occult without classic CNV before (left) and 15 weeks after anti-VEGF (vascular endothelium growths factor) treatment (right).

without classic choroidal neovascularization (Figure 3.7 left top, middle, bottom). In addition to a normal appearance of the NFL, GCL and IPL and INL, the photoreceptor layer is strongly comprised, due to a serous detachment. Ultrahigh resolution OCT enables visualization of the occult membrane underneath the RPE as well as the outer membrane of Bruch's membrane, indicating intra-Bruch's choroidal neovascularization for the first time (arrows). In all three cross-sections highly reflective particles in the level of the outer photoreceptor layer which could be isolated RPE cells or damaged photoreceptors could be differentiated by ultrahigh resolution OCT. Fifteen weeks later the effect of therapy treatment can clearly be visualized with ultrahigh resolution ophthalmic OCT (Figure 3.7 right top, middle, bottom). The PR complex has recovered; some subtle serous detachments as well as the occult membrane are still present.

Finally, Figure 3.8 demonstrates the potential of ophthalmic ultrahigh resolution OCT to not only provide additional information about the status of the photoreceptor layer in patients with macular hole for the decision of surgical intervention but also to monitor the effect of this intervention and investigate its outcome. A 65-year-old women presented with a decrease of visual acuity in her right eye, Snellen visual acuity had dropped from 1.0 to 0.3, Watzke-Allen sign was positive. Examination of the right eye revealed a stage 2 macular hole (Figure 3.8 top right). UHR OCT shows a complete tissue defect through all retinal layers. The vitreous adhesion, causing disruption and a marginal defect of the inner retinal layers can be seen well. Large intraretinal cysts seem to be located in the ONL, and there is a complete absence of the PR layer at the

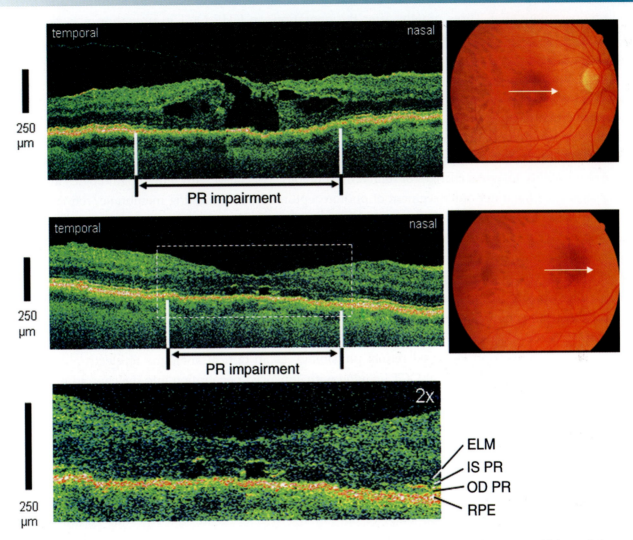

Fig. 3.8: Monitoring of surgical intervention with *in vivo* ultrahigh resolution OCT: (Top left) Horizontal ultrahigh-resolution optical coherence tomographic image; bars and arrows indicating extent of photoreceptor impairment well beyond the margin of the macular hole. (Top right) Preoperative fundus photo with macular hole and surrounding fluid cuff, arrow indicating horizontal scan. (Middle left) Horizontal ultrahigh-resolution optical coherence tomographic image; bars and arrows indicating extent of residual postoperative photoreceptor impairment 3 months following macular hole surgery. (Middle right) Postoperative fundus picture with clinically closed macular hole, arrow indicating horizontal scan. (Bottom) magnification of middle left with labeling of retinal layers: the outer retina remains abnormal 3 months after surgery; IS PR, inner segments of photoreceptors; OS PR, = outer segments of photoreceptors; RPE, retinal pigment epithelium.

center of the hole. The structure of the PR layer, especially the IS PR and OS PR as well as the high reflective layer between these two layers, seems to be altered far beyond the full thickness tissue defect. This alteration extends even outside the area of the intraretinal cysts, indicating an impairment of the PR layer extending peripherally to the cystoid changes of the ONL (Figure 3.8 top left). In this eye, a vitrectomy with intraoperative posterior vitreous separation and intraocular tamponade with C_3F_8 gas in a 12.5% concentration was performed. No peeling of the inner limiting membrane was performed. After 3 weeks and complete resorption of the air/gas bubble, the macular hole appeared closed on clinical examination (Figure 3.8 middle right). Visual acuity, however, was 0.3 and was therefore almost unchanged compared to the preoperative value. Three months after the operation, an UHR OCT examination was performed (Figure 3.8 middle left). The hole appears closed by a complete bridge of tissue. At the center, however, small cystoid spaces in the outer retinal layers can be seen (Figure 3.8, middle left and middle bottom). The appearance and the size of the PR layer impairment are almost unchanged to the preoperative picture (Figure 3.8, middle left). Therefore, although the hole is closed on clinical appearance, a normal architecture of the outer retinal layers, especially the PR layer, had not been restored.

Ultrahigh resolution ophthalmic OCT enables unprecedented visualization of all major intraretinal layers which had previously only been possible with histopathology. Clear visualization of all the major intraretinal layers and the ability to assess changes of retinal morphology associated with retinal pathologies in an early stage, especially in the inner outer segment of photoreceptors/external limiting membrane/retinal pigment epithelium complex, promises to have a significant impact on the diagnosis, investigation and better understanding of pathogenesis as well as the evaluation of novel therapy approaches of a variety of macular diseases. The hypothesis is that intraretinal structures, that are relevant for the diagnosis and monitoring of early stages of eye diseases, can be resolved by the proposed optical biopsy version of OCT.

Recent developments of ophthalmic UHR OCT include high speed,[20-22] three dimensional retinal imaging, using broadband super luminescent diode light sources,[23] combining adaptive optics and UHR OCT,[24] spatially resolved spectroscopic OCT,[25] functional imaging as a non-invasive method alternative to electrical retinal recordings for probing depth resolved retinal physiology as an optical analogue to electrophysiological measurements in the retina, as well as OCT imaging with enhanced penetration into the choroid by employing novel wavelength regions. Using state of the art laser technology, including ultrabroad bandwidth femtosecond solid state lasers, fiber lasers and photonic crystal fibers based light sources, ultrahigh resolution OCT in the 600–1060 nm wavelength region enabled enhanced penetration into the choroid.[26] Furthermore, OCT could be used in this wavelength region for the first time to perform non-invasive, depth resolved optical probing of light stimulated intraretinal physiological responses to function as an optical analogue to electrophysiological measurements in the retina.

In addition, a compact closed-loop adaptive optics (AO) system, based on a real-time Hartmann-Shack wave-front sensor at 30 Hz and a 37 element low-cost micro machined membrane deformable mirror, was interfaced to an UHR OCT system, based on a commercially available OCT instrument.[24] Correction of ocular aberrations for a 3.68 mm pupil diameter enabled a significant improvement of the OCT transverse resolution from 20 μm to about 5-10 μm in addition to the 3 μm axial resolution. This is a 2-3 time improvement as compared to UHR OCT systems used so far, that employed a 1 mm beam diameter without AO. Furthermore, a significant UHR OCT signal to noise ratio improvement of up to 9 dB using AO, as compared to uncorrected ocular aberrations, could be achieved.

Finally, *in vivo* ultrahigh resolution, high speed (25000 A-scans/second) retinal imaging obtained with Fourier domain (FD) OCT employing a specially developed, commercially available, compact, broad bandwidth Titanium: sapphire laser[13] could be achieved.[20-22] Similar *in vivo* OCT sensitivity performance as well as visualization of intraretinal layers, especially the inner and outer segment of the photoreceptor layer, was achieved by ultrahigh resolution FDOCT as compared to standard ultrahigh resolution OCT and a 40 times higher data acquisition speed of FDOCT, enabling *in vivo* three-dimensional ultrahigh resolution retinal imaging.[20-22]

It is unlikely that OCT will replace histology or other existing ophthalmic diagnostic modalities. However, from the viewpoint of screening and diagnosis of diseases, the proposed version of OCT might enable significantly new insight in the pathogenesis and therapy control of several retinal diseases. The unique features of this developed technology would enable a broad range of research and clinical applications, which might not only complement many of the existing ophthalmic imaging technologies available today, but also potentially reveal previously unseen, intraretinal changes.

REFERENCES

1. Drexler W, Morgner U, Kärtner FX, et al. In vivo ultrahigh resolution optical coherence tomography. Opt Lett. 1999;24:1221-1223.
2. Drexler W, Morgner U, Ghanta RK, et al. New technology for ultrahigh resolution optical coherence tomography of the retina. In: The Shape of Glaucoma, Eds.: Lemij H, Schuman JS. Kugler Publications, 2000:75-104.
3. Drexler W, Morgner U, Ghanta RK, et al. Ultrahigh resolution ophthalmologic optical coherence tomography. Nature Medicine 2001;7:502-507.
4. Drexler W, Sattmann H, Hermann B, et al. Enhanced visualization of macular pathology using ultrahigh resolution optical coherence tomography. Arch Ophthalmol. 2003;121:695-706.
5. Drexler W. Ultrahigh resolution optical coherence tomography. Journal Biomed Optics. 2004;9: 47-74.
6. Huang D, Swanson EA, Lin CP, et al. Optical Coherence Tomography. Science. 1991; 254:1178-1181.
7. Hee MR, Izatt JA, Swanson EA. Optical coherence tomography of the human retina. Arch Ophthalmol. 1995;113:325-332.
8. Schuman JS, Puliafito CA, Fujimoto JG. Optical coherence tomography of ocular disease. Slack Inc, Thorofare, New Jersey. 2004.
9. Kowalevicz AM, Schibli TR, Kärtner FX, Fujimoto JG. Opt Lett. 2002;27:2037.
10. Uemura S, Torizuka K. Jpn J Appl Phys. 2000;39:3472.
11. Sorokina I, Sorokin E, Wintner E, et al. Opt Lett. 1997;22:1716.
12. Wagenblast PC, Morgner U, Grawert F. Opt Lett. 2002;27:1726.
13. Unterhuber A, Hermann B, H. Sattmann H, et al. Compact, low cost Ti:Al$_2$O$_3$ laser for in vivo ultrahigh resolution optical coherence tomography. Opt Lett. 2003;28:905-907.
14. Glosmann M, Hermann B, Schubert C, et al. Histological correlation of pig retina radial stratification with ultrahigh resolution optical coherence tomography. Invest Ophthalmol Vis Sci. 2003 ;44:1696-1703.
15. Anger EM, Hermann B, Schubert C, et al. Ultrahigh resolution optical coherence tomography of the monkey fovea. Identification of retinal sub layers by correlation with semithin histology sections. Exp Eye Res. 2004;78:1117-1125.
16. Ko TH, Fujimoto JG, Duker JS, et al. Comparison of Ultrahigh- and Standard-Resolution Optical Coherence Tomography for Imaging Macular Hole Pathology and Repair. Ophthalmology. 2004;111:2033-2043.
17. Ergun E, Hermann B, Wirtitsch M, et al. Assessment of Central Visual Function in Stargardt's disease/Fundus Flavimaculatus with Ultrahigh-Resolution Optical Coherence Tomography. Invest Ophthalmol Vis Sci. (in press).
18. Wollstein G, Paunescu LA, Ko TH, et al. Ultrahigh-Resolution Optical Coherence Tomography in Glaucoma. Ophthalmology. (in press).
19. Gass JDM. Reappraisal of Biomicroscopic Classification of Stages of Development of a Macular Hole. Am J Ophthalmol. 1995;199:6:752-759.
20. Leitgeb RA, Drexler W, Unterhuber A, et al. Ultrahigh resolution Fourier domain optical coherence tomography. Optics Expr. 2004;12:2157-2165.
21. Wojtkowski M, V.J. Srinivasan VJ, T.H. Ko TH, et al. Ultrahigh-resolution, high-speed, Fourier domain optical coherence tomography and methods for dispersion compensation. Optics Expr. 2004;12:2404-2422.
22. Cense B, Nassif NA, Chen TC, et al. Ultrahigh-resolution high-speed retinal imaging using süectral-domain optical coherence tomography. Optics Expr. 2004;12:2435-2447.
23. Ko TH, Adler DC, Fujimoto JG, et al. Ultrahigh resolution optical coherence tomography imaging with broadband super luminescent diode light source. Optics Expr. 2004;12:2112-2119.
24. Hermann B, Fernández EJ, Unterhuber A, et al. Adaptive optics ultrahigh resolution optical coherence tomography. Opt Lett. 2004;29:1-3.
25. Hermann B, Bizheva K, Unterhuber A, et al. Precision of extracting absorption profiles from weakly scattering media with spectroscopic optical coherence tomography. Opt Exp. 2004;12:1677-1688.
26. Unterhuber A, Povazay B, Bizheva K, et al. Advances in broad bandwidth light sources for ultrahigh resolution optical coherence tomography. Physics in Medicine and Biology. 2004;49:1235-1246.

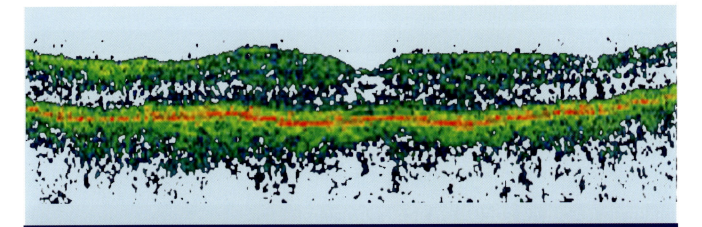

CHAPTER
4

Diabetic
Macular Edema

Alain Gaudric,
Pascale Massin, Ali Erginay

INTRODUCTION

The quantitative assessment of macular edema was one of the first uses of optical coherence tomography (OCT). In a series of 45 patients, Hee and associates[1] concluded in 1995 that cross-sectional images of the macula appeared to be "useful for objectively monitoring retinal thickness with high resolution in patients with macular edema. It may eventually prove to be a sensitive diagnostic test for the early detection of macular thickening in patients with diabetic retinopathy." Now ten years later, OCT is widely used to detect and monitor diabetic macular edema, using the scan profile and macular mapping.

DIABETIC MACULAR EDEMA ON SCAN PROFILES

The scan profile allows the appraisal of intraretinal changes, of the shape of the inner boundary of the thickened macula, and of the presence of possible subretinal detachment or incomplete vitreomacular separation, findings which are often missed by clinical examination alone. The scan profile mode of OCT now allows remarkably accurate definition of the different characteristics of diabetic macular edema, such as diffuse swelling, cystoid cavities, and hard exudates, all of which are clearly visible on OCT scans.

Intraretinal Changes

Diffuse Swelling

Diffuse swelling appears as a thickening of the retina without definite cystic spaces. The outer plexiform layer and outer nuclear layer are often the most prone to thickening and hyporeflectivity (Figs 4.1A to G).[2]

Cystoid Cavities

Cystoid cavities are hyporeflective spaces of various sizes, mainly located in the outer retina (Henle fiber and outer plexiform layers), and sometimes also in the inner plexiform layer. In the most advanced stages of diabetic macular edema, one or several large central cysts are responsible for significant thickening of the foveola. However, it should be borne in mind that these hyporeflective spaces, which, in bidirectional scans look like individual "cysts", would probably look as if they were interconnected in a three-dimensional representation (Figs 4.2 to 4.14).[3]

Optical coherence tomography is very useful to determine whether edema threatens or involves the macular center. In some cases, the edges of the macula may be thickened, even though the foveal center retains a normal contour (Figs 4.2 and 4.14). Macular thickening may be asymmetric, especially in focal edema, and may only involve a sector of the macular area (Figs 4.14 and 4.15). Therefore, the mean macular thickness calculated for each area may not exactly reflect the topography of the edema, which may involve less than an entire area, or on the contrary, encroach upon two areas.

Foveolar Detachment

In some cases, diabetic macular edema is combined with a foveolar detachment which was not detected or even suspected on biomicroscopy. In such cases, the macula usually thickens significantly and contains prominent cystoid cavities. (Figs 4.7 to 4.9). However, extrafoveal focal edema may also result in the migration of subretinal fluid to the subretinal space, despite the absence of major foveal cystic changes or thickening

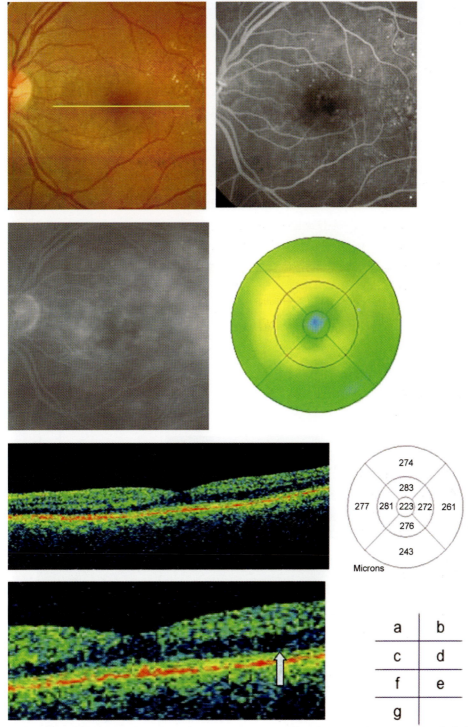

Figs 4.1A to G: Non-cystoid diffuse macular edema in moderate non-proliferative diabetic retinopathy. A: Color fundus photograph showing microaneurysms, punctuate hemorrhages and a few scattered hard exudates. B: Fluorescein angiography, early phase. Note the numerous microaneurysms and minimal enlargement of the foveal avascular zone. C: Fluorescein angiography, late phase. Diffuse leakage is visible. D and E: Retinal thickness map; the color code indicates moderate diffuse macular thickening. Mean thickness values are at the upper limit of normal. F: Horizontal 6 mm linear scan. The macular profile seems normal, except for the foveal depression, which is shallower than usual, indicating a diffuse swelling of the macula. G: Detail. Hyporeflective space in the outer nuclear layer (arrow), indicating accumulation of intraretinal fluid. The visual acuity of this eye is 20/20

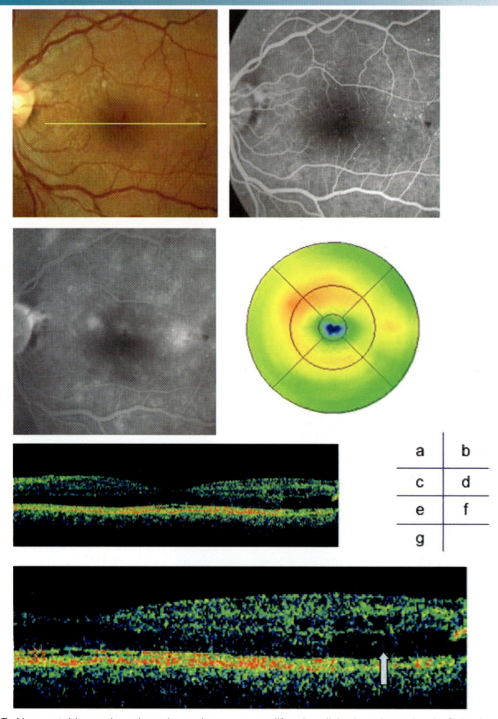

Figs 4.2A to F: Non-cystoid macular edema in moderate non-proliferative diabetic retinopathy. A: Color fundus photograph showing an irregular retinal reflex. Punctuate hemorrhages and minimal hard exudates are visible. B: Fluorescein angiography, early phase showing numerous microaneurysms and a small area of capillary closure, temporal to the macula. C: Fluorescein Angiography, late phase. Note the diffuse leakage in the macular area. D: Retinal thickness maps; despite diffuse perimacular thickening, the foveal center has remained almost normal (dark blue). E: Horizontal 6 mm scan. The foveal pit contour is normal. The microcystic changes temporal to the macula correspond to the area of focal leakage. F: detail: note the large cystic spaces in the outer nuclear layer (ONL). Smaller cysts are also present in the inner retinal layers. The visual acuity of this eye is 20/32.

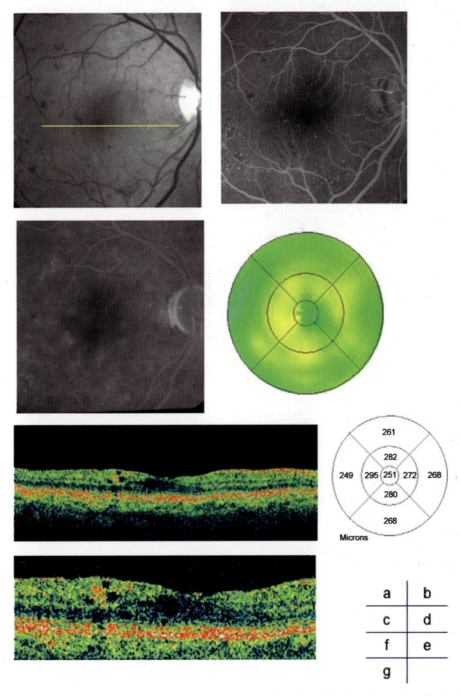

Figs 4.3A to G: Early cystoid macular edema in moderate non-proliferative diabetic retinopathy. A: Red-free photograph: showing numerous punctate hemorrhages in the posterior pole. B: Fluorescein angiography, early phase. Many microaneurysms are visible. C: Fluorescein angiography, early phase; mild diffuse macular leakage, without a cystoid appearance. D and E: Retinal thickness maps show diffuse, moderate macular thickening, with flattening of the foveal depression. Mean thickness of the central area is slightly increased (251 μm). F: Horizontal 6 mm scan disclosing slight moderate thickening of the macula and flattening of the foveal depression. There is a cystoid cavity in the temporal part of the fovea, and numerous microcystic changes are visible which were not seen on fluorescein angiography. G: Detail showing the cystoid spaces. The visual acuity of this eye is 20/25.

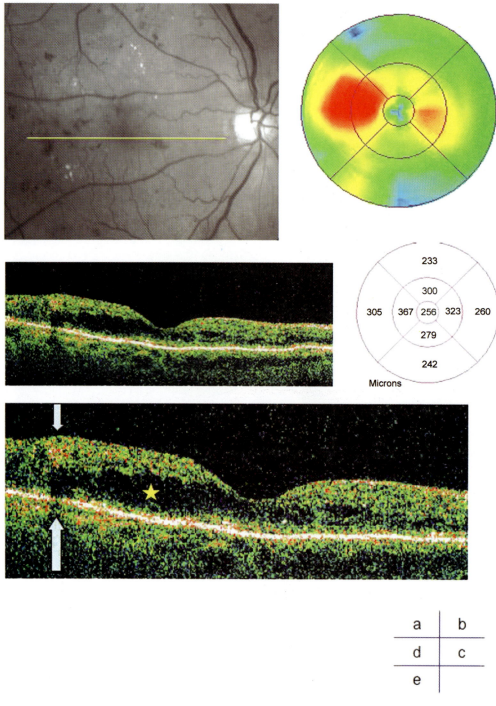

a	b
d	c
e	

Figs 4.4A to E: Macular edema in moderate non-proliferative diabetic retinopathy A: Red-free photograph of the posterior pole showing intraretinal hemorrhages, microaneurysms, and a few hard exudates. B: Retinal thickness maps; color map shows two foci of retinal thickening, respectively on the temporal and nasal sides of the macula. Central foveolar thickness is normal (182 µm) but foveal thickness (central 1000 µm) is greater than normal (256 µm) D: Horizontal 6 mm scan; retinal thickening is more prominent on the temporal than nasal side of the macula. Despite diffuse macular thickening, the foveal pit is still present. E: detail; an inner intraretinal hemorrhage gives focal hyper-reflectivity and an underlying shadow (between the two arrows); note the diffuse outer swelling in the outer nuclear layer (star). The visual acuity of this eye is 20/25

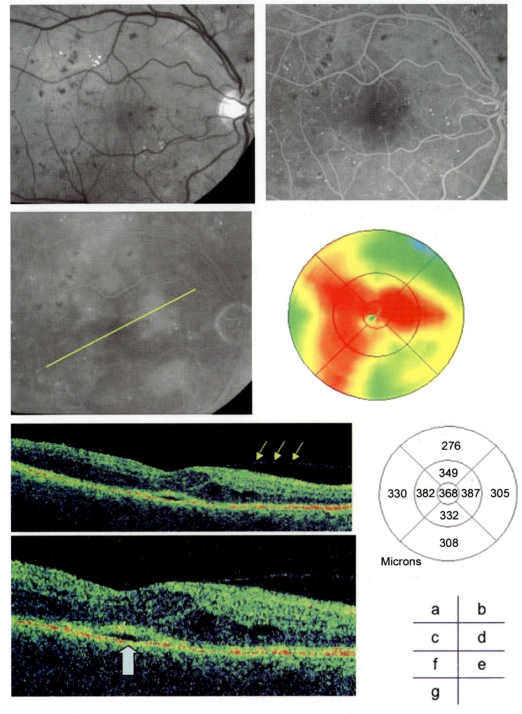

Figs 4.5A to G: Macular edema in moderate non-proliferative diabetic retinopathy. A: Red-free photograph of the posterior pole showing intraretinal hemorrhages, microaneurysms, and hard exudates. B and C: Fluorescein angiography, early and late phases, showing mild cystoid macular edema. D and E: Retinal thickness maps; color map shows diffuse macular thickening. Central macular thickness has increased to 368 μm F: Horizontal 6mm scan; retinal thickening is more prominent on the nasal side of the macula. The posterior hyaloid is only partially detached on this side (yellow arrows) G: Detail; note the intraretinal cystic spaces in a moderately thickened retina and the presence of a small shallow foveolar detachment (large arrow). The visual acuity of this eye is 20/25.

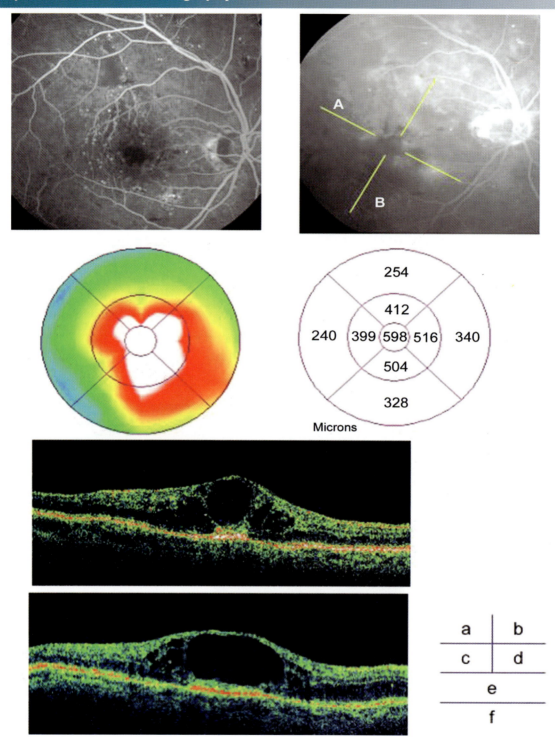

Figs 4.6A to F: Severe cystoid macular edema in severe non-proliferative diabetic retinopathy. A: Fluorescein angiography, early phase, showing areas of capillary non-perfusion. B: Fluorescein angiography, late phase, showing cystoid macular edema (lines a and b refer to the direction of the linear scans below). C and D: Retinal thickness maps; color map shows diffuse macular thickening. Central macular thickness has increased to 598 µm. E: 6 mm scan (A): a large central foveal cyst is surrounded by smaller cysts, resulting in significant macular thickening. F: 6 mm scan (B); on a perpendicular scan, the central cyst seems larger. The visual acuity of this eye is 20/125

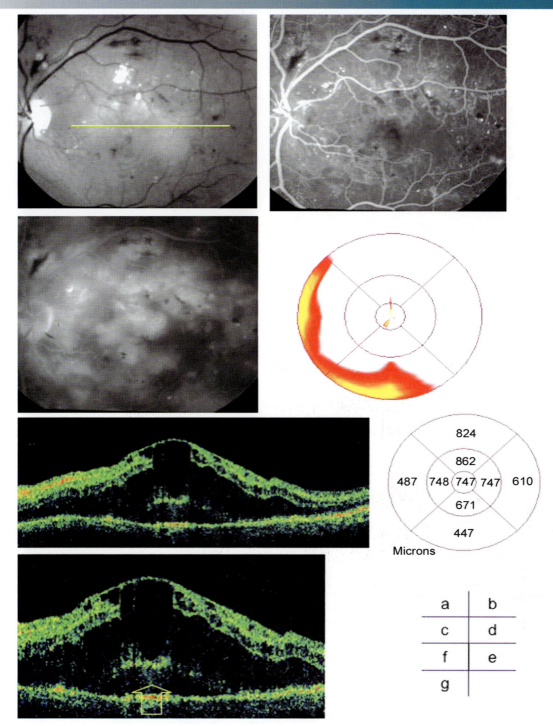

Figs 4.7A to G: Severe cystoid macular edema in mild proliferative diabetic retinopathy. A: Red-free photograph of the posterior pole showing intraretinal hemorrhages and hard exudates. B: Fluorescein angiography, early phase ; note the areas of capillary non-perfusion, intraretinal microvascular anomalies, and early preretinal new vessels. C: Fluorescein angiography, late phase disclosing the severe cystoid macular edema. D and E: Retinal thickness maps; color map shows severe macular thickening. Central average thickness has increased to 747 µm. F: Horizontal 6 mm scan; a large central foveal cyst surrounded by smaller ones has resulted in significant macular thickening. G: Detail; note that the intraretinal cystic spaces have mainly developed in the outer retinal layers. A small foveolar detachment is present (large arrow). The visual acuity of this eye is 20/100.

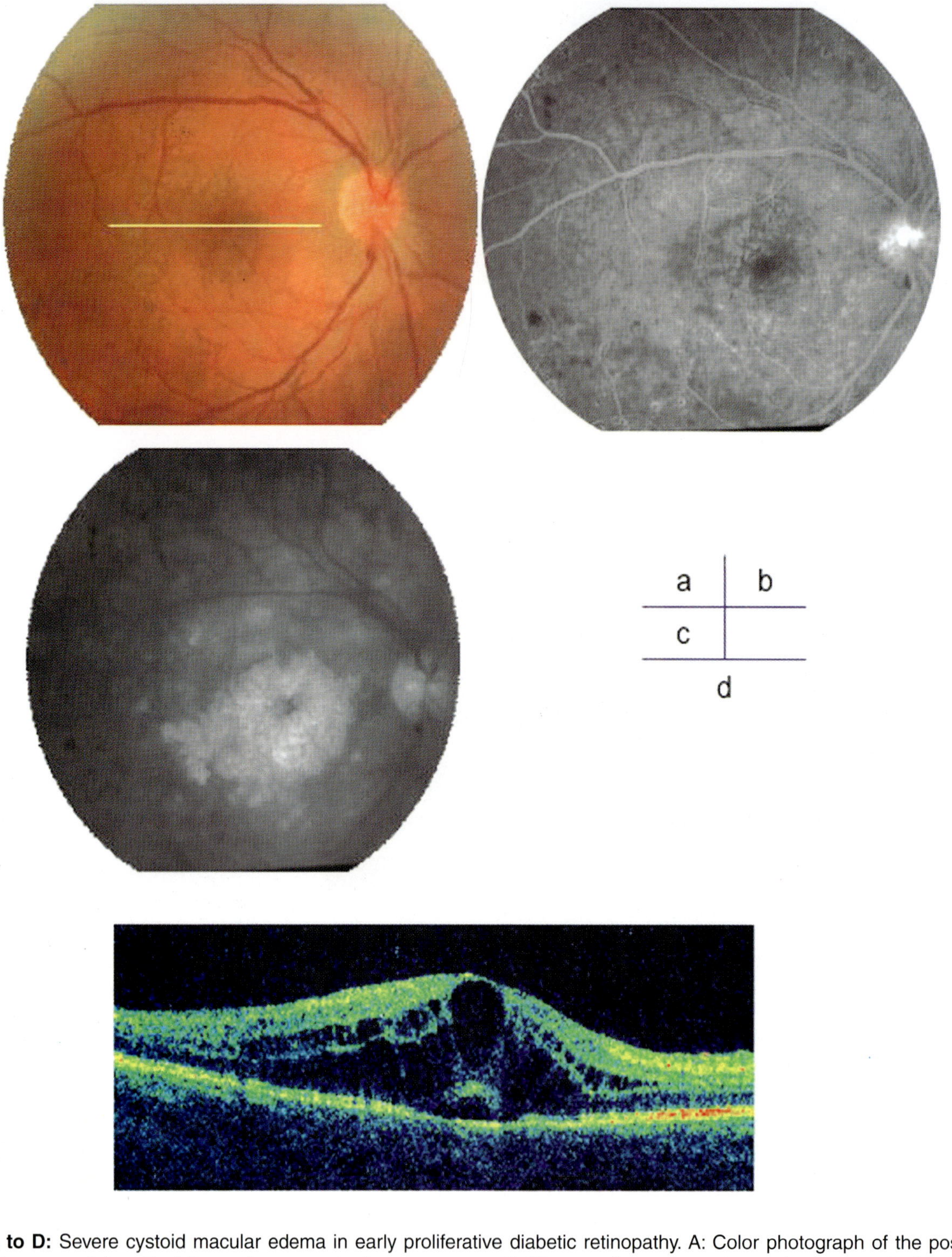

Figs 4.8A to D: Severe cystoid macular edema in early proliferative diabetic retinopathy. A: Color photograph of the posterior pole showing some intraretinal hemorrhages and microaneurysms. B: Fluorescein angiography, early phase note the diffuse capillary dilation and small disc new-vessels. C: Fluorescein angiography, late phase, shows severe diffuse cystoid macular edema. C: Horizontal 6 mm scan; a large central foveal cyst is surrounded by smaller ones in the outer nuclear and plexiform layers; a small foveolar detachment is present. The visual acuity of this eye is 20/400

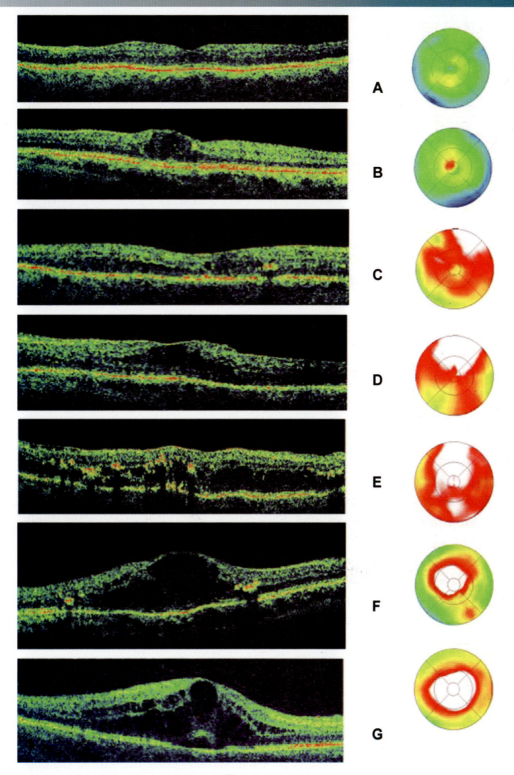

Figs 4.9A to G: The increasing severity of diabetic macular edema on OCT (from A to G) A: Minor diffuse retinal thickening. B: Central foveal cyst, but minor thickening of the macular area. C: Foveal thickness is less than in b, but the macular area thickening is more diffuse. D to F: Severe cystoid macular edema, with hyper-reflective hard exudates. G: Severe cystoid macular edema with foveal detachment.

(Figs 4.16A to E). In that case the foveal detachment is not usually due to any vitreoretinal traction.[4-6] It was seen in 15% of eyes with diabetic macular edema by Otani and associates.[5] The pathogenesis and functional consequences of foveal detachment combined with cystoid macular edema are still unknown. However, in a personal series of 78 eyes with macular edema examined by OCT, the presence of foveal elevation did not correlate with poorer visual acuity, compared to other cases with the same macular thickening.[7]

Hard Exudates

Hard exudates appear as hyper-reflective intraretinal deposits, mostly located in the outer plexiform layer of the retina. They mask the reflectivity of the underlying tissue.[4, 5, 8] They may accumulate in the fovea, in which case the macula is often thickened by edema (Figs 4.11 and 4.12). However, in other cases, the foveal thickness is normal or nearly normal although the exudates surrounding the focal edema accumulate in the fovea. This is not surprising, if one considers that the exudates deposit occurs at the limit of the area of fluid reabsorption (Figs 4.13 to 4.15). In these cases, OCT helps to distinguish between resorption exudates and exudates surrounding an active focus of edema (Figs 4.15A to F).

Centrofoveal exudates have different appearances on OCT. Some of them accumulate in the inner foveola at the border of an area of retinal thickening. VA may be only moderately impaired in these cases (Figs 4.17 and 4.18). Very different are the subfoveal plaques of exudates. They form a subfoveal deposit and are associated with atrophy of the macular tissue, which explains the poor vision of the eyes affected (Figs 4.19A to C).

Inner Retinal Boundary

In scans passing through the macular center, the shape of the inner retinal boundary indicates the severity of central macular edema.

The earliest sign of foveolar edema on OCT scans is the *flattening of the foveal pit* (Figs 4.3, 4.9 A to C). When macular edema is definitely present, the inner retinal boundary tends to be dome-shaped (Figs 4.6 to 4.9). A dome-shaped profile is more frequently observed when the posterior hyaloid remains attached to the macular center, i.e. detached from the macular area except at the foveolar center (Figs 4.22A and B). However, this convex profile may also exist if the posterior hyaloid is detached (Figs 4.7A to G).

In rare cases, the macular center rises steeply and exhibits concave slopes. This is typically the case when a thick, hyper-reflective, taut posterior hyaloid is attached to the top of the elevated macular center, and causes tractional diabetic macular edema (Figs 4.23, 4.24 and 4.26).[9-11]

Lastly, macular edema may also be combined with an epiretinal membrane, which may result in superficial retinal folds; OCT-3 has enhanced epiretinal membrane visibility (Figs 4.24 and 4.25).

Posterior Hyaloid

The posterior hyaloid is only visible on OCT when it is partly or slightly detached from the retinal surface. As OCT-3 has a 4 mm deep field, a posterior hyaloid detachment from the retinal surface of more than 2 mm may not be visible if the retinal scan is in the center of the box. Lowering the scan to the bottom of the box may enable a detached posterior hyaloid to be visualized 3 to 3.5 mm above the retinal plane.

There are in fact two reasons why the posterior hyaloid may be not visible on OCT scans: either it is completely attached to the retinal surface or it is completely detached and too far from that surface. Therefore, when the posterior hyaloid is not visible at the surface on an OCT scan, it is necessary to ascertain, from the fundus biomicroscopy whether or not the Weiss ring is detached, in order to determine the status of the vitreomacular junction. Optical coherence tomography is especially useful for detecting incomplete or shallow detachments of the posterior hyaloid, which previously were not usually detectable.

Perifoveolar Vitreous Detachment with a Normal Posterior Hyaloid

In about half the cases of diabetic macular edema, the posterior hyaloid is detached from the retinal surface in the perifoveolar area but remains attached to the foveolar center. This configuration gives the posterior hyaloid its typical double convexity on cross-sectional scans (Figs 4.21 and 4.22). Sometimes the detachment is asymmetric and more pronounced nasally than temporally (Figs 4.5 and 4.21). In a three-dimensional image, this biconvex appearance would correspond to a posterior hyaloid detachment over the posterior pole, whose limit would describe a circle concentric to the temporal vessels and tangent to the optic disc. Such detachment would exhibit umbilication at its center due to vitreofoveolar adherence.

This appearance is not different from the initial stages of posterior vitreous detachment, described by Uchino in healthy subjects,[12] and shown by Ito[13] in fellow eyes of eyes with idiopathic macular holes. However, it may increase the thickness of a pre-existing macular edema.[14]

Perifoveolar Vitreous Detachment with a Thick Posterior Hyaloid

In rare cases, i.e. about 1% or less, the partially detached posterior hyaloid looks much thicker and more hyper-reflective than usually; it is also less curved and often straight and taut over the macular area[10, 11] (Figs 4.23 and 4.26). In other cases, however, it may retain its biconvexity (Figs 4.24A to C). The reason for this thickening of the posterior hyaloid is unclear. It could be due to the lining of the posterior hyaloid by a layer of fibrosis originating in the retina or optic disc, as a sequela of fibrovascular proliferation; in for instance, in proliferative diabetic retinopathy. In case of non-proliferative diabetic retinopathy, the cause of this thickening is unknown. Posterior hyaloid traction may also be combined with an epiretinal membrane which causes or increases macular thickening (Figs 4.23 to 4.25).

Pre-retinal Hemorrhage

Pre-retinal hemorrhages may completely mask the underlying features (Figs 4.27A and B). Intraretinal hemorrhages, on the contrary are rarely visible on OCT scans, as their reflectivity is weak.

Lamellar Hole

Lamellar hole may be the end stage of longstanding macular edema with central cyst, combined with vitreomacular traction (Figs 4.28A to C). In rare cases, the evolution of diabetic macular edema may also lead to a full-thickness hole. Full-thickness macular hole may even occur as an end stage of cystoid macular edema combined with vitreous traction.

CAN TRACTIONAL MACULAR EDEMA BE DEFINED ON OPTICAL COHERENCE TOMOGRAPHY SCANS?

It is difficult to answer this question. Optical coherence tomography provides a static representation of the macular profile and cannot indicate the presence of forces affecting the macular surface.

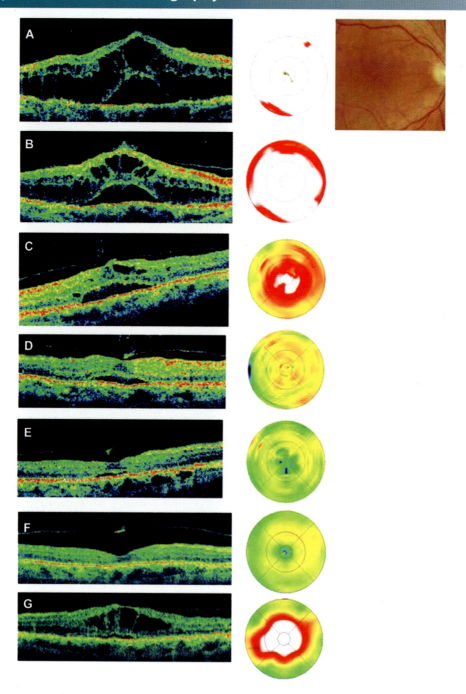

Figs 4.10A to G: Evolution of diffuse cystoid macular edema after injection of 4 mg intravitreal triamcinolone acetonide. A: Severe cystoid macular edema, with foveal detachment before injection. Right color fundus photograph. visual acuity : 20/400. Center average thickness: 805 μm. B: Two days after intravitreal triamcinolone acetonide: Center average thickness: 767 μm. C: Seven days after intravitreal triamcinolone acetonide: Center average thickness: 477μm. D: Two weeks after intravitreal triamcinolone acetonide. Center average thickness: 314 μm. E: Three weeks after intravitreal triamcinolone acetonide: Center average thickness: 264 μm. F: Two months after intravitreal triamcinolone acetonide: Center average thickness is now almost normal (225 μm). Foveal detachment has progressively stabilized. The posterior hyaloid is detached from the macular surface. Visual acuity has improved to 20/100. G: Five months after intravitreal triamcinolone acetonide: macular edema has recurred; Center average thickness: 633 μm. VA: 20/400.

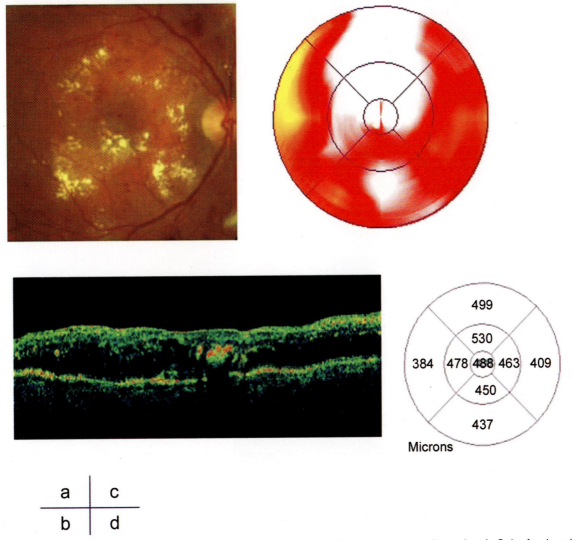

Figs 4.11A to D: Severe macular edema with hard exudates in non-proliferative diabetic retinopathy. A: Color fundus photograph showing several rings of hard lipid exudates, which join in the fovea. B: Horizontal 6 mm scan showing diffuse swelling and thickening of the macula, and the accumulation of hard exudates in the outer part of the fovea. C and D: Retinal thickness map showing that retinal thickening is maximal in the circinate hard exudates. Foveal thickness is 488 μm.

However, there are some examples indicating that biconvex perifoveal detachment of the posterior hyaloid is not a stable situation, as this detachment usually progresses with time.[12, 13, 15] Once the posterior hyaloid is detached from the macula except for the foveolar center, the last step is the avulsion of the adhesion to the center, resulting in a change in the profile of the posterior hyaloid from biconvex to dome shape. This evolution suggests that in such cases, forces come into play which detaches the posterior hyaloid from the retinal surface. Note, however, that during the progression of idiopathic posterior vitreous detachment, such forces do not, in normal subjects, result in any visible change in the OCT profile of the macula. In diabetic macular edema it is, therefore, difficult to interpret images showing a change in the posterior hyaloid profile as evidence of significant traction on the macula.

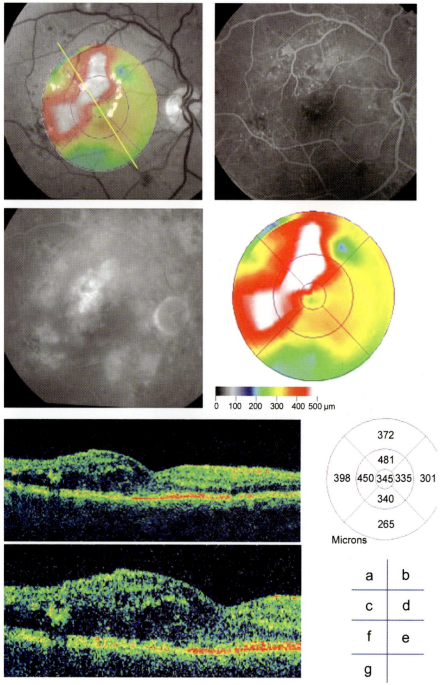

Figs 4.12A to G: Severe macular edema with hard lipid exudates in non-proliferative diabetic retinopathy. A: Red-free fundus photograph with superimposition of the retinal thickness map. The maximum area of thickening on the color map corresponds to the center of the circinate exudates. B and C: Fluorescein angiography shows multiple microaneurysms and late diffuse macular leakage. D and E: Retinal macular map; retinal thickening is greatest on the temporal side of the macula. The focal topography of retinal thickening indicates the area to be treated by focal/grid laser photocoagulation. Foveal thickness measured 345 µm. The macular thickness color code indicates that the retinal thickness at the center is about 300 µm, and that it reaches 400 and even 500 µm at the temporal periphery of the fovea. F: Horizontal 6 mm scan, showing asymmetrical macular thickening, mainly involving the temporal part of the macula. G: Detail showing the hyper-reflectivity of certain hard exudates in the outer retina, temporal to the fovea. These highly reflective spots shadow the underlying backscattering. Only the temporal part of the foveal center has greatly thickened, as also visible on D. The visual acuity of this eye is 20/100.

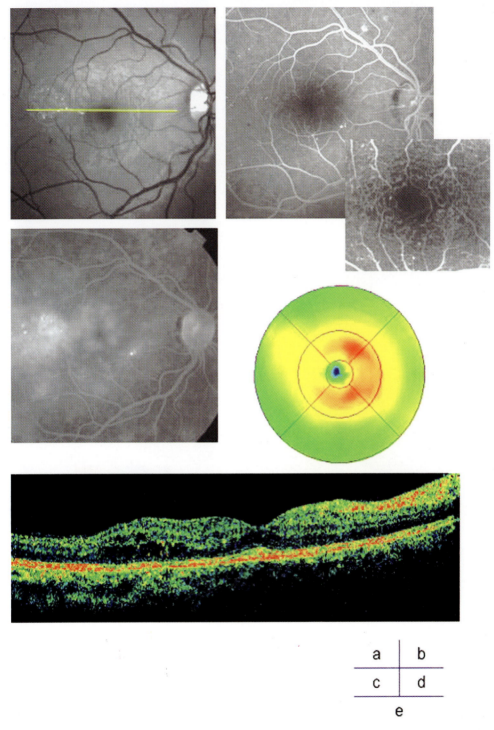

a	b
c	d
e	

Figs 4.13A to E: Mild macular edema with minimal hard exudates in non-proliferative diabetic retinopathy. A: Red-free fundus photograph shows a few exudates temporal to the fovea. B and C: Fluorescein angiography early phase: Note the dilation of the macular capillary bed , microaneurysms and capillary occlusions. Late phase angiography shows diffuse macular leakage. D: Retinal macular map showing moderate diffuse macular thickening. Center average thickness at the center is 261 μm. E: Horizontal OCT scan showing retinal thickening temporal to the macula, mainly involving the outer retina. Visual acuity is 20/25.

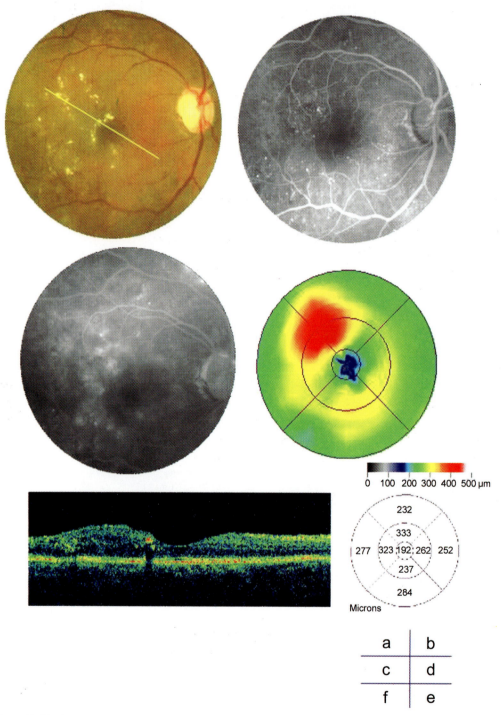

Figs 4.14A to F: Moderate macular edema with multifocal hard exudates in non-proliferative diabetic retinopathy. A: Color fundus photograph showing numerous hard lipid exudates encroaching on the fovea. B and C: Fluorescein angiography showing perifoveal and multifocal leakage in the macular area. D and E: Retinal macular map shows that focal retinal thickening is at its maximum in the superotemporal part of the fovea. The color thickness code indicates that foveolar thickness is in the normal range (blue). The center average thickness is 196 μm. F: Oblique retinal scan: extrafoveal retinal thickening and deposition of hard lipid exudates at the temporal edge of the macula, at the limit of retinal thickening. The foveal pit has retained a nearly normal profile. Visual acuity is 20/32.

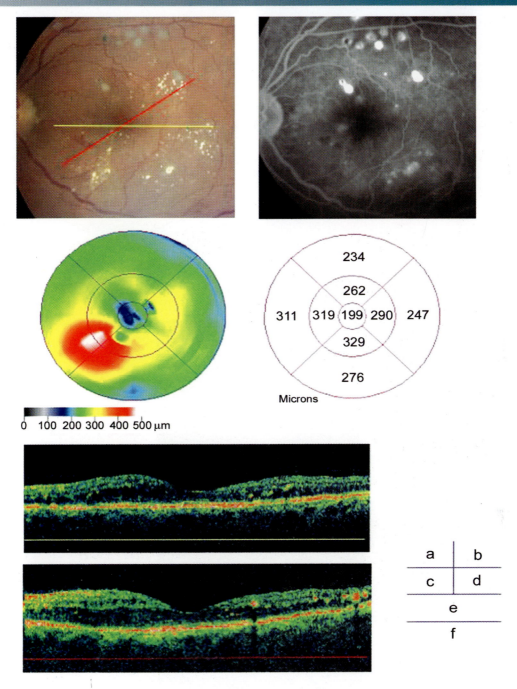

Figs 4.15A to F: Moderate macular edema with multifocal hard exudate in non-proliferative diabetic retinopathy. A: Color fundus photograph showing numerous hard lipid exudates threatening the fovea. Yellow and red lines correspond to the linear scans in E and F. B: Fluorescein angiography showing minimal perifoveal leakage, and previous laser scars. C and D: Retinal macular map shows that focal retinal thickening is maximal on the inferonasal side of the macula. The color thickness code indicates that foveolar thickness is in the normal range (blue). Center average thickness is 199 μm. Therefore, additional focal laser treatment should be primarily directed to the inferonasal sector of the macular area. The exudates located temporally may be on the way to spontaneous regression. Note also that, although color map indicates areas of retinal thickening greatest than 400 and even 500 μm, average thickness map displays only thickness values of 311 to 329 μm. E and F: Horizontal and oblique retinal scans showing that macular thickening is mainly located nasally; retinal thickness is nearly normal temporally, despite the presence of intraretinal hard exudates. Visual acuity is 20/25.

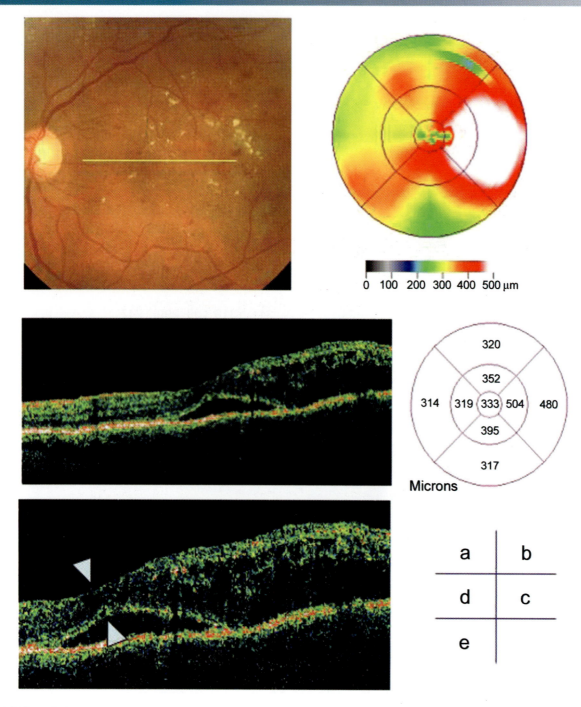

Figs 4.16A to E: Moderate macular edema with multifocal hard exudates combined with foveal detachment, in non-proliferative diabetic retinopathy. A: Color fundus photograph showing two supero-temporal rings of hard exudates threatening the foveal center. B and C: Retinal macular map shows that focal retinal thickening is maximal in temporal part of the macula. The color thickness code indicates that the foveola has thickened (green-yellow). Center average thickness is 333 µm. D and E: Horizontal retinal scan and detail: in the temporal area, the macula edema is maximal in the outer retina, although small retinal cysts are also present in the inner layers. This edema is in continuity with a foveal detachment, which was not detectable on fundus examination or a retinal map. The true central foveal thickness, measured by calipers, is 208 µm . Visual acuity is 20/63. The visual prognosis is good: macular thickness should return to normal after focal laser treatment.

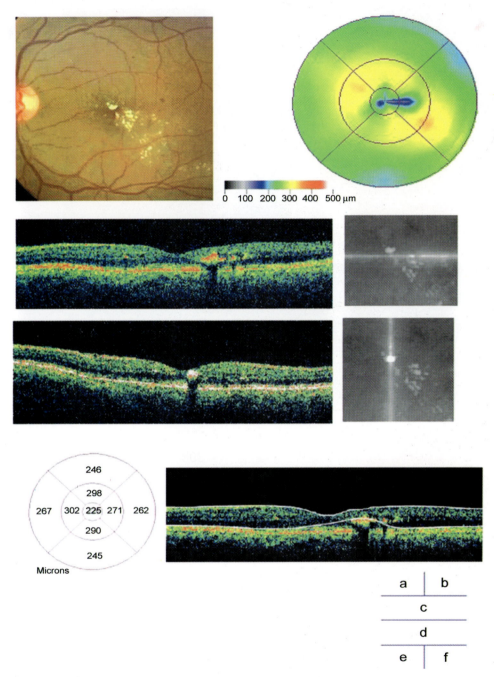

Figs 4.17A to F: Apparently severe macular edema. Hard exudates involving the center of the macula in non-proliferative diabetic retinopathy. A: Color fundus photograph showing temporoinferior hard exudates involving the foveal center. B and E: Retinal macular map showing two areas of moderate focal retinal thickenin G: the superonasal and inferotemporal areas of the macula. The latter area corresponds to the circinate hard exudates. The color code tends to show that the thickness of the foveal center and temporal parafoveal zone is normal. C and D: Horizontal retinal scan showing hard intraretinal exudates on the temporal edge of the macula. The vertical scan passes exactly through hard exudates involving the foveal center. F: Analysis of the horizontal scan of the mapping shows an artifact due to the presence of a hard exudate, which explains the misleadingly normal appearance of the temporal parafoveal area.

Despite the presence of a central intraretinal hard exudate, and probably because the fovea has in fact moderately thickened, visual acuity is 20/25. The visual prognosis should be good after focal laser photocoagulation.

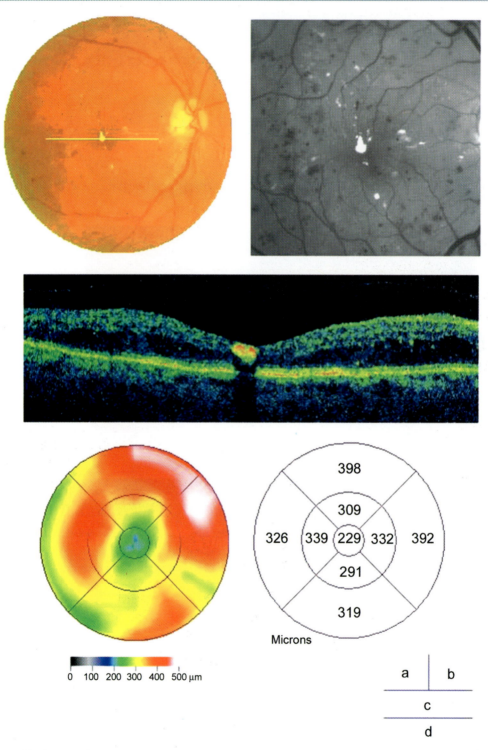

Figs 4.18A to D: Apparently severe macular edema. Hard exudates involving the center of the macula, in non-proliferative diabetic retinopathy. A and B: Color and red-free photographs showing microhemorrhages, microaneurysms and scattered hard exudates involving the foveal center. C: Horizontal retinal scan showing hard intraretinal exudates in the inner portion of the foveal center. These exudates mask the underlying retinal pigment epithelium and choriocapillaris layers. D: Retinal macular map showing diffuse macular thickening, mainly extrafoveal. Center average thickness has only increased slightly (229 μm). Visual acuity is 20/25, but in the absence of treatment, foveal function is certainly threatened

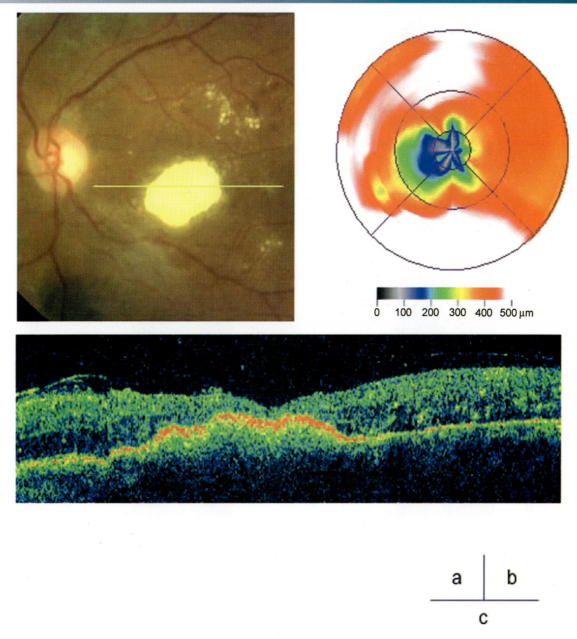

Figs 4.19A to C: Severe macular edema with a subfoveal plaque of lipid exudates in non-proliferative diabetic retinopathy. A: Color photograph showing a compact yellow subfoveal plaque of hard lipid exudates. B: Retinal macular map showing diffuse retinal thickening, except at the fovea, which seems atrophic, despite an artifactual pattern. C: Horizontal retinal scans showing the hyper-reflectivity and thickness of subfoveal hard exudates. The underlying retinal tissue is indeed atrophic.

On the other hand, a thick, hyper-reflective, taut posterior hyaloid does usually indicate vitromacular traction. One sign of this traction is the shape of the macular elevation combined with the hyper-reflective posterior hyaloid: thus, the slope of the macula tends to be convex instead of the usual concave appearance of macular edema (Figs 4.23 and 4.24). The combination of a hyper-reflective, thick posterior hyaloid adhering to an elevated foveal center, and convex slopes of the thickened macula is strongly suggestive of tractional diabetic macular edema (Figs 4.24A to C).

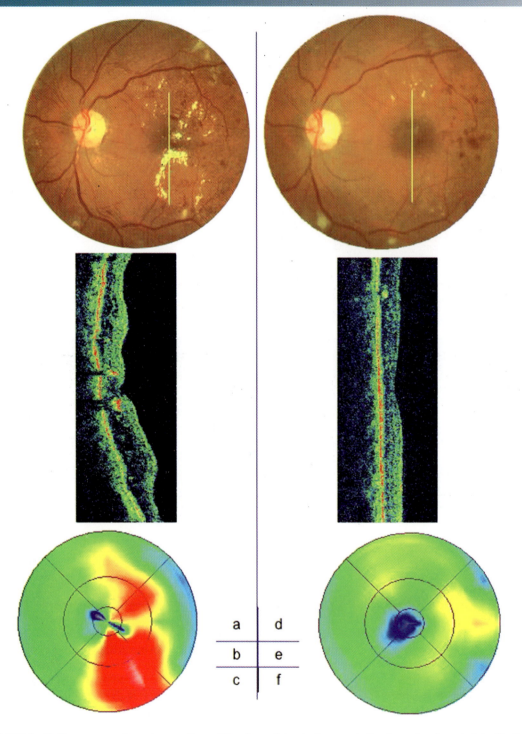

Figs 4.20A to F: Severe macular edema with multifocal exudates before and after laser treatment. A to C: Before laser, fundus color photograph shows two rings of hard exudates encroaching on the fovea; on a vertical retinal scan, diffuse macular thickening as well as hyper-reflective hard exudates are visible near the foveal center. Retinal macular map shows that retinal thickening is maximal at the center of circinate hard exudates. Center average thickness is 253 µm. D to F: Four months after focal laser treatment directed at the center of exudative rings, fundus photograph shows the disappearance of hard exudates; on a vertical retinal scan, the macular profile is almost normal. Retinal macular scan shows almost normal values for macular thickness. Center average thickness is now 176 µm.

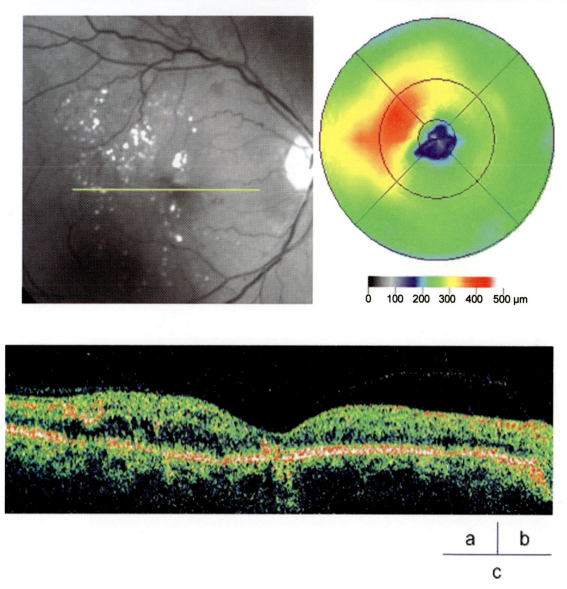

Figs 4.21A to C: Partial posterior hyaloid detachment in a case of moderate macular edema. A: Red-free photograph shows hard exudates encroaching on the fovea. B: Retinal macular map shows that central average thickness is still normal. C: Horizontal retinal scan showing persistence of the foveal pit and thickening of the temporal part of the macula. The posterior hyaloid is partly detached from the macular surface, more nasally than temporally; it is thin and displays low reflectivity. This partial detachment has not caused any deformation of the fovea

ASSESSMENT OF MACULAR EDEMA ON RETINAL MAP ANALYSIS

There are two kinds of retinal map analysis which provide complementary information: the color map and the mean thickness map.

The color map gives a topographic representation of retinal thickness calculated from the values measured on each linear scan, so that the values between two linear scans are extrapolated and not measured.

The mean thickness map gives the average retinal thickness in each of the 9 different sectors of the macula. The average sectorial retinal thickness is calculated from the measures constituting the linear scans.

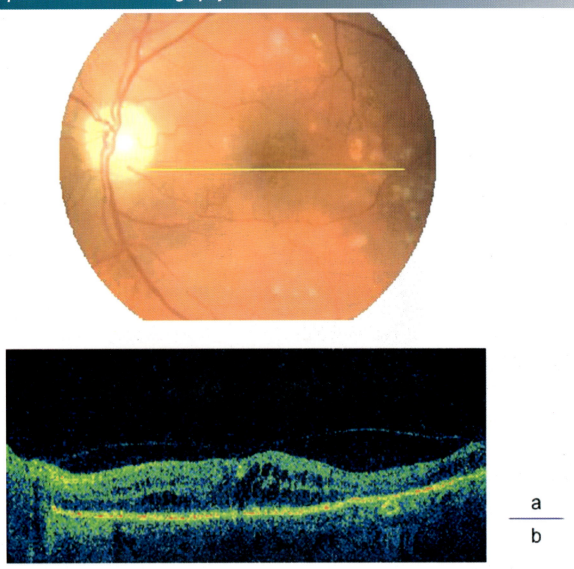

Figs 4.22A and B: Partial posterior hyaloid detachment in a case of diffuse cystoid macular edema. A: Color fundus photograph showing perimacular laser scars. No hard exudates are any longer present. B: 9 mm horizontal retinal scan showing partial detachment of the posterior hyaloid, which has remained thin and normally reflective. The macula has been thickened by cystic spaces. The posterior hyaloid remains attached to the elevated foveal center

The pattern of the 9 different sectors of the macular map for which the average retinal thickness is measured was modeled on the macular edema pattern of the Early Treatment of Diabetic Retinopathy Study (ETDRS), and is therefore especially well suited to the assessment of diabetic macular edema .

Mean foveal thickness refers to the average of retinal thickness values in the central 1000 microns central disc, and central foveal thickness refers to the average of 6 values of retinal thickness at the intersection of the six radial scans.

The color map shows small variations in each sector and gives semi-quantitative indications of local retinal thickness by means of a color code. The mean thickness map gives the average retinal thickness values of each sector. In this representation, an area of retinal thickening smaller than a sector may be underestimated, lost in the thickness average of the sector (Figs 4.15A to F).

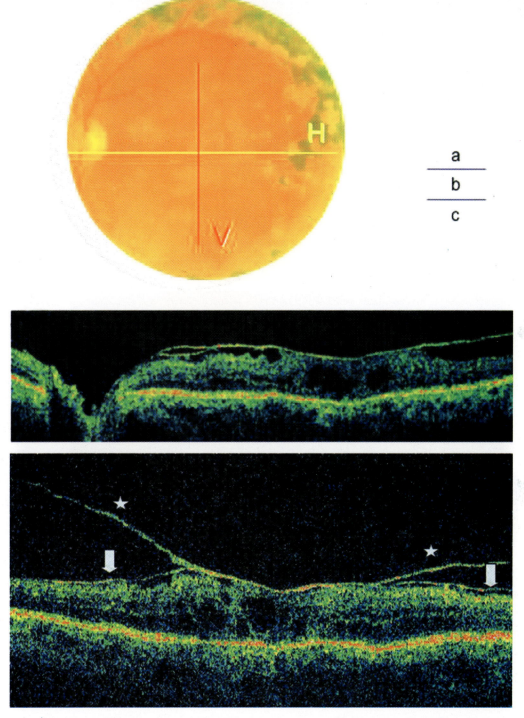

Figs 4.23A to C: Tractional diabetic macular edema in an eye with proliferative diabetic retinopathy, treated by panretinal photocoagulation. A: Color fundus photography showing laser scars at the periphery of the posterior pole. Lines H and V show the direction of the cross-sectional scans below. B: Horizontal retinal scan showing diffuse thickening of the macula, superficial retinal folds, and a large area of adherence between of a preretinal thick, hyper-reflective, taut, epiretinal tissue to the macular center. C: Vertical retinal scan shows that this epiretinal tissue in fact consists of the thickened, taut, incompletely detached posterior hyaloid (stars) and of an epiretinal membrane (arrows) which adheres both to the retinal surface and the posterior hyaloid. Visual acuity is 20/200, and macular surgery is advised to remove this epiretinal traction.

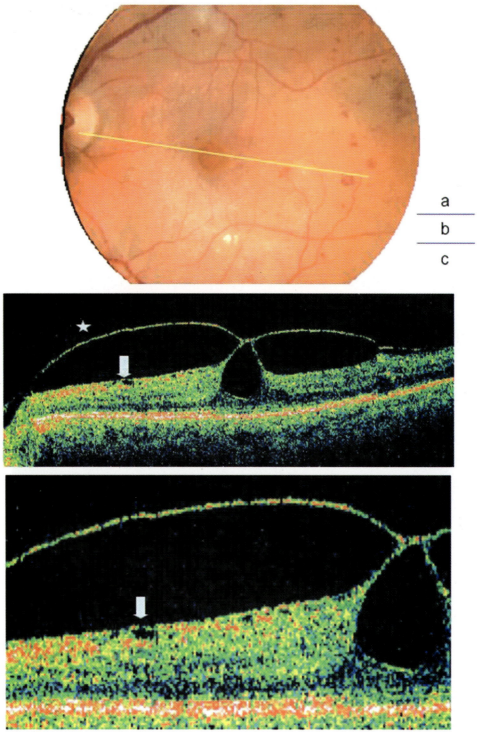

Figs 4.24A to C: Tractional diabetic macular edema in an eye with severe non-proliferative diabetic retinopathy. A: Color fundus photography showing what looks like a hole in the macula, surrounded by a glistening reflex. Numerous intraretinal hemorrhages are present. B: 9 mm retinal scan showing an incompletely detached, thick, hyper-reflective posterior hyaloid (arrow) still attached to the optic disc, the foveal center, and the border of the posterior pole. An epiretinal membrane is also present, and adheres to the retinal surface, causing small superficial retinal folds (arrow). See detail in C. The hole-like appearance on fundus photography is in fact due to the presence of a large foveal cyst. Visual acuity is still 20/50, but only pars plana vitrectomy can preserve or improve vision in this case.

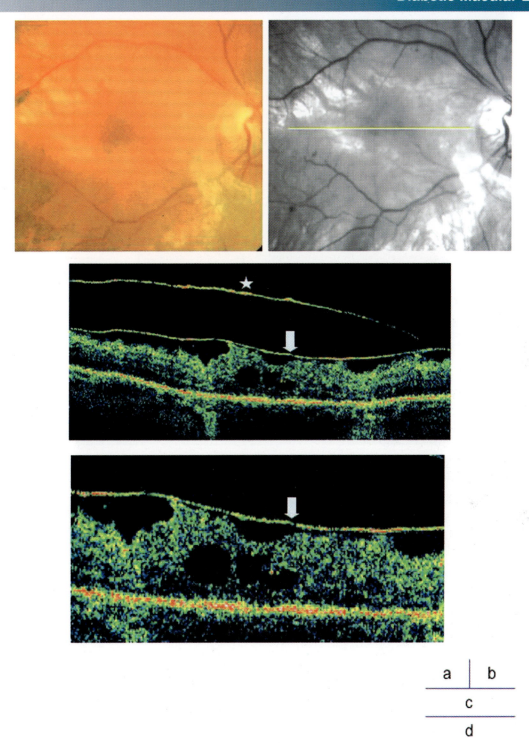

Figs 4.25A to D: Epiretinal membrane and diabetic macular edema, in an eye with proliferative diabetic retinopathy treated by panretinal photocoagulation. A and B: Color and red-free photographs showing retinal folds in the macula and an opaque epiretinal membrane near the optic disc. C and D (detail) : Horizontal retinal scan showing cystic changes in a thickened folded retina. An epiretinal membrane (arrow) adheres to the top of the retinal folds. The posterior hyaloid (star) is partially detached from the retina but adheres to the epiretinal membrane near the disc. Visual acuity is 20/200. Pars plana vitrectomy and epiretinal peeling might improve vision, depending on the amount of damage to the macula caused by long-standing macular edema.

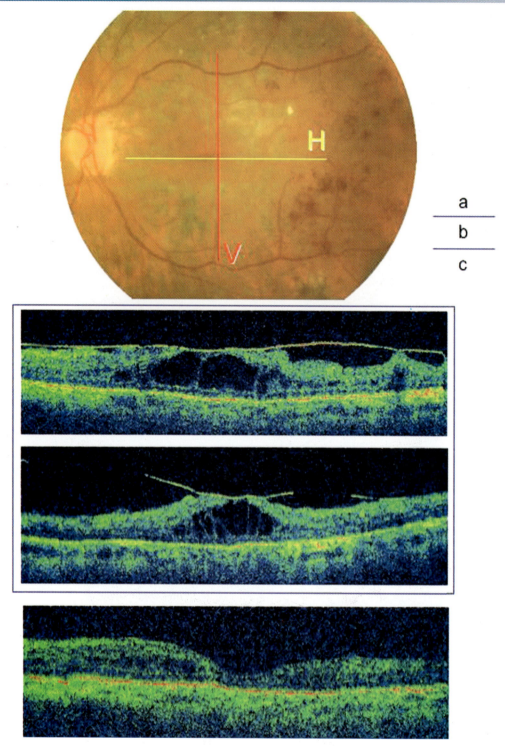

Figs. 4.26A to C: Tractional diabetic macular edema before and after surgery, in proliferative diabetic retinopathy treated by panretinal photocoagulation. A: Color fundus photograph showing a whitish reflex in the macular area. Numerous intraretinal hemorrhages are present. H and V respectively indicate horizontal and vertical retinal scans. B: Horizontal and vertical retinal scans show a thickened posterior hyaloid partially detached from the posterior pole and exerting traction on the fovea, which exhibits large intraretinal cystic cavities. C: Two months after pars plana vitrectomy and posterior hyaloid detachment, the macular profile has almost returned to normal. Visual acuity is improved from 20/400 to 20/100.

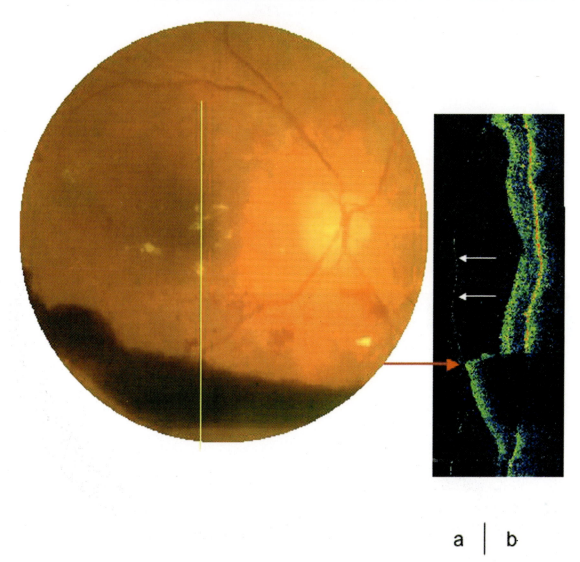

a | b

Figs 4.27A and B: Preretinal hemorrhages in proliferative diabetic retinopathy. A: Color fundus photograph showing a preretinal hemorrhage. B: Optical coherence tomography scan shows the horizontal level of the hemorrhage, limited by the posterior hyaloid (white arrows)

REPRODUCIBILITY AND RELIABILITY

It has been shown with both OCT-1 and Stratus OCT-3 that mean retinal thickness measurement is highly reliable and reproducible in the different areas of OCT mapping, both in normal subjects and in diabetic patients with macular edema.[16, 17] Several methods have been proposed to assess the variations in sectorial mean thickness.[18,19]

LIMITATIONS AND PITFALLS

Accuracy of retinal thickness measurement according to ETDRS zone.

Retinal thickness in each zone is calculated as the average of the values measured on the portions of axis passing through that zone. It is, therefore, obvious that there are fewer points per surface unit in the outer

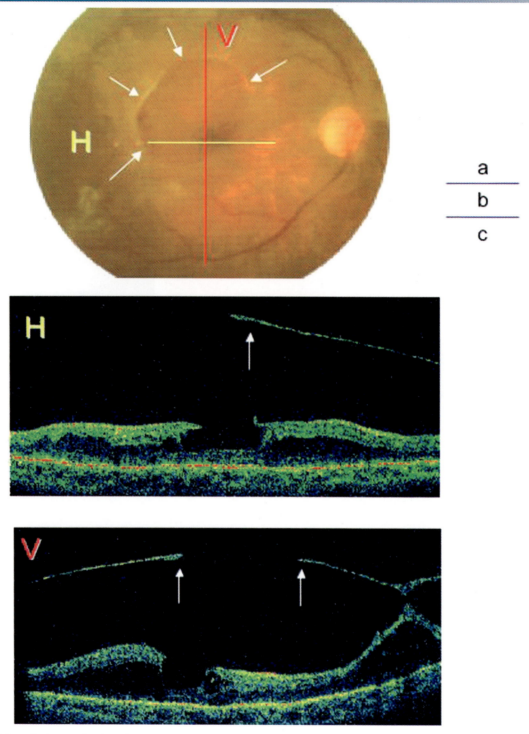

Figs 4.28A to C: A macular lamellar hole resulting from macular edema and vitreomacular traction. A: Color fundus photograph showing a hole in the thick detached posterior hyaloid (arrows). H and V indicate respectively the directions of the horizontal and vertical retinal scans. B: Horizontal 6 mm retinal scan showing a lamellar macular hole in a thickened macula. Note the partially detached thickened posterior hyaloid (arrow). C: 9 mm vertical retinal scan showing a lamellar hole in the partially detached posterior hyaloid (arrows), which is still attached to the inferotemporal retinal vein. The lamellar hole probably occurred during the posterior hyaloid detachment

rings than in the innermost ring (1,250 measures per mm^2 in zone 1, 317/mm^2 in zone 2 and only 141/mm^2 in zone 3). Consequently, more values are extrapolated in the outermost rings of the mapping than in the central one. However, this theoretical limitation does not prevent OCT mapping from being at least as sensitive as stereophotography or biomicroscopy for the detection of areas of focal or diffuse edema. There is also a good correlation between OCT and fluorescein angiography for the detection of areas of leakage (see below).

Limitations Dependent on Patient Fixation

At the central point of the macula and in the 1 mm central area, the reproducibility of retinal thickness measurement is excellent in normal subjects. The 1 mm central area is the most sensitive to variations in fixation, because retinal thickness varies constantly from the foveolar center to the edge of the macula. However, even in eyes with significant macular thickening and poor vision, whose fixation may be unstable, it has been shown that the retinal thickness values in this central area are very reliable.[17, 20] This might be partly because when the central macula is thickened, the inner retinal boundary loses its concavity or acquires a flat or dome shape, so that small variations in fixation do not result in significant changes in mean retinal macular thickness.

In the most peripheral zones of the mapping, slight instability of the central fixation does not lead to significant changes in thickness, because retinal thickening in these zones is relatively uniform.

Limitations due to Artifacts

Artifacts occurring on one or several scans may impair macular mapping. This can be avoided by replacing the artifactual scan by a new one, or if the artifact persists, in deleting the scan to carry out the mapping. There are various causes of artifacts: a partially detached posterior hyaloid may be mistaken for the inner retinal boundary, hard exudates may interfere with the detection of the outer retinal boundary (Figs 4.17A to F), or subfoveal detachment may alter the detection of the outer retinal boundary.

Lastly, it is now obvious that the OCT-3 software includes an erroneous definition of the outer retinal boundary, which in normal eyes is located at the level of the posterior photoreceptor signal and not of the retinal pigment epithelium.[21] This error tends to result in overestimation of macular thickening compared to baseline, as in macular edema the photoreceptor line often alters, so that the software then detects the retinal pigment epithelium boundary correctly, adding 20 to 40 µm to its baseline value.

COMPARISON OF OPTICAL COHERENCE TOMOGRAPHY WITH BIOMICROSCOPY, STEREO PHOTOGRAPHY, AND FLUORESCEIN ANGIOGRAPHY

Optical coherence tomography has been compared to the three other types of examinations above, for its ability to detect minor changes, and to locate areas of retinal thickening precisely.

Optical Coherence Tomography and Biomicroscopy

It is now well established that optical coherence tomography is more sensitive than slit-lamp biomicroscopy for the detection of small changes in retinal thickness.[22-24] In addition, OCT is clearly better than the other types of fundus examination, as it alone can show shallow posterior hyaloid detachment, or foveal detachment underlying cystoid macular edema.

OCT is also more sensitive than biomicroscopy in identifying vitreoretinal adhesions associated with macular disease.[25]

Optical Coherence Tomography and Stereophotography

The data obtained from fundus stereophotographs and OCT mapping for the detection and quantification of diabetic macular edema have only been compared in one study using the first generation of OCT. The degree of agreement between subjective and objective assessments of retinal thickening by stereophotos and OCT respectively was very good, indicating that changes in diabetic macular edema can be accurately and prospectively measured with OCT.[26]

Optical Coherence Tomography and Fluorescein Angiography

There is usually a good correlation between the features of OCT and fluorescein angiography in clinically significant diabetic macular edema.[17, 27] However, in some cases, the appearance of cystoid macular edema on fluorescein angiography may be undetectable on OCT. [28, 29] We have also observed such cases in which cystoid cavities were not associated with macular thickening. More frequently, small areas of macular leakage shown by fluorescein angiography may correspond to insignificant zones of retinal thickening on OCT (Figs 4.29A to H). On the other hand, OCT alone would miss the diagnosis of macular ischemia which is only shown by fluorescein angiography (Figs 4.30A to D).

OPTICAL COHERENCE TOMOGRAPHY AND TREATMENTS FOR DIABETIC MACULAR EDEMA

Laser Photocoagulation

Laser photocoagulation of macular edema is usually based on fundus biomicroscopy, which shows the areas of retinal thickening, and on fluorescein angiography, which shows the leaky microvascular anomalies. Optical coherence tomography mapping is an excellent adjunct to fundus photograph, or fluorescein angiography, for detecting the areas to treat. It might replace fluorescein angiography in the follow-up of photocoagulation (Figs 4.20A to F).

Pars Plana Vitrectomy

Pars plana vitrectomy is used to treat both tractional and non tractional diabetic macular edema. The benefit of pars plana vitrectomy for tractional macular edema has been clearly shown by many publications and is widely accepted (Figs 4.26A to C). However, there is still some controversy about the middle and long-term usefulness of vitrectomy for non-tractional diffuse diabetic macular edema. The role of OCT in distinguishing tractional from non-tractional diabetic macular edema is essential, although the signs of vitreomacular traction (a hyper-reflective, thickened posterior hyaloid adhering to the top of the macular edema, whose shape is altered by the traction) are not completely accepted.

Intravitreal Drugs

The use of intravitreal drugs such as corticosteroids or anti-VEGF has increased the use of OCT for monitoring the effect of these treatments and helping to reach decisions regarding retreatment. These intravitreal

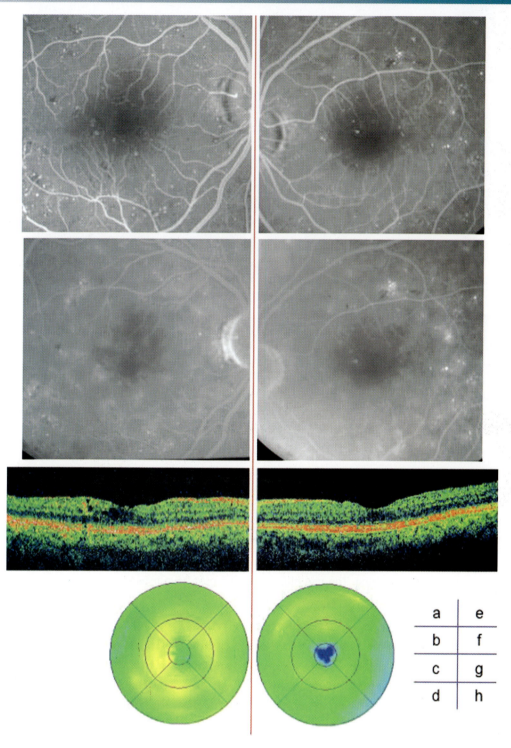

Figs 4.29A to H: Fluorescein angiography and OCT in both eyes of a patient with minimal non-proliferative diabetic retinopathy. VA is 20/25 in both eyes. Early and late stages of fluorescein angiography showing in a few microaneurysms and mild late leakage in both eyes (RE: A and B ; LE: E and F). Horizontal retinal scans show the presence of intraretinal cystic spaces in RE (C). The foveal profile in LE is normal (G).Center average thickness has slightly increased in RE (251 μm), but is normal in LE (187 μm). In this case, OCT has detected early macular edema in one eye, although on fluorescein angiography the intensity of dye leakage was similar in both eyes.

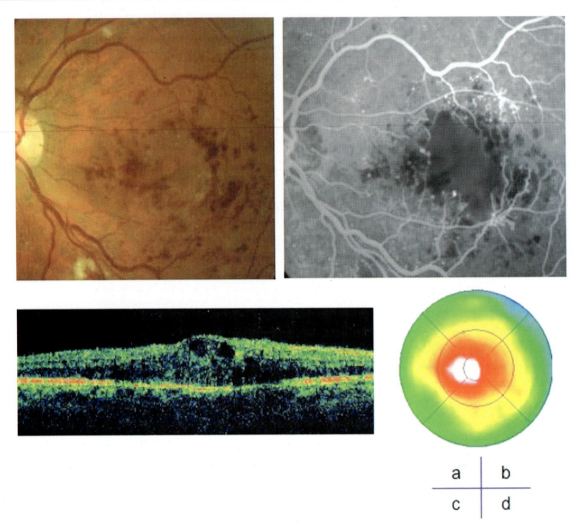

Figs 4.30A to D: Fluorescein angiography and OCT in a case of ischemic maculopathy. Visual acuity is 20/400. A: Color fundus photograph showing numerous dot hemorrhages in the macula. B: Fluorescein angiography shows extensive non-perfusion of macular capillaries, in an area of about 2 disc diameters. C and D: Horizontal retinal scan and center average thickness show significant macular edema and retinal thickening. The use of OCT alone would have missed the ischemic component of this edema

drugs indeed exert a favorable effect on the hydration of the retina, especially of the posterior pole. Their effect in reducing macular thickness or volume precedes the improvement of visual acuity. Conversely, a recurrence of macular thickening often precedes visual acuity impairment. In these cases, OCT mapping is a useful indicator of the anatomic efficacy of the drug (Fig. 4.10). It has also been shown that measurement of macular thickness by OCT may serve as a pharmacodynamic criterion for non-invasive assessment of the pharmacokinetics of intravitreal triamcinolone.[30]

REFERENCES

1. Hee MR, Izatt JA, Swanson EA, et al. Optical coherence tomography of the human retina. Arch Ophthalmol. 1995;113:325-332.
2. Yamamoto S, Yamamoto T, Hayashi M, Takeuchi S. Morphological and functional analyses of diabetic macular edema by optical coherence tomography and multifocal electroretinograms. Graefe's Arch Clin Exp Ophthalmol. 2001;239:96-101.

3. Antcliff RJ, Marshall J. The pathogenesis of edema in diabetic maculopathy. Semin Ophthalmol. 1999;14:223-232.
4. Puliafito CA, Hee MR, Lin CP, et al. Imaging of macular diseases with optical coherence tomography. Ophthalmology. 1995;102:217-229.
5. Otani T, Kishi S, Maruyama Y. Patterns of diabetic macular edema with optical coherence tomography. Am J Ophthalmol. 1999;127:688-693.
6. Yamamoto T, Hitani K, Tsukahara I, et al. Early postoperative retinal thickness changes and complications after vitrectomy for diabetic macular edema. Am J Ophthalmol. 2003;135:14-19.
7. Catier A, Tadayoni R, Paques M, et al. Optical coherence tomography characterization of macular edema according to various etiology. Am J Ophthalmol. 2005; In press.
8. Otani T, Kishi S. Tomographic findings of foveal hard exudates in diabetic macular edema. Am J Ophthalmol. 2001;131:50-54.
9. Imai M, Iijima H, Hanada N. Optical coherence tomography of tractional macular elevations in eyes with proliferative diabetic retinopathy. Am J Ophthalmol. 2001;132:81-84.
10. Kaiser PK, Riemann CD, Sears JE, Lewis H. Macular traction detachment and diabetic macular edema associated with posterior hyaloidal traction. Am J Ophthalmol. 2001;131:44-49.
11. Massin P, Duguid G, Erginay A, et al. Optical coherence tomography for evaluating diabetic macular edema before and after vitrectomy. Am J Ophthalmol. 2003;135:169-177.
12. Uchino E, Uemura A, Ohba N. Initial stages of posterior vitreous detachment in healthy eyes of older persons evaluated by optical coherence tomography. Arch Ophthalmol. 2001;119:1475-1479.
13. Ito Y, Terasaki H, Suzuki T, et al. Mapping posterior vitreous detachment by optical coherence tomography in eyes with idiopathic macular hole. Am J Ophthalmol. 2003;135:351-355.
14. Gaucher D, Tadayoni R, Erginay A, et al. Optical coherence tomography assessment of the vitreoretinal relationship in diabetic macular edema. Am J Ophthalmol. 2005;in press.
15. Haouchine B, Massin P, Gaudric A. Foveal pseudocyst as the first step in macular hole formation: a prospective study by optical coherence tomography. Ophthalmology. 2001;108:15-22.
16. Browning DJ, Fraser CM. Intraobserver variability in optical coherence tomography. Am J Ophthalmol. 2004;138:477-479.
17. Goebel W, Kretzschmar-Gross T. Retinal thickness in diabetic retinopathy: a study using optical coherence tomography (OCT). Retina. 2002;22:759-767.
18. Browning DJ, Fraser CJ. Regional patterns of sight-threatening diabetic macular edema. Am J Ophthalmol. 2005;140:117-124.
19. Chan A, Duker JS. A standardized method for reporting changes in macular thickening using optical coherence tomography. Arch Ophthalmol 2005;123:939-943.
20. Massin P, Vicaut E, Haouchine B, et al. Reproducibility of retinal mapping using optical coherence tomography. Arch Ophthalmol. 2001;119:1135-1142.
21. Ko TH, Fujimoto JG, Duker JS, et al. Comparison of ultrahigh- and standard-resolution optical coherence tomography for imaging macular hole pathology and repair. Ophthalmology. 2004;111:2033-2043.
22. Hee MR, Puliafito CA, Wong C, et al. Quantitative assessment of macular edema with optical coherence tomography. Arch Ophthalmol. 1995;113:1019-1029.
23. Brown JC, Solomon SD, Bressler SB, et al. Detection of diabetic foveal edema: contact lens biomicroscopy compared with optical coherence tomography. Arch Ophthalmol. 2004;122:330-335.
24. Browning DJ, McOwen MD, Bowen RM, Jr, O'Marah TL. Comparison of the clinical diagnosis of diabetic macular edema with diagnosis by optical coherence tomography. Ophthalmology. 2004;111:712-715.
25. Gallemore RP, Jumper JM, McCuen BW, et al. Diagnosis of vitreoretinal adhesions in macular disease with optical coherence tomography. Retina. 2000;20:115-120.
26. Strom C, Sander B, Larsen N, et al. Diabetic macular edema assessed with optical coherence tomography and stereofundus photography. Invest Ophthalmol Vis Sci. 2002;43:241-245.
27. Kang SW, Park CY, Ham DI. The correlation between fluorescein angiographic and optical coherence tomographic features in clinically significant diabetic macular edema. Am J Ophthalmol. 2004;137:313-322.
28. Antcliff RJ, Stanford MR, Chauhan DS, et al. Comparison between optical coherence tomography and fundus fluorescein angiography for the detection of cystoid macular edema in patients with uveitis. Ophthalmology. 2000;107:593-599.
29. Hirakawa H, Iijima H, Gohdo T, Tsukahara S. Optical coherence tomography of cystoid macular edema associated with retinitis pigmentosa. Am J Ophthalmol. 1999;128:185-191.
30. Audren F, Tod M, Massin P, et al. Pharmacokinetic-pharmacodynamic modeling of the effect of triamcinolone acetonide on central macular thickness in patients with diabetic macular edema. Invest Ophthalmol Vis Sci. 2004;45:3435-3441.

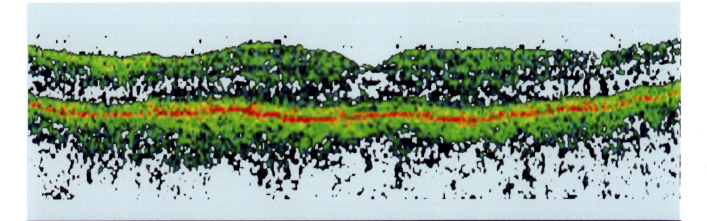

CHAPTER
5

Retinal Vein Occlusion

Robert F See, Sharon Fekrat

INTRODUCTION

Retinal venous occlusive disease trails only diabetic retinopathy as a leading retinal vascular cause of visual morbidity.[1] It may present as a smaller macular branch vein occlusion or a larger central retinal vein occlusion.

BRANCH RETINAL VEIN OCCLUSION

Branch retinal vein occlusion (BRVO) occurs when blood flow through a branch of the central retinal vein is interrupted. The severity of ocular morbidity from this disease varies greatly depending on the location and extent of the occlusion as well as the development of complications such as macular edema, epiretinal membrane, neovascularisation of the disc and elsewhere, traction retinal detachment, and vitreous hemorrhage.

A BRVO may cause acute painless vision loss if the vein occlusion is large and/or affecting the macula, or may be asymptomatic if the involved branch is small or more peripheral. Clinical findings include sectoral venous dilation and tortuosity accompanied by intraretinal hemorrhage and macular edema, usually distal to an arteriovenous crossing that marks the site of occlusion (Fig. 5.1A). Over time, the hemorrhage and edema may resolve, and the ophthalmoscopic findings may be subtle.

The common adventitial sheath at the crossing site of the branch artery and branch vein may play a role in the pathogenesis of the BRVO. At this site, atherosclerosis causes thickening and hardening of the arterial wall which compresses the underlying vein. The turbulence caused at the crossing may lead to clot formation and occlusion of the branch vein. The venous blood stagnates, and the increasing pressure in the arterial system causes the thinner, weaker veins to break and bleed in the affected distribution. As the blood column slows, it leads to decreased arterial perfusion of the retina. This can lead to retinal ischemia in the distribution of the affected artery. The vitreous may also play a role in compression of susceptible arteriovenous crossing sites.[2-5]

The risk of retinal neovascularisation is greatest in eyes with more than 5 disc areas of non-perfusion on fluorescein angiography and usually develops in the first 6 to 12 months. The Branch Vein Occlusion Study (BVOS) demonstrated that 40% of untreated eyes will develop neovascularisation.[6] If left untreated, 60% of these will develop a vitreous hemorrhage. Therefore, once neovascularisation is documented, the area of non-perfusion should receive scatter laser photocoagulation.

During the first year following a BRVO, macular edema may resolve spontaneously with improvement in visual acuity in 36% of eyes.[7] After one year, the chances of visual improvement are much less likely. The BVOS recommended waiting at least 3 months for spontaneous resolution of the edema before considering grid pattern laser photocoagulation.[7] Only eyes with perfused edema and visual acuity 20/40 or worse are candidates for grid pattern laser. No laser is recommended for eyes with ischemic macular edema (Fig. 5.1B). Intravitreal triamcinolone acetonide may improve macular edema in eyes with either perfused or non-perfused edema; however, these reports include only a small number of patients with limited follow-up.[8]

In the past, vitrectomy has been reserved for eyes with vitreous hemorrhage or traction retinal detachment. There is more interest now in the role of the vitreous in eyes with persistent macular edema. Early reports have demonstrated improvement in visual acuity and retinal thickness following vitrectomy.[3-5, 9] Arteriovenous sheathotomy can be performed in conjunction with vitrectomy. During this procedure, the common adventitial sheath at the arteriovenous crossing is cut, relieving venous compression by the overlying branch artery. Venous flow through the branch vein may be restored once the external compression is relieved, and this may then lead to either displacement of the thrombus or subsequent recanalization.[10-12] Further study of this technique is warranted.

CENTRAL RETINAL VEIN OCCLUSION

Central retinal vein occlusion (CRVO) is a retinal vascular condition that may cause significant ocular morbidity. It commonly affects men and women equally and occurs predominantly in persons over the age of 65 years.[13-15] Younger individuals who present with a clinical picture of a CRVO may have an underlying inflammatory etiology.[16-18]

Central retinal vein occlusion classically presents with acute painless loss of vision in the affected eye. Intraretinal hemorrhages and dilated/tortuous retinal veins in all four quadrants are the hallmark of CRVO. The hemorrhages radiate from the optic nerve head and may result in the classic "blood and thunder" appearance. Optic nerve head swelling, cotton-wool spots, and macular edema are also present to varying degrees (Fig. 5.2A). A CRVO is classified by the Central Vein Occlusion Study (CVOS) based on the perfusion status of the retina as determined by fluorescein angiography (Fig. 5.2B). A non-perfused or ischemic CRVO has 10 or more disc areas of retinal capillary non-perfusion on fluorescein angiography. Generally, these eyes display more intraretinal hemorrhage, as well as retinal and disc edema, than perfused CRVOs.

Histopathologic studies have found that the main site of occlusion is in the central retinal vein proximal to the lamina cribrosa.[19] Here, the vein may be susceptible to occlusion due to arteriosclerosis of the adjacent central retinal artery, inflammation, or movement of the lamina cribrosa due to changes in intraocular pressure. Hemodynamic alterations in blood viscosity or blood flow may also play a role.[20]

Over time, the fundus appearance changes, and the intraretinal hemorrhage may slowly reabsorb. Optociliary shunt vessels, epiretinal membranes and anterior segment or posterior neovascularisation may develop in the chronic phase of the disease. Macular edema is almost always present and often persists even after the intraretinal hemorrhage reabsorbs.

A careful history, including a medical history of hypertension, diabetes, or heart disease, and a personal or family history of thrombosis or a hypercoagulable state, should be obtained. A systemic work-up is usually not indicated in persons older than 60 years of age with one affected eye and risk factors for CRVO such as hypertension or glaucoma.[21,22] In persons with no known risk factors and/or with bilateral and sequential CRVOs, an initial evaluation should include blood pressure, complete blood count, lipid profile, and fasting plasma homocysteine level.[23] Referral to a hematologist for additional evaluation may be beneficial in select cases.

An initial complete ophthalmic examination should be performed on both eyes. The iris and angle should be carefully examined prior to pupillary dilation for neovascularisation at each visit. Fluorescein angiography is not routinely obtained but may be performed to determine the perfusion status of the eye in preparation for therapeutic intervention.

The CVOS was designed to determine the role of laser photocoagulation in CRVO. Grid pattern argon laser photocoagulation in eyes with perfused macular edema and 20/50 acuity or worse was not found to significantly change the mean visual acuity and is not recommended for macular edema in eyes with CRVO.[24] The CVOS demonstrated no advantage to prophylactic pan-retinal photocoagulation in eyes with non-perfused CRVO and without any anterior segment neovascularisation. Therefore, it is recommended that pan-retinal photocoagulation only be performed for identified neovascularization. Ninety percent of neovascularisation will regress in 1-2 months following pan-retinal photocoagulation. Prophylactic pan-retinal photocoagulation should be reserved for eyes with a non-perfused CRVO and risk factors for developing iris and angle neovascularisation (male gender, short duration of CRVO, extensive retinal non-perfusion, and extensive retinal hemorrhage) where monthly follow-up is not possible.[25]

Creation of a laser-induced chorioretinal anastomosis in eyes with perfused CRVO may allow transretinal retrograde flow of venous blood from the occluded retinal venous system into the choroidal circulation and prevent the conversion of the CRVO to ischemic perfusion status. Improvements in visual acuity following anastomosis formation may be due to decreased macular edema and/or improved perfusion of the retinal vessels following this procedure.[26,27]

The use of corticosteroids in eyes with CRVO is targeted at treating the macular edema. Although systemic corticosteroids have been used to treat associated inflammatory disease in younger persons with CRVO, they have minimal role in the treatment of the macular edema. Intravitreal delivery of corticosteroids, such as triamcinolone acetonide, has been shown to reduce macular edema and improve visual acuity and retinal thickness by volumetric OCT.[28] The National Eye Institute sponsored SCORE Study is underway to further evaluate the role of intravitreal triamcinolone in eyes with macular edema associated with CRVO and BRVO.

Vitrectomy may be indicated in eyes with complications of CRVO such as a non-clearing vitreous hemorrhage. Removal of epiretinal membranes and fibrovascular tissue along with pan-retinal endolaser photocoagulation can be combined with vitrectomy surgery; however, visual outcomes may be limited due to the extent of underlying retinal non-perfusion.[29,30]

Radial optic neurotomy (RON) at the time of vitrectomy surgery involves making a radial incision at the nasal edge of the optic nerve, thereby incising the lamina cribrosa and relaxing the surrounding scleral ring. This may relieve the compression of the central retinal vein by the artery as they pass together through the lamina cribrosa. Retinal hemorrhage, venous congestion, and macular edema may improve with resultant improvement in visual acuity following RON surgery. However, published results with this technique involve small numbers of patients with limited follow-up, and this technique requires further study to fully define its role in the management of CRVO.[31,32]

OPTICAL COHERENCE TOMOGRAPHY

The gold standard for evaluating macular edema has been fluorescein angiography. More recently, OCT has become an important tool in the management of eyes with macular edema due to branch or central retinal vein occlusion. Optical coherence tomography has demonstrated the ability to detect macular edema that is not appreciable by ophthalmoscopy or fluorescein angiography in various disease processes, including retinal vein occlusion.[33-36] It can also better define the axial distribution of fluid that is observed as thickening of the macula on exam (Fig. 5.2C).[35]

Serous retinal detachment has been reported as an under recognized cause of visual morbidity in eyes with retinal venous occlusive disease, contributing to photoreceptor atrophy from prolonged serous detachment of the fovea. Spaide and associates[34] have found that 71% of eyes with BRVO had an accompanying serous foveal retinal detachment with or without overlying cystoid macular edema.

Better definition of the anatomy with OCT may allow treatment to be directed at contributing causes for the visual dysfunction. Individuals with macular edema and/or serous foveal retinal detachment may be initially treated with a more conservative approach, such as an intravitreal steroid injection. Optical coherence tomography findings of a concurrent mechanical cause such as an associated epiretinal membrane (Fig. 5.3E) or traction on the disc may lead to an earlier surgical intervention.

Epiretinal membrane formation can be a cause of visual morbidity in eyes with BRVO. Battaglia Parodi and associates[37] found epiretinal membrane formation to be more common in nasal branch vein occlusions, particularly following pan-retinal photocoagulation. The authors theorized that this may be due to incomplete separation of the posterior hyaloid and/or the increase in prevalence of vitreous hemorrhage in nasal BRVO. Epiretinal membranes secondary to BRVO are well demonstrated by OCT and are more likely to have areas of focal adhesion to the retina compared to the diffuse adhesion of idiopathic membranes.[38] Advanced knowledge of the configuration of the epiretinal membrane may aid in surgical planning.

Optic disc traction is a recently recognized finding associated with ischemic CRVO.[39] Optical coherence tomography can determine the configuration of the traction as well as accompanying subretinal fluid better than biomicroscopy. Earlier intervention may be indicated to prevent optic atrophy due to disc traction and secondary changes in laminar flow through the peripapillary blood vessels or retinal atrophy due to prolonged detachment of the macula.[39]

Optical coherence tomography plays a major part in monitoring the response to treatment interventions in eyes with retinal vein occlusion. It allows the ophthalmologist to directly follow and assess the response after treatment of macular edema, associated epiretinal membrane, or optic disc traction.[40] Macular thickness can be measured by serial volumetric analysis, and the retinal cross sections allow patients to better understand their response to treatment (Figs 5.2C and 5.2D).

INTERESTING CASE EXAMPLES

Case 1

A 46-year-old man presented with a visual acuity of 20/125 and dilated/tortuous vessels with retinal hemorrhages in all four quadrants (Fig. 5.3A). Fluorescein angiography showed a perfused CRVO without any neovascularisation (Fig. 5.3B). The OCT scan through the fovea demonstrated cystoid macular edema and subfoveal fluid (Fig. 5.3C) with a foveal thickness of 803 ± 184 microns (Fig. 5.3D). Over the next 11 months, intravitreal triamcinolone acetonide (4 mg) was injected twice without improvement in cystoid macular edema or visual acuity. Pars plana vitrectomy combined with radial optic neurotomy and intravitreal triamcinolone acetonide was performed. Four months after surgery, the best-corrected visual acuity improved to 20/64. An OCT demonstrated resolution of the subretinal fluid and improvement in the macular edema (Fig. 5.3E) with a foveal thickness of 375 ± 10 microns. (Fig. 5.3F). An epiretinal membrane had developed (Fig. 5.3E) and the patient underwent a second vitrectomy procedure to remove the membrane. Five months after vitrectomy and epiretinal membrane peel, the best-corrected visual acuity was 20/40, and the OCT confirmed the absence of the epiretinal membrane with improved edema (Fig. 5.3G) and a foveal thickness of 176 ± 8 microns (Fig. 5.3H).

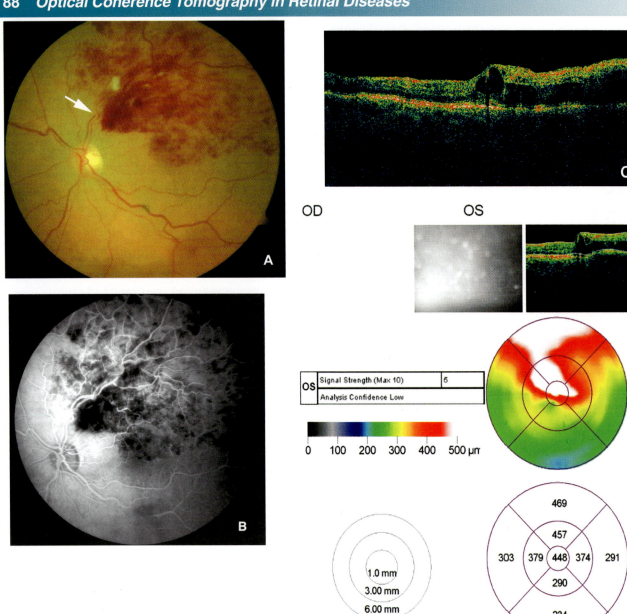

OD   OS

Figs 5.1A to D: An 84-year-old female with hypertension had decreased vision in the left eye for one week. Her best-corrected visual acuity was 20/70 OS. The retina demonstrated typical findings of BRVO (A) with intraretinal hemorrhages and cotton wool spots distal to an arteriovenous crossing (arrow). Fluorescein angiography showed capillary non-perfusion and delayed venous filling in the involved area (B). An OCT scan along the 90° meridian showed the normal inferior macula on the left and the involved retina, thickened with intraretinal hemorrhage and edema, on the right (C). The macular thickness map showed an increased mean retinal thickness in the superior quadrant 457 microns (3.00 mm ring) and 469 microns (6.0 mm ring) compared to 290 microns and 234 microns in the unaffected inferior quadrant (D).

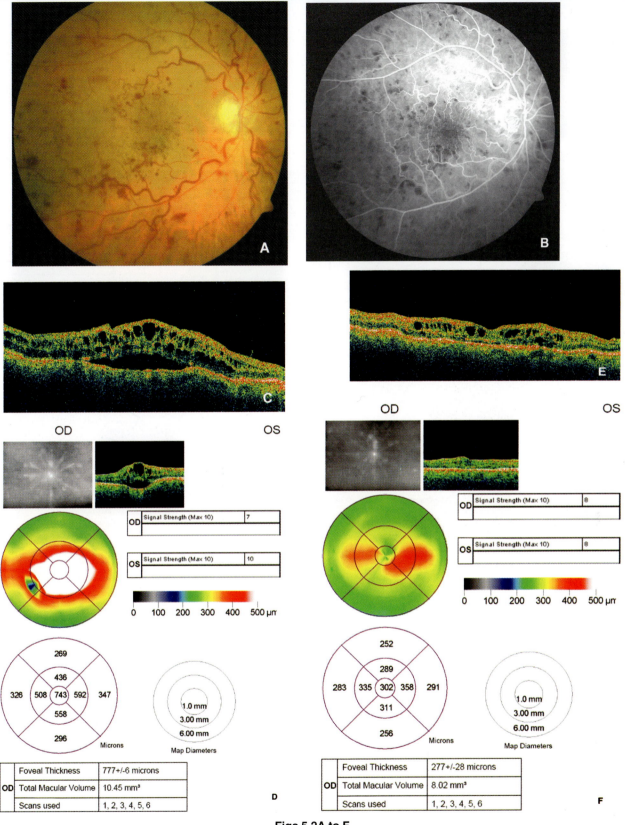

Figs 5.2A to F

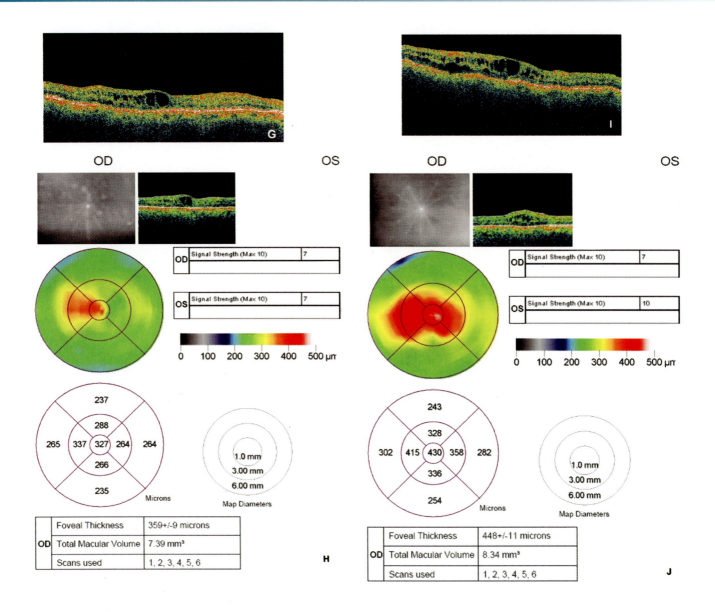

Figs 5.2A to L: A 78-year-old man with hypertension, coronary artery disease and bilateral open angle glaucoma presented with painless loss of vision in his right eye for three weeks. His best-corrected visual acuity was 20/126. Examination of the right eye revealed intraretinal hemorrhages and dilated/tortuous veins in all four quadrants. There was thickening of the central macula without an epiretinal membrane, and there was no neovascularisation (A). There was delayed filling of the retinal venous system on the fluorescein angiogram, and the retinal capillaries were perfused (B). An OCT scan through the fovea along the 5° meridian showed the retinal thickening to be secondary to cystoid macular edema as well as foveal serous retinal detachment (C). The macular thickness map of the right eye showed markedly thickened retina with a foveal thickness of 777 ± 6 microns and total macular volume of 10.45 mm³ compared to the unaffected left eye, 156 ± 5 microns and 6.2 mm³ (D). Neither the visual acuity nor the OCT appearance of the fovea improved during the next two months of observation, and the patient underwent intravitreal triamcinolone acetonide injection. Two months after the injection, the visual acuity improved to 20/80 and a repeat OCT (5° meridian) demonstrated resolution of the subretinal fluid and improvement in the cystoid macular edema (E) with a corresponding decrease in the foveal thickness, 227 ± 28 microns, and total macular volume, 8.02 mm³ (F). The visual

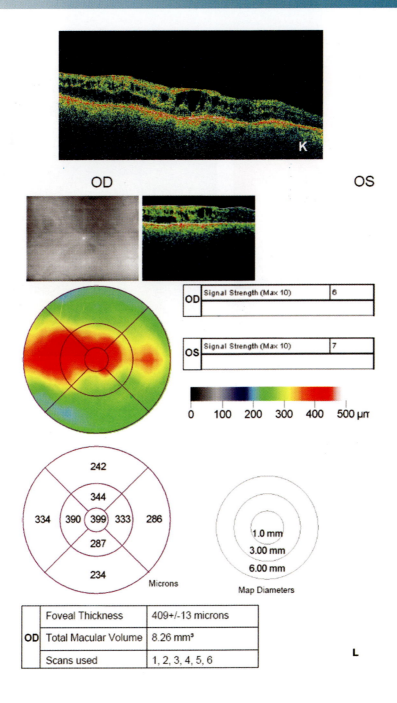

acuity remained stable through nine months post-injection and serial OCT scans (5° meridian) at four (G), seven (I) and nine months (K) post-injection demonstrated persistent cystoid macular edema without subretinal fluid. The corresponding macular thickness maps (H, J and L) demonstrate a stable foveal thickness and total macular volume.

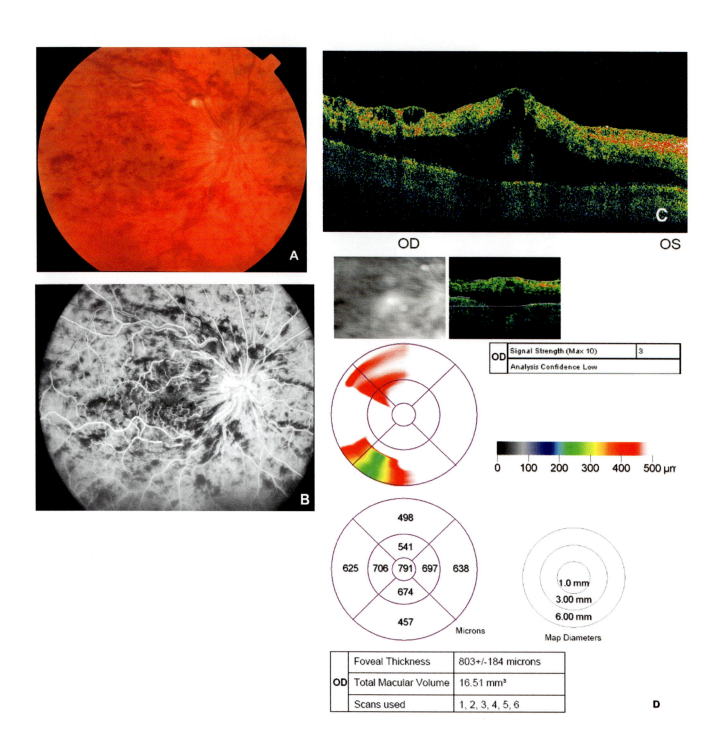

Figs 5.3A to D

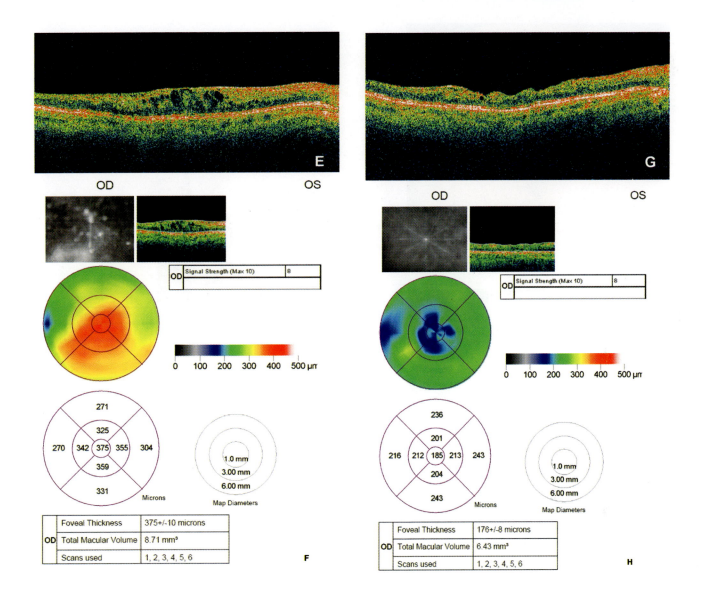

Figs 5.3A to H: A 46 year old man presented with a visual acuity of 20/125 and dilated/tortuous vessels with retinal hemorrhages in all four quadrants (A). Fluorescein angiography showed a perfused CRVO without any neovascularisation (B). The OCT scan through the fovea along the 5° meridian demonstrated cystoid macular edema and subfoveal fluid (C) with a foveal thickness of 803 ± 184 microns and total macular volume of 16.51 mm³ (D). Over the next 11 months, intravitreal triamcinolone acetonide (4 mg) was injected twice without improvement in cystoid macular edema or visual acuity. Pars plana vitrectomy combined with radial optic neurotomy and intravitreal triamcinolone acetonide was performed. Four months after surgery, the best-corrected visual acuity improved to 20/64. An OCT (5° meridian) demonstrated resolution of the subretinal fluid and improvement in the macular edema (E) with a foveal thickness of 375 ± 10 microns and total macular volume 8.71 mm³ (F). An epiretinal membrane had developed (E) and the patient underwent a second vitrectomy procedure to remove the membrane. Five months after vitrectomy and epiretinal membrane peel, the best corrected visual acuity was 20/40, and the OCT confirmed the absence of the epiretinal membrane with improved edema (G) and a foveal thickness of 176 ± 8 microns and a total macular volume of 6.43 mm³ (H).

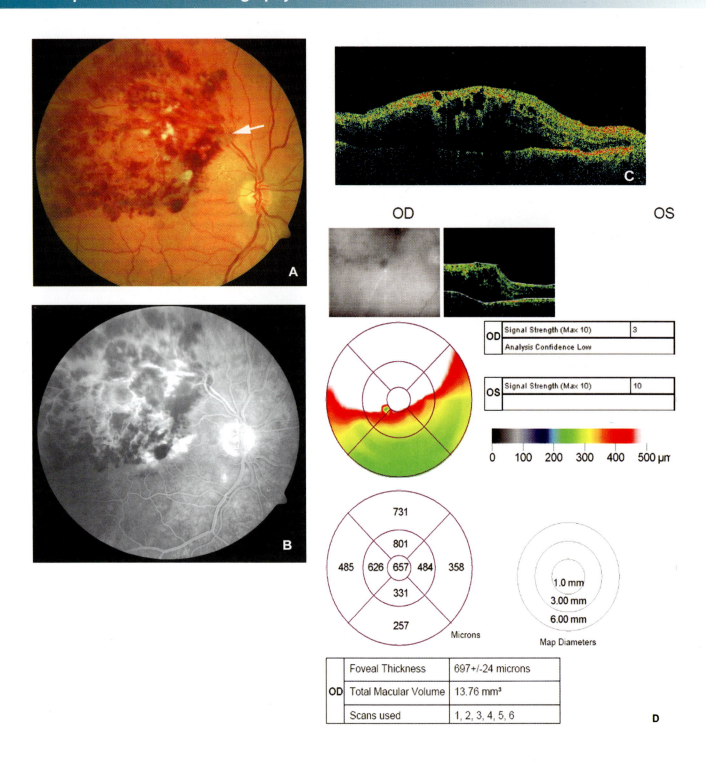

OD   OS

OD	Signal Strength (Max 10)	3
	Analysis Confidence Low	

OS	Signal Strength (Max 10)	10

0   100   200   300   400   500 μm

731

801

485   626   657   484   358

331

257

Microns

1.0 mm
3.00 mm
6.00 mm

Map Diameters

OD	Foveal Thickness	697+/-24 microns
	Total Macular Volume	13.76 mm³
	Scans used	1, 2, 3, 4, 5, 6

Figs 5.4A to D

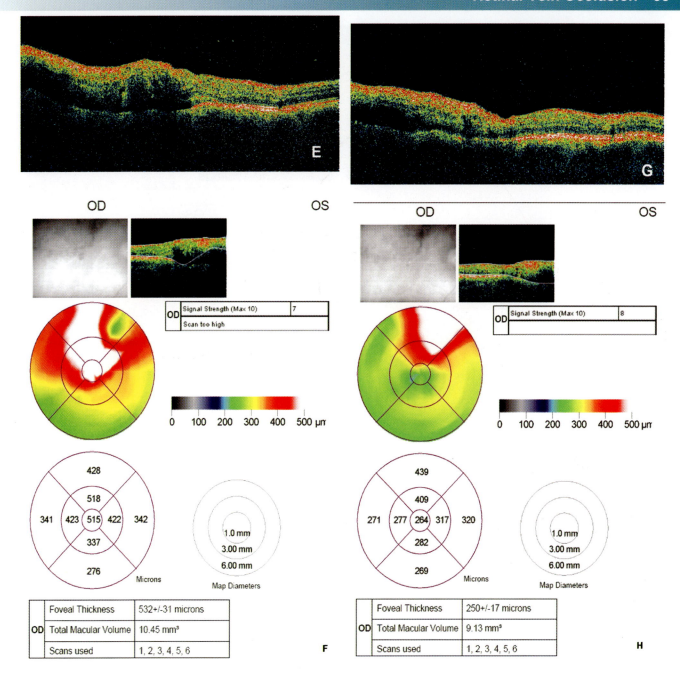

Figs 5.4A to J: A 52-year-old man with a history of hypertension and coronary artery disease presented with five weeks of decreased vision OD. The visual acuity was 20/250 OD and the patient described an inferonasal visual field defect. Examination revealed a BRVO along the superotemporal arcade (A) with characteristic intraretinal hemorrhages, venous tortuosity and cotton wool spots distal to an arteriovenous crossing (arrow). Areas of capillary non-perfusion were seen on fluorescein angiography (B). Optical coherence tomography demonstrated cystoid macular edema and accompanying serous retinal detachment (C). The foveal thickness was 697 ± 24 microns, and the total macular volume was 13.76 mm³ (D). An intravitreal triamcinolone acetonide (4 mg) injection was performed. One week after injection the visual acuity improved to 20/100, and an

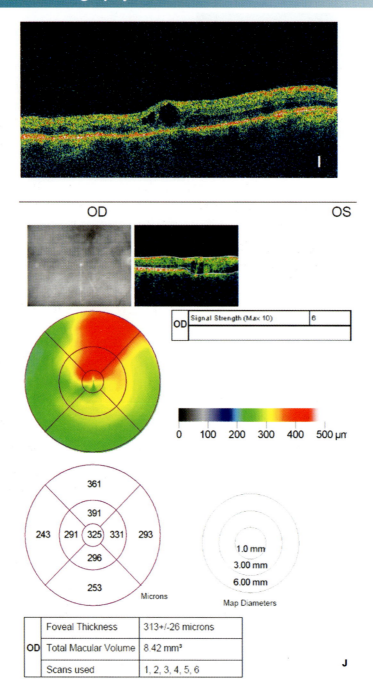

OCT of the macula along the 270° meridian (E) showed resolution of the serous fluid and a marked decrease in foveal thickness, measuring 532 ± 31 microns, and total macular volume, 10.45 mm³ (F). One month post-injection the visual acuity was still 20/100 and the OCT (270° meridian) demonstrated further resolution of the cystoid macular edema (G). The macular thickness map also showed a decrease in foveal thickness, 250 ± 17 microns, and total macular volume, 9.13 mm³ (H). At 3 months post-injection, the vision had declined to 20/160 and the OCT showed recurrent cystoid macular edema (I). The foveal thickness was increased, 313 ± 26 microns, however, the total macular volume was decreased, 8.42 mm³, attributable to improvement in the edema between the 3 mm and 6 mm rings in the superior quadrant (J)

Case 2

A 52-year-old man with a history of hypertension and coronary artery disease presented with five weeks of decreased vision OD. The visual acuity was 20/250 OD and the patient described an inferonasal visual field defect. Examination revealed a BRVO along the superotemporal arcade (Fig. 5.4A) with characteristic intraretinal hemorrhages, venous tortuosity and cotton wool spots. Areas of capillary non-perfusion were seen on fluorescein angiography (Fig. 5.4B). Optical coherence tomography demonstrated cystoid macular edema and accompanying serous retinal detachment (Fig. 5.4C). The foveal thickness was 697 ± 24 microns (Fig. 5.4D). An intravitreal triamcinolone acetonide (4 mg) injection was performed. One week after injection the visual acuity improved to 20/100, and an OCT of the macula (Fig. 5.4E) showed resolution of the serous fluid and a marked decrease in foveal thickness, measuring 532 ± 31 microns (Fig. 5.4F). One month post-injection, the visual acuity was still 20/100 and the OCT demonstrated further resolution of the cystoid macular edema (Fig. 5.4G). The macular thickness map also showed a decrease in foveal thickness, 250 ± 17 microns (Fig. 5.4H). At 3 months post-injection, the vision had declined to 20/160 and the OCT showed recurrent cystoid macular edema (Fig. 5.4I). The foveal thickness was increased, 313 ± 26 microns, however, the total macular volume was decreased, attributable to improvement in the edema between the 3 mm and 6 mm rings in the superior quadrant (Fig. 5.4J).

REFERENCES

1. Clarkson JG. Central Retinal Vein Occlusion, 3 ed. In: Schachat AP (Ed.) Retina. St.Louis: Mosby, 2001:1368-1375.
2. Saika S, Tanaka T, Miyamoto T, Ohnishi Y. Surgical posterior vitreous detachment combined with gas/air tamponade for treating macular edema associated with branch retinal vein occlusion: retinal tomography and visual outcome. Graefe's Arch Clin Exp Ophthalmol. 2001; 239:729-732.
3. Amirikia A, Scott IU, Murray TG, et al. Outcomes of vitreoretinal surgery for complications of branch retinal vein occlusion. Ophthalmology. 2001;108:372-376.
4. Ando N. Vitrectomy for ischemic maculopathy associated with retinal vein occlusion. Vail Vitrectomy Meeting. Vail, 2000.
5. Kurimoto M, Takagi H, Suzuma K. Vitrectomy for macular edema secondary to retinal vein occlusion: evaluation by retinal thickness analyzer. Jpn J Ophthalmol. 1999;53:717-720.
6. Branch Vein Occlusion Study Group. Argon laser scatter photocoagulation for prevention of neovascularization and vitreous hemorrhage in branch vein occlusion. A randomized clinical trial. Arch Ophthalmol. 1986;104:34-41.
7. The Branch Vein Occlusion Study Group. Argon laser photocoagulation for macular edema in branch vein occlusion. Am J Ophthalmol. 1984; 98:271-282.
8. Chen SD, Lochhead J, Patel CK, Frith P. Intravitreal triamcinolone acetonide for ischaemic macular oedema caused by branch retinal vein occlusion. Br J Ophthalmol. 2004; 88:154-155.
9. Saika S, Tanaka T, Miyamoto T. Surgical posterior vitreous detachment combined with gas/air tamponade for treating macular edema associated with branch retinal vein occlusion: retinal tomography and visual outcome. Graefe's Arch Clin Exp Ophthalmol. 2001; 239:729-732.
10. Shah GK, Sharma S, Fineman MS, et al. Arteriovenous adventitial sheathotomy for the treatment of macular edema associated with branch retinal vein occlusion. Am J Ophthalmol. 2000;129:104-106.
11. Shah GK. Adventitial sheathotomy for treatment of macular edema associated with branch retinal vein occlusion. Curr Opin Ophthalmol. 2000;11:171-174.
12. Opremcak EM, Bruce RA. Surgical decompression of branch retinal vein occlusion via arteriovenous crossing sheathotomy: a prospective review of 15 cases. Retina. 1999;19:1-5.
13. The Central Vein Occlusion Study Group. Baseline and early natural history report: the Central Vein Occlusion Study. Arch Ophthalmol. 1993;111:1087-1095.
14. Hayreh SS, Zimmerman MB, Podhajsky P. Incidence of various types of retinal vein occlusion and their recurrence and demographic characteristics. Am J Ophthalmol. 1994;117:429-441.
15. Mitchell P, Smith W, Chang A. Prevalence and associations of retinal vein occlusion in Australia: the Blue Mountains Eye Study. Arch Ophthalmol. 1996; 114:1243-1247.
16. Fong AC, Schatz H. Central retinal vein occlusion in young adults. Surv Ophthalmol. 1993;38:88.
17. Fekrat S, Finkelstein D. Venous Occlusive Disease, 1st ed. In Regillo CD, Brown GC, Flynn HW (eds): Vitreoretinal disease: The essentials. New York: Thieme, 1999: 117-131.
18. Gutman FA. Evaluation of a patient with central retinal vein occlusion. Ophthalmology. 1983;90:481-483.
19. Green W, Chan C, Hutchins G, Terry J. Central retinal vein occlusions: a prospective histopathologic study of 29 eyes in 28 cases. Retina. 1981;1:27-55.

20. Hayreh SS. Central retinal vein occlusion. Ophthalmol Clin North Am. 1998;11:559-590.
21. Sperduto RD, Hiller R, Chew E, et al. Risk factors for hemiretinal vein occlusion: comparison with risk factors for central and branch retinal vein occlusion: the eye disease case-control study.[comment]. Ophthalmology. 1998;105:765-771.
22. Anonymous. Risk factors for central retinal vein occlusion. The Eye Disease Case-Control Study Group. Arch Ophthalmol. 1996;114:545-554.
23. Cahill M, Karabatzaki M, Meleady R, et al. Raised plasma homocysteine as a risk factor for retinal vascular occlusive disease. Br J Ophthalmol. 2000;84:154-157.
24. The Central Vein Occlusion Study Group. Evaluation of grid pattern photocoagulation for macular edema in central vein occlusion. Ophthalmology. 1995;102:1425-1433.
25. The Central Vein Occlusion Study Group. A randomized clinical trial of early panretinal photocoagulation for ischemic central vein occlusion. The Central Vein Occlusion Study Group N Report. Ophthalmology. 1995;102:1434-1444.
26. Fekrat S, Goldberg MF, Finkelstein D. Laser-induced chorioretinal venous anastomosis for nonischemic central or branch retinal vein occlusion.[comment]. Arch Ophthalmol. 1998;116:43-52.
27. Fekrat S, de Juan E, Jr. Chorioretinal venous anastomosis for central retinal vein occlusion: transvitreal venipuncture. Ophthal Surg Lasers. 1999;30:52-55.
28. Park CH, Jaffe GJ, Fekrat S. Intravitreal triamcinolone acetonide in eyes with cystoid macular edema associated with central retinal vein occlusion. Am J Ophthalmol. 2003;136:419-425.
29. Lam HD, Blumenkranz MS. Treatment of central retinal vein occlusion by vitrectomy with lysis of vitreopapillary and epipapillary adhesions, subretinal peripapillary tissue plasminogen activator injection, and photocoagulation. Am J Ophthalmol. 2002;134:609-611.
30. Yeshaya A, Treister G. Pars plana vitrectomy for vitreous hemorrhage and retinal vein occlusion. Ann Ophthalmol. 1983;15:615-617.
31. Weizer JS, Stinnett SS, Fekrat S. Radial optic neurotomy as treatment for central retinal vein occlusion. Am J Ophthalmol. 2003;136:814-819.
32. Opremcak EM, Bruce RA, Lomeo MD, et al. Radial optic neurotomy for central retinal vein occlusion: a retrospective pilot study of 11 consecutive cases. Retina. 2001;21:408-415.
33. Apushkin MA, Fishman GA, Janowicz MJ. Monitoring cystoid macular edema by optical coherence tomography in patients with retinitis pigmentosa. Ophthalmology. 2004;111:1899-1904.
34. Spaide RF, Lee JK, Klancnik JK, Jr., Gross NE. Optical coherence tomography of branch retinal vein occlusion. Retina. 2003;23:343-347.
35. Antcliff RJ, Stanford MR, Chauhan DS, et al. Comparison between optical coherence tomography and fundus fluorescein angiography for the detection of cystoid macular edema in patients with uveitis. Ophthalmology. 2000;107:593-599.
36. Kang SW, Park CY, Ham DI. The correlation between fluorescein angiographic and optical coherence tomographic features in clinically significant diabetic macular edema. Am J Ophthalmol. 2004;137:313-322.
37. Battaglia Parodi M, Iacono P, Di Crecchio L, et al. Clinical and angiographic features in nasal branch retinal vein occlusion. Ophthalmologica. 2004;218:210-213.
38. Mori K, Gehlbach PL, Sano A, et al. Comparison of epiretinal membranes of differing pathogenesis using optical coherence tomography. Retina. 2004;24:57-62.
39. Rumelt S, Karatas M, Pikkel J, et al. Optic disc traction syndrome associated with central retinal vein occlusion. Arch Ophthalmol. 2003;121:1093-1097.
40. Ip MS, Kumar KS. Intravitreous triamcinolone acetonide as treatment for macular edema from central retinal vein occlusion. Arch Ophthalmol. 2002;120:1217-1219.

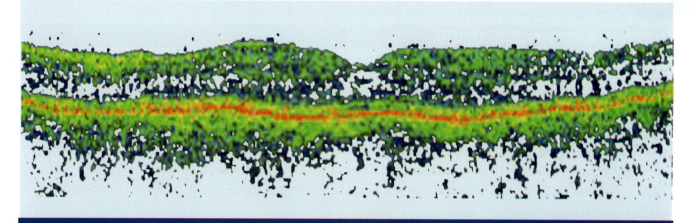

CHAPTER

6

Retinal Artery Occlusion and Retinal Arterial Macroaneurysm

Keisuke Mori

RETINAL ARTERY OCCLUSION

Retinal artery occlusion is a relatively common etiology for sudden vision loss in aged adults. The embolization and thrombosis are the common cause of arterial obstruction.[1-3] The ophthalmic artery is the first branch of the internal carotid artery so that embolic material from either the heart or the carotid arteries has a direct route to the eye. Other possible mechanisms and/or trigger of occlusion are vasculitis, spasms, circulatory collapse and raised intraocular pressure during the surgery.[2,4,5] Retinal artery occlusion is frequently associated with systemic abnormalities. Two-thirds of patients with retinal artery occlusion have associated systemic arterial hypertension, one-fourth have diabetic mellitus and also one-fourth have cardiac valvular disease.[1]

The clinical feature of retinal artery occlusion depends on the size and location of the obstructed vessel and its severity and distribution. Retinal arterial occlusive disease includes central retinal artery occlusion (CRAO), branch retinal artery occlusion (BRAO), cilioretinal artery occlusion and occlusion of precapillary arterioles (cotton-wool spots) based on the location of affected vessel and its distribution. Approximately 57% of retinal artery obstructive diseases are CRAO, and 38% is BRAO and 5% is cilioretinal artery occlusion.[6] The visual prognosis of BRAO and cilioretinal artery occlusion is generally good, but visual field defects usually remain.

The retina of patients with CRAO appears as whitening or opacification as a result of cloudy swelling due to intracellular edema, especially in the macular area (posterior pole) where the inner retinal structure is thickest. Since the central fovea (foveola) lacks these layers, the orange-red appearance is evident in the central fovea in contrast to the surrounding opaque retina (cherry red spot). The retinal arteries are thinned and are associated with irregularities in caliber. Segmentation or boxcarring of the blood column can be seen in both arterioles and venules.

In 20-25% of eyes with CRAO, a portion of the papillomacular bundle is supplied by one or more cilioretinal arterioles from the ciliary circulation.[6] If the cilioretinal sparing in papillomacular bundle reaches the foveola, the central vision may be preserved.

Optical Coherence Tomography

Histopathologically, the neuronal cells in the inner retina become edematous during the first few hours after artery occlusion. The intracellular swelling accounts for the whitening or opacification of the affected retina observed ophthalmoscopically.[7] The retinal opacification usually resolves within 4 to 6 weeks.

The optical coherence tomography (OCT) images of ischemic retina due to CRAO and BRAO correlate with the histopathological findings of acute retinal ischemia cited above. The affected area demonstrates increased thickness and reflectivity in the inner retina. The marked difference from retinal edema due to other retinal vascular disease such as retinal vein occlusion or diabetic maculopathy is lack of areas or cystic spaces of low reflectivity due to fluid accumulation. After the resolution of retinal cloudy edema inner retina becomes atrophic and thin, which is characteristic of OCT findings of chronic CRAO or BRAO.

Interesting Case Examples

Case 1. Central Retinal Artery Occlusion

A 73-year-old male noticed sudden visual loss in his right eye 36 hours earlier. His right eye vision was counting fingers. Fundus examination revealed whitening or opacification, as a result of retinal intracellular edema in the posterior pole. Opacification was significant with cilioretinal arteries sparing one-fourth the papillomacular bundle (Fig. 6.1A). A longitudinal echogram of right internal carotid artery demonstrated the atherosclerotic plaque which might have been the origin of the embolus in the central retinal artery (Fig. 6.1B). Fluorescein angiogram, showed cilioretinal arteries (Figs 6.1C and D). A vertical OCT scan showed enhanced reflectivity with mild increase of inner retinal thickness without cystic spaces of low reflectivity due to fluid accumulation (Fig. 6.1E). A horizontal OCT scan demonstrated cilioretinal arteries sparing in papillomacular bundle (Fig. 6.1F).

Case 2. Branch Retinal Artery Occlusion

A 61-year-old male reported sudden onset of superior visual field loss in his right. His right visual acuity was 20/200. Fundus examination revealed cloudy swelling of the retina present in the distribution of the occluded artery running through inferior macula (Fig. 6.2A). Fluorescein angiogram, at 8 minutes and 20 seconds showed segmentation or boxcarring of the blood column in the occluded inferior branch (Fig. 6.2B). A vertical OCT scan showed the inferior retina with increased reflectivity and thickness in contrast with normal superior retina (Fig. 6.2C).

RETINAL ARTERIAL MACROANEURYSM

The retinal arterial macroaneurysm is fusiform or round dilation of retinal arteriole in the posterior pole. The macroaneurysm generally affects a patient older than sixties, who is usually associated with hypertension and arteriosclerotic cardiovascular diseases.[8]

The patient with macroaneurysm is asymptomatic if there is no complication in the macular area, but becomes symptomatic when the macroaneurysm complicates with retinal edema, exudation and hemorrhage. The clinician may have a problem in diagnosing a case with the massive hemorrhage which masks the macroaneurysm. In that case fluorescein angiography may also fail to show the macroaneurysm because of the blockage by surrounding preretinal hemorrhage. Bleeding from the macroaneurysm may occur in subretinal, intraretinal, preretinal (beneath posterior hyaloid or internal limiting membrane), intravitreous or combined. The clinician can strongly presume the macroaneurysm if the case is associated with hemorrhages in multiple levels. Indocyanine green (ICG) angiography may be also helpful in delineating the macroaneurysm with preretinal hemorrhage because of spectral properties of ICG dye.

Laser photocoagulation directly to the macroaneurysm is still controversial. Several series of reports demonstrated possible role of laser treatment for the macroaneurysm.[9,10] Many investigators and clinicians consider direct laser photocoagulation if the retinal edema and lipid exudation is involving the macula. However, recent study of long-term visual outcome of macroaneurysms demonstrated visual prognosis was better in untreated cases when compared to laser-treated cases.[11] Recently, submacular surgery with tissue plasminogen activator-assisted thrombolysis has been proposed for subretinal hemorrhage removal in the cases with macroaneurysms.[12, 13]

Optical Coherence Tomography

The retinal arterial macroaneurysm may be associated with vitreous, preretinal (beneath posterior hyaloid or internal limiting membrane), intraretinal, subretinal hemorrhage, or combined. Optical coherence

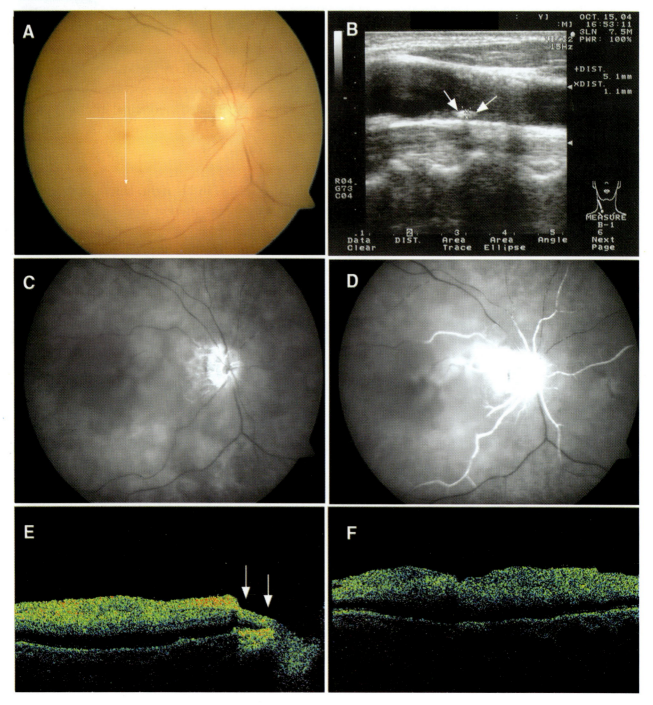

Fig. 6.1: A: Fundus photograph. Whitening or opacification as a result of retinal intracellular edema in the posterior pole is significant with cilioretinal arteries sparing one-fourth the papillomacular bundle. B: A longitudinal echogram of right internal carotid artery demonstrates the atherosclerotic plaque (arrow) which may be the origin of the embolus in the central retinal artery. C: Fluorescein angiogram, 23. 4 seconds after injection. Cilioretinal arteries are evident. D: Fluorescein angiogram, 1 minute and 16 seconds. E: A vertical OCT scan shows enhanced reflectivity with mild increase of inner retinal thickness without cystic spaces of low reflectivity due to fluid accumulation. F: A horizontal OCT scan demonstrates cilioretinal arteries sparing in papillomacular bundle (arrows).

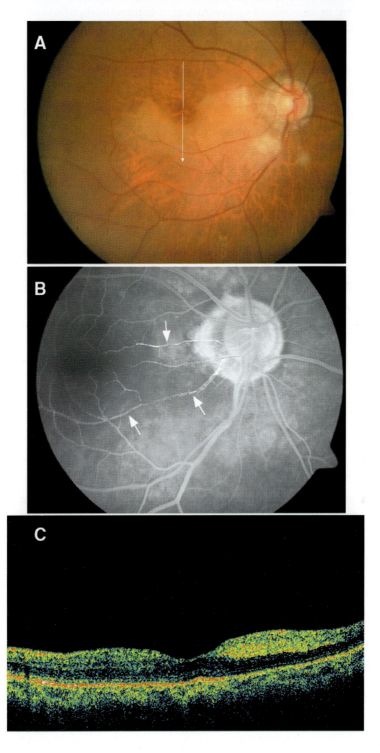

Fig. 6.2: A: Fundus photograph. Retinal cloudy swelling is present in the distribution of the occluded artery running through inferior macula. B: Fluorescein angiogram, 8 minutes and 20 seconds. Note segmentation or boxcarring of the blood column in the occluded inferior branch (arrows). C: A vertical OCT scan. The inferior retina with increased reflectivity and thickness (arrowheads) contrast with normal superior retina.

tomography provides an 'in vivo' direct visualization of intraretinal pathology with unprecedented resolution if the hemorrhage is posterior to the retina. Intraretinal morphological alterations associated with the macroaneurysm commonly are retinal edema and exudation. Optical coherence tomography demonstrates retinal edema associated with the macroaneurysm as diffuse retinal thickening and elevation with cystic spaces of low reflectivity as a result of fluid accumulation. Hard exudates are highly backscattering, usually shown as small high reflective dots or areas with shadow of deeper retinal structures. Optical coherence tomography provides information of location in layers of these pathologies. Cystic space of fluid accumulation and retinal exudation are generally located in the inner and outer plexiform layers. Optical coherence tomography provides follow-up information of these pathologies and response to therapeutic interventions.

If the hemorrhage is anterior to the retina, the details of retinal structure are masked by high backscattering of hemorrhage. The preretinal hemorrhage sometimes merges imperceptibly with the retina. Optical coherence tomography can occasionally distinguish hemorrhages beneath internal limiting membrane from posterior hyaloid since the internal limiting membrane tends to be more reflective than the posterior hyaloid.

Interesting Case Examples

Case 1. Retinal Arterial Macroaneurysm

A 67-year-old female had a history of progressive blurred vision in her left eye. Her vision measured 20/200. Laser photocoagulation directed toward the arterial macroaneurysm was performed. One month after laser vision improved to 20/60.

Fundus photograph before laser shows an arterial macroaneurysm along the arteriole superotemporal to the fovea, complicating retinal edema and exudation (Fig. 6.3A). Fluorescein angiogram, 32 second after injection is shown in Fig. 6.3B. An oblique OCT scan (5 mm) crossing the macroaneurysm and the parafovea demonstrated diffuse retinal thickening and elevation with cystic spaces of low reflectivity as a result of fluid accumulation. Small high reflective dots, representing intraretinal exudation, located at the level corresponding to outer plexiform layer are shown in Fig. 6.3C. A horizontal OCT scan crossing fovea delineated serous retinal detachment with intraretinal exudation (Fig. 6.3D). A macular horizontal cross-sectional image one month after the treatment depicted decreased retinal edema and relative increase of intraretinal exudation (Fig. 6.3E).

Case 2. The Retinal Arterial Macroaneurysm with Massive Hemorrhage

An 80-year-old female noticed sudden visual loss in her right eye. Her right eye visual acuity was 4/200. Neodymium: YAG laser was delivered to internal limiting membrane to open trapped hemorrhage overlying the macula.[14,15] The treatment resulted in rapid and marked clearing of hemorrhage. Two months after laser treatment mild foveal edema with intraretinal exudation was still persistent and visual acuity improved moderately to 20/60.

Fundus examination before the treatment showed an arterial macroaneurysm along the arteriole superotemporal to the fovea, complicating preretinal and subretinal hemorrhages (Fig. 6.4 A). Fluorescein angiogram demonstrated hyperfluorescence of the macroaneurysm (Fig. 6.4 B). A vertical OCT scan delineated preretinal hemorrhage as a dome-shaped, highly elevated, highly reflective zone beneath the internal limiting membrane. The detail of retinal structure of inferior macula was masked by high backscattering of hemorrhage (Fig. 6.4 C). Fundus photograph immediately after Nd: YAG laser

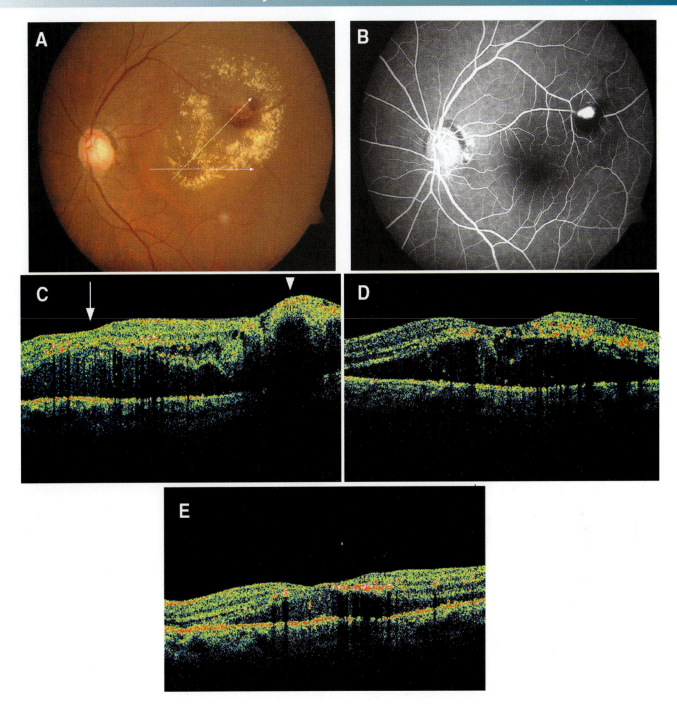

Fig. 6.3: A: Fundus photograph before laser shows an arterial macroaneurysm along the arteriole superotemporal to the fovea, complicating retinal edema and exudation. B: Fluorescein angiogram, 32 second after injection. C: An oblique OCT scan (5 mm) crossing the macroaneurysm (arrowhead) and the parafovea (arrow) demonstrates diffuse retinal thickening and elevation with cystic spaces of low reflectivity as a result of fluid accumulation. Small high reflective dots, representing intraretinal exudation, located at the level corresponding to outer plexiform layer. D: A horizontal OCT scan crossing fovea delineates serous retinal detachment with intraretinal exudation. E: A macular horizontal cross-sectional image one month after the treatment depicts decreased retinal edema and relative increase of intraretinal exudation.

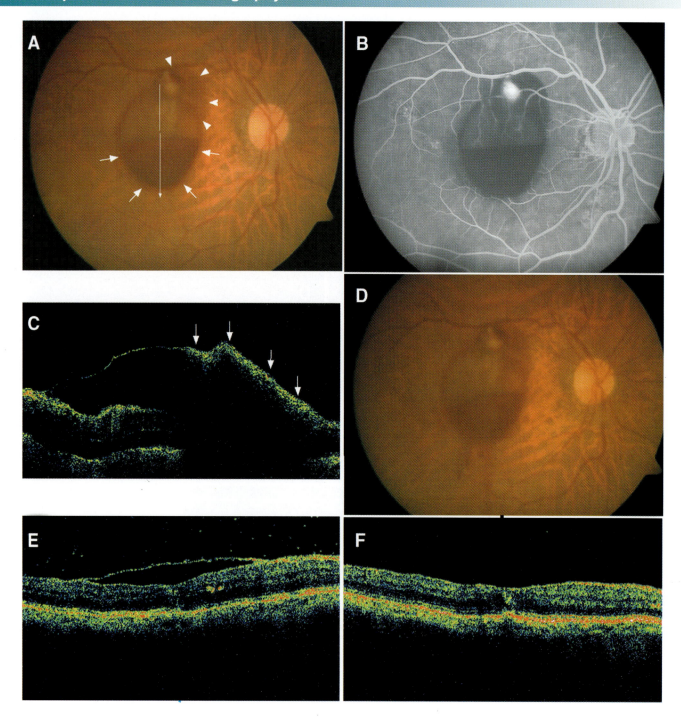

Fig. 6.4: A: Fundus photograph before the treatment shows an arterial macroaneurysm along the arteriole superotemporal to the fovea, complicating preretinal (arrowheads) and subretinal (arrows) hemorrhages. B: Fluorescein angiogram demonstrates hyperfluorescence of the macroaneurysm. C: A vertical OCT scan delineates preretinal hemorrhage as a dome-shaped, highly elevated, highly reflective zone beneath the internal limiting membrane (arrows). The detail of retinal structure of inferior macula is masked by high backscattering of hemorrhage. D: Fundus photograph immediately after Nd:YAG laser membranotomy. Vertical OCT cross-sections 7-day E: and 2-month F: after the treatment. Please notice rapid clearing of premacular hemorrhage. However, mild foveal edema with intraretinal exudation is delineated by OCT.

membranotomy is shown in Fig. 6.4D. Vertical OCT cross-sections 7-day (Fig. 6.4E) and 2-month (Fig. 6.4 F) after the treatment showed rapid clearing of premacular hemorrhage. However, mild foveal edema with intraretinal exudation was delineated by OCT.

REFERENCES

1. Brown GC, Magargal LE. Central retinal artery obstruction and visual acuity. Ophthalmology. 1982;89: 14-19.
2. Gold D. Retinal arterial occlusion. Trans Sect Ophthalmol Am Acad Ophthalmol Otolaryngol. 1977;83: 392-408.
3. Perraut LE, Zimmerman LE. The occurrence of glaucoma following occlusion of the central retinal artery: A clinicopathologic report of six new cases with a review of the literature. Arch Ophthalmol. 1959; 61: 845-865.
4. Appen RE, Wray SH, Cogan DG. Central retinal artery occlusion. Am J Ophthalmol. 1975;79: 374-381.
5. Silberberg DH, Laties AM. Occlusive migraine. Trans Pa Acad Ophthalmol Otolaryngol. 1974;27: 34-38.
6. Brown GC, Shields JA. Cilioretinal arteries and retinal arterial occlusion. Arch Ophthalmol. 1979;97: 84-92.
7. Yanoff M, Fine BS. Ocular Pathology: A Text and Atlas. 3rd ed. Philadelphia, JB Lippincott 1989:383-400.
8. Robertson DM. Macroaneurysms of the retinal arteries. Trans Am Acad Ophthalmol Otolaryngol. 1973;77: 55-67.
9. Lewis RA, Norton EW, Gass JD. Acquired arterial macroaneurysms of the retina. Br J Ophthalmol 1976;60: 21-30.
10. Mainster MA, Whitacre MM. Dye yellow photocoagulation of retinal arterial macroaneurysms. Am J Ophthalmol. 1988;105:97-98.
11. Brown DM, Sobol WM, Folk JC, Weingeist TA. Retinal arteriolar macroaneurysms: long-term visual outcome. Br J Ophthalmol. 1994;78:534-538.
12. Peyman GA, Nelson NC Jr, Alturki W, et al. Tissue plasminogen activating factor assisted removal of subretinal hemorrhage. Ophthalmic Surg. 1991;22:575-582.
13. Humayun M, Lewis H, Flynn HW Jr, et al. Management of Submacular hemorrhage associated with retinal arterial macroaneurysms. Am J Ophthalmol. 1998;126:358-361.
14. Tassignon MJ, Stempels N, Van Mulders L. Retrohyaloid premacular hemorrhage treated by Q-switched Nd-YAG laser. A case report. Graefes Arch Clin Exp Ophthalmol. 1989;227:440-442.
15. Raymond LA. Neodymium: YAG laser treatment for hemorrhages under the internal limiting membrane and posterior hyaloid face in the macula. Ophthalmology 1995;102:406-411.

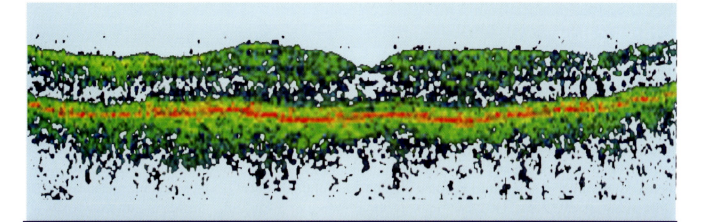

C H A P T E R

7

Age-Related Macular Degeneration and Choroidal Neovascularisation

Gisèle Soubrane, Gabriel Coscas

INTRODUCTION

The International community in a published classification has identified two phases in age-related macular degeneration: *age-related maculopathy* including all type of drusen and retinal pigment epithelium disturbances and *age-related macular degeneration* including the exudative (or neovascular) form and the atrophic form (with extra or juxtafoveal atrophic patches). Fluorescein angiography (FA) remains the gold standard for diagnosis and distinction of these two forms. Leakage is the key symptom of choroidal new vessels (CNV) in the exudative form. Optical coherence tomography (OCT) examination provides useful informations about quantification of retinal thickness and accumulation of fluid in between or within the retinal layers. In addition, in selected cases, OCT may identify the presence of neovascular membrane, fibrous tissue or vitreoretinal adherence or traction. Optical coherance tomography could become a useful tool for follow-up with or without treatment.

AGE-RELATED MACULOPATHY

Soft Drusen

Soft drusen are considered the most significant marker of the initial stage of age-related maculopathy. Modification in their aspect is an indicator of the risk of developing choroidal neovascularisation (CNV). Hard drusen are considered as a sign of begnin ageing, usually not detectable on OCT possibly due to their small size.

Clinically, their shape is irregular, their size larger than 63 microns with indistinct margins, and fairly pale color. The largest drusen are usually situated closest to the fovea, while smaller soft drusen and hard drusen remain in the outer macula. (Fig. 7.1A).

On fluorescein angiography in the early phase, soft drusen are hypofluorescent and almost invisible. *In the late and very late phase*, they gradually stain and become hyperfluorescent. (Fig. 7.1B)

On ICG angiography (ICG-A) with a conventional fundus camera, drusen are faintly hypofluorescent and visible only when they are rather large. With SLO-ICG imaging soft drusen are dark or hypofluorescent in the early phase. This aspect persists until the *late phase*. Mid-phase ICG-A demonstrates a more prominent blocking effect or hypofluorescence from the drusen against the persistent moderate hyperfluorescence of the background. (Fig. 7.1C). *In the inversion phase* (as choroidal vessels are no longer visible), the soft drusen are very distinct, and their dimensions, number, and confluence are more clearly seen. Any progressive hyperfluorescence within the soft drusen area should immediately suggest choroidal neovascularisation

On OCT, soft drusen are easily recognized as localized multiple elevation of the hyper-reflective band of the retinal pigment epithelium -Bruch's membrane-choriocapillaris complex. During progression of the disease, their elevation might increase in size, in height and become confluent or indistinct. Drusen themselves have moderate reflectivity (green in color), with no shadowing backwards to choroid. There is no sub-retinal nor intra-retinal fluid accumulation. The different retinal layers remain normally organized (Fig. 7.1D). A normal morphology of the overlying neurosensory retina with no change in thickness of the sensory retina and with conservation of the parallelism of the different reflective bands is observed.

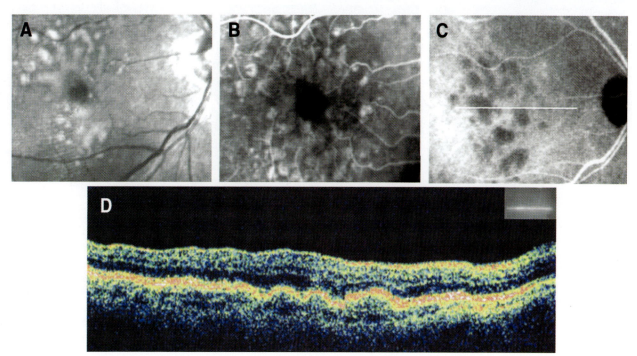

Fig. 7.1: Soft drusen. (A) Red-free photograph : Numerous macular soft drusen partially confluent. (B) FA: Late-staining drusen. (C) SLO-ICG-A : Late phase: Soft drusen of various sizes, small or large, and confluent, persistent in the late phase. (D) OCT: Corrugated iron like elevations of the retinal pigment epithelium-Bruch's membrane complex, with no shadowing towards the choroid.

The natural history of soft drusen is variable. They become progressively larger and confluent, of irregular shape (Fig. 7.2). At that stage, drusen usually occupy a large area in the posterior pole. Pigmentary changes of variable density develop in association with the confluent drusen and induce a sharp posterior shadowing. These findings are the characteristics of "high-risk drusen": numerous, large, confluent drusen with pigmentary changes.

Then, confluent drusen could subsequently form *drusenoid pigment epithelial detachment (PED)* (Fig. 7.3). Its shape is typically slightly irregular with a bumpy surface. Hyper-pigmentation gradually forms a radiating pigment figure. It is surrounded by several large soft drusen and many small drusen located more peripherally (Fig. 7.3A).

OCT examination will show an irregular elevation of the retinal pigment epithelium-Bruch's membrane complex, more extensive and larger than soft drusen. The drusenoid PED has moderate hyper-reflectivity. There is limited or no shadowing towards the choroid (Fig. 7.3C).

Drusenoid PED have usually a slow natural history, with progressive enlargement and confluence. Gradually, it generally begins to collapse, evolving towards atrophy, which is the most common outcome. Progression to CNV may also be observed but less frequently.

At this stage, OCT appears useful to identify soft drusen in conjunction with fluorescein angiography and even more with SLO-ICG angiography on which soft drusen disclose permanent hypofluorescence. The additional informations provided by OCT include their density, their thickness, their confluence and their exact location in relation to the fovea. Any change with increasing thickness due to either intraretinal or to

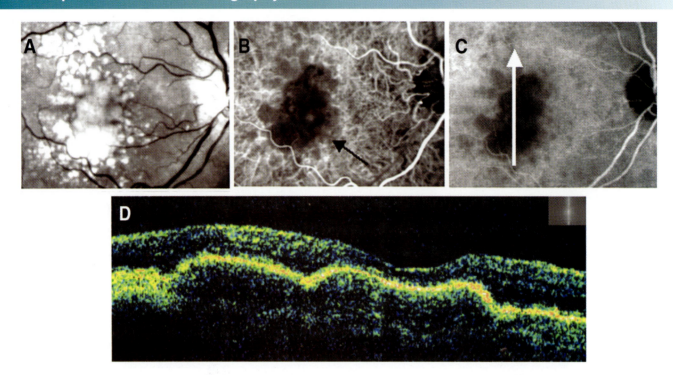

Fig. 7.2: Confluent soft drusen (A and B) Red-free photograph and FA: Confluent drusen or moderate drusenoid pigment epithelial detachment, relatively well demarcated and surrounded by many drusen small or large. No signs of CNV. (C) SLO-ICG : The confluent drusen are dark and well delimited. Neither hyperfluorescence nor signs of the presence of CNV are evident at this stage. (D) OCT : Irregular elevation of the retinal pigment epithelium band due to larger confluent drusen, with no shadowing towards the choroid.

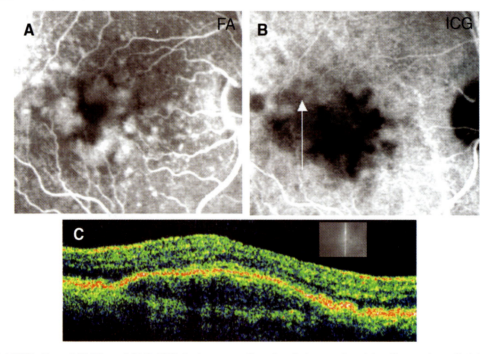

Fig. 7.3: Drusenoid PED (A and B) FA and SLO-ICG-A : Large confluent soft drusen, involving the center with late staining in FA and hypofluorescence in ICG-A. (C) OCT : Smooth elevation of the retinal pigment epithelium-Bruch's membrane-choriocapillaris band with moderate reflectivity and no shadowing.

subretinal accumulation of fluid is suggestive of proliferation of choroidal new vessels that OCT can detect even at a very early and localized stage not only on thickness mapping but also on systematic sections (as the raster scanning)

AGE-RELATED MACULAR DEGENERATION (AMD)

Geographic Atrophy

Dry (atrophic, non-neovascular) AMD is one of the two main clinical types of AMD of equal incidence than wet AMD. Atrophic AMD is characterized by progressive loss of central vision due to loss of retinal pigment epithelium cells with atrophy of the chorio-capillaris and death of central photoreceptors. Atrophic AMD is also defined by the absence of exudation and neovascularisation.

Geographic atrophy may result of a number of possible manifestations (Fig. 7.4A and 7.5A):
- Presence, extension, and *progressive coalescence* of small areas of atrophy of the retinal pigment epithelium and the overlying photoreceptors.
- *Drusen regression* resulting into small atrophic areas initially isolated and perifoveal, gradually enlarging around the fovea. The central sparing may persist for variable time.
- Atrophy secondary to a *retinal pigment epithelium tear* with retraction of the retinal pigment epithelium.
- *Flattening of elevated retinal pigment epithelium* and disappearance of any accumulated material (fluid or drusenoid PED or pseudovitelliform dystrophy).

Clinically, hypopigmentation or depigmentation of the retinal pigment epithelium with clear-cut areas of atrophy, with or without pigmentary migration and drusen, may be seen on biomicroscopic examination, depending on the extent and location of the lesions. Loss of visual acuity initially moderate may become severe.

On fluorescein angiography, atrophic areas induce progressive transmission defect (window defect) that persists in the late phase and remain well demarcated without leakage. Auto-fluorescence studies have shown that accumulation of hypofluorescent material around the atrophic areas is suggestive of the eventual progression of the disease (Fig. 7.5B).

On ICG, the masquage by the normal retinal pigment epithelium is markedly attenuated in infrared light. Nevertheless, the atrophic areas enhance the contrast of the underlying crossing, rarefied, but still perfused, choroidal vessels (Fig. 7.4C, 7.5E). Late-phase ICG-A demonstrates relative hypofluorescence of all atrophic areas (Fig. 7.5F).

When CNV occurs as a complication of atrophic AMD, it develops at the margin of the atrophic areas mostly on the foveal side. These CNV are clearly visible on ICG angiography.

On OCT, an atrophic area manifests as (Fig. 7.4D and 7.5G):
- a decrease in thickness of the neurosensory retina
- a disappearance of the hyporeflective band corresponding to the photoreceptors
- an increased hyper-reflectivity of the retinal pigment epithelium-Bruch's membrane-choroicapillaris extending back towards the underlying choroid.

The atrophic lesion may be of varying extent with clear-cut limits. When the central macula is involved, the foveal depression is flattened and the neurosensory retina progressively thinned confirms the existence of retinal pigment epithelium atrophy observed with the other imaging methods.

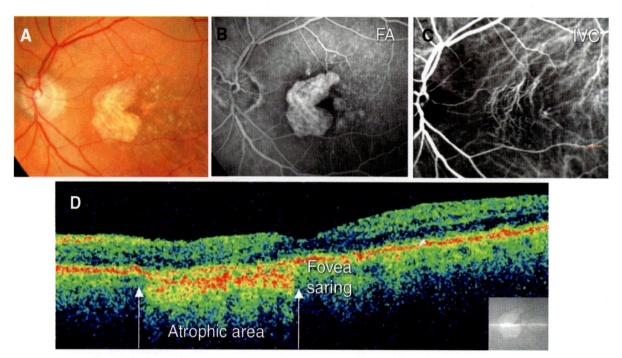

Fig. 7.4: Atrophic AMD with foveal sparing (A) Color : Extensive, irregular, discolored, and well-demarcated area in the nasal part of the macula, with sparing of the temporal zone, which contains drusen. The preserved xanthophyll pigment in the foveal center appears dark. (B and C) FA and ICG-A : Progressive abnormal hyperfluorescence of the atrophic area (window defect), sparing the foveal center. On ICG-A, Enhanced visibility of choroidal vessels in the atrophic area, with fewer branches. (D) OCT : Hyper-reflective band extending towards the choroid with retinal thinning throughout the atrophic area.

Optical coherance tomography will help:
- to confirm the presence of any atrophic area
- to show relative thinning of the sensory retina
- to analyze at the border of any scar the presence of CNV or the post laser recurrence of neovascularization.

The additional information provided by OCT is the degree of thinning of the neurosensory retina and the possible sparing of the fovea. The eventual association, particularly at the border of area, of exudation is suggestive of CNV proliferation.

Exudative Age-Related Macular Degeneration

Optical coherance tomography is of major interest in exudative maculopathy in providing on one hand, indirect signs, strongly suggestive of leaking vessels and, on the other hand, direct signs of CNV.

The indirect signs, difficult to visualize on FA but obvious on OCT scans include :
- increase in retinal thickness due to accumulation of either subretinal or intraretinal fluid
- decrease or even disappearance of the foveal depression
- detachment of the neurosensory retina
- detachment of the retinal pigment epithelium (serous, hemorrhagic or fibrovascular) resulting sometimes in a retinal pigment epithelium tear.

The direct signs due to choroidal new vessels themselves are well-imaged on FA but discrete on OCT and require a precise analysis of perfectly focused sections. Optical coherance tomography scans are best oriented

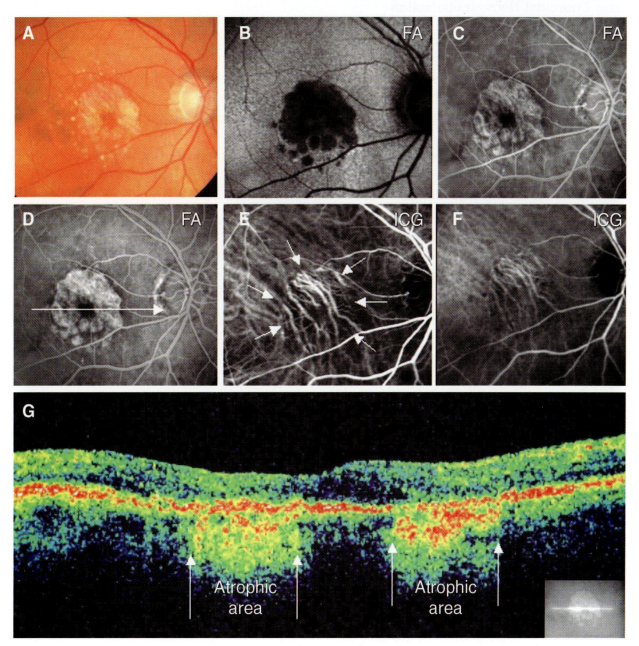

Fig. 7.5: Geographic atrophy with foveal sparing. (A and B) Color and auto-fluorescence demonstrate a perifoveal, beagle-like, slightly irregular but well-demarcated discolored area. In its center, a small, darker area of preserved xanthophyll pigment is seen. Absence of auto-fluorescence of all the atrophic area (B). (C and D) On FA, progressive hyperfluorescence and window defect with central sparing. Several soft drusen can be seen in the inferior region. (E and F) ICG angiography : Large choroidal vessels cross the area of atrophy. (G) OCT : Throughout the atrophic area, hyper-reflectivity extending deep towards the choroid with retinal thinning. The central area, which is spared, presents abnormal retinal pigment epithelium-Bruch's membrane band with back shadowing at this level.

by the features observed on fluorescein and ICG angiography. Optical coherance tomography will confirm the CNV and will precise the topography of the new vessels, their exact extent, their relation with the RPE and the neurosensory retina and their degree of activity. The indications for treatment are based on confrontation of imaging techniques.

Classic Choroidal Neovascularisation

The classic form of CNV is the typical variant of exudative AMD. It requires urgent treatment. There are several treatment options (direct laser photocoagulation, photodynamic therapy with verteporfine and intra-vitreal anti-angiogenics drugs). These treatments need very close follow up. Imaging technics and OCT are particularly useful for the best management.

Clinically, reduction of visual acuity and metamorphopsia are highly suggestive of CNV and fundus examination reveals characteristic exudative changes (fluid, hemorrhages, lipids).

On fluorescein angiography, classic CNV present characteristic features: well demarcated area of bright localized hyperfluorescence in the early phase (sometimes showing as a neovascular network) (Fig. 7.6A and 7A) giving rise to an intense leakage on mid and late phase which extends beyond the initial boundaries.

On ICG angiography, the filling of the neovascular net occurs early contrasting against the hypofluorescent macular background (Fig. 7.6C). In the late venous phase, usually a rapid wash-out occurs mainly in the center of the lesion; staining or leakage is minimal and limited. ICG- A might demonstrate the extent of the hyperfluorescent area that is due to associated occult CNV emphasing the need for the confrontation of the three imaging modalities.

On OCT, active classic CNV will be disclose direct and indirect exudative symptoms :

The *direct signs* are not always clearly defined corresponding to the dimension, location, shape and the stage of progression of CNV (associated occult CNV, fibrosis, hemorrhage...).

Typically, classic CNV disclose as a hyper-reflective, fusiform area of thickening, above and adjacent to the retinal pigment epithelium usually separated by a thin less reflective band (Fig. 7.9). The shadowing underneath the retinal pigment epithelium towards the choroid is usually marked (Fig. 7.6).

The indirect exudative signs associate increase of thickness of the sensory retina due to intra-retina fluid accumulation (Fig. 7.8A), flattening of the foveal depression (Fig. 7.8B). Conversely, the eventual persistence of the foveal depression provides additive landmarks for the exact location and extension of the CNV Detachment and elevation of the neuro-sensory retina may be associated without or with cystic spaces (Fig. 7.8C). Retinal pigment epithelium detachment (serous or hemorrhagic) may be present if classic CNV are associated with occult CNV.

- The exudative reaction may be accentuated and elevated in active classic CNV (Fig. 7.7) or usually more limited as spontaneous fibrosis progressively develops (Fig. 7.10).

Post-treatment outcome may demonstrate either obliteration (Fig. 7.9) or persistence of CNV and/or exudation without or with extension or recurrence.

The correlation between the presence or absence of *leakage* in FA, degree of *perfusion* in ICG and amount of intra- or sub-retinal *fluid* in OCT give very useful informations for the best management during follow up.

The OCT features are complementary to those of FA and ICG for selection of treatment options and their evaluation. The location of classic CNV in relation to the center of the fovea is an essential factor for treatment indication. Immediately after laser photocoagulation, after PDT with verteporfin or after transpupillary thermotherapy, OCT discloses a moderate to major intraretinal accumulation of fluid. This rapid response is due to either the breakdown of the external retinal barrier, or to retinal necrosis, or to inflammatory reaction, or to all of these mechanisms. Progressively the acute response will resolve. Four weeks after PDT meticulous analysis of the presence (or disappearance) of sub-retinal and intra-retinal fluid might be of clinical relevance for indication of retreatment.

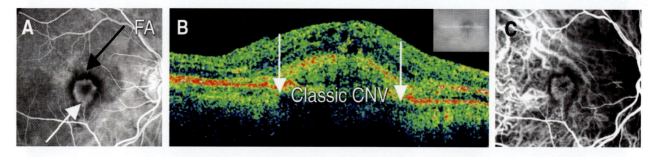

Fig. 7.6: Recent-onset typical classic CNV. (A) FA : Small (one disc diameter) "cartwhell"-shaped hyperfluorescence (white arrow) surrounded by hyper-pigmented ring (black arrow),that will be masqued by late leakage. (B) OCT: Intra-retinal fluid accumulates and forms cystic spaces in the sensory retina. Classic CNV presents as a hyper-reflective band anterior to the RPE, separated by a less reflective area and inducing posterior shadowing in the area between the arrows. (C) ICG-A : Rapid filling of the CNV with late staining (hyperfluorescence). The aspect is similar to that of the image seen on FA but on late-phase ICG, there is minimal leakage.

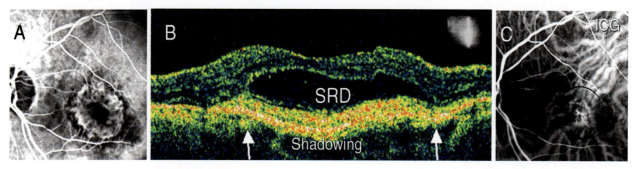

Fig. 7.7: Very active classic CNV. (A) FA : Lacy pattern or "cartwheel" shaped early hyperfluorescence. (B) OCT: Fluid accumulation in the sensory retina results in increased thickness. There is a large subfoveal retinal detachment (SRD) due to fluid accumulation. The hyper-reflective fusiform band of classic CNV is separated by a less reflective band from the posterior retinal pigment epithelium. This type of CNV induces moderate posterior shadowing (arrows). (C) ICG-A: Very rapid filling of the CNV and its afferent and efferent vessels, crossing over choroidal veins allows precise assessment of its extent and is followes by a rapid "wash-out".

Occult Choroidal Neovascularisation

Occult CNV is the most frequent type of CNV in AMD (60 to 85%). The term "occult" emphasizes that this type of CNV is difficult to visualize, analyze, and localize on fluorescein angiography. The essential advantage of ICG angiography is that it allows detection and localization of the occult CNV nearly always, analysis of the filling and staining pattern of the neovascular network and degree of activity of CNV.

Occult CNV has a variable natural history.with different presentation and progression :

- The initial stage might be *almost asymptomatic* for many months or years (which explains why it was initially called "dormant" CNV). It is evidenced during follow-up mostly in second eyes as a late staining plaque on ICG (Fig. 7.11).
- The *symptomatic phase* will result either from slow progression with deterioration of visual acuity, metamorphopsia, accumulation of lipids and enlargement of the lesion (Fig. 7.12 and 7.13) or from sudden acute episodes of exacerbation (sometimes as subretinal hematoma) (Fig. 7.14). The development of a serous PED is an alternative way of progression to a fibrovascular PED and a large disciform scar.

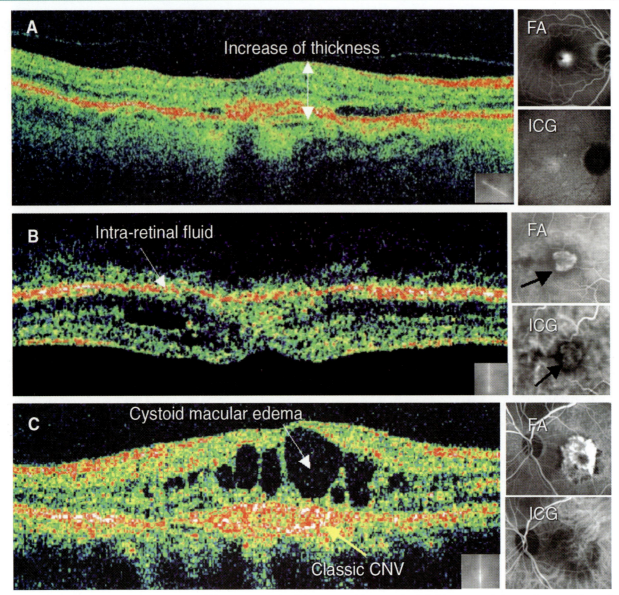

Fig. 7.8: Exudative AMD, indirects signs (A) Increase of thickness and intra-retinal fluid accumulation with small juxta-foveal intra-retinal cyst. (B) Progressive flattening of foveal depression associated with intra-retinal fluid accumulation and increase of thickness of the sensory retina. (C) Accentuated increase of thickness of the sensory retina associated with cystoid macular edema and large foveal cyst.

- In addition, classic CNV proliferate within the occult CNV and may result in various combinations (Fig. 7.15) (*predominantly or minimally occult*).

Early diagnosis is thus essential, as the treatment of advanced occult CNV remains extremely difficult, despite considerable recent progress in this area.

Typical Occult Choroidal Neovascularisation

On FA, the occult CNV have poorly demarcated boundaries in the early and mid phase frames with late leakage from an undetermined source in the *late phase frames* (type II of the MPS classification). When progressing, hemorrhages, lipids and growth of the neovascular lesion will occur.

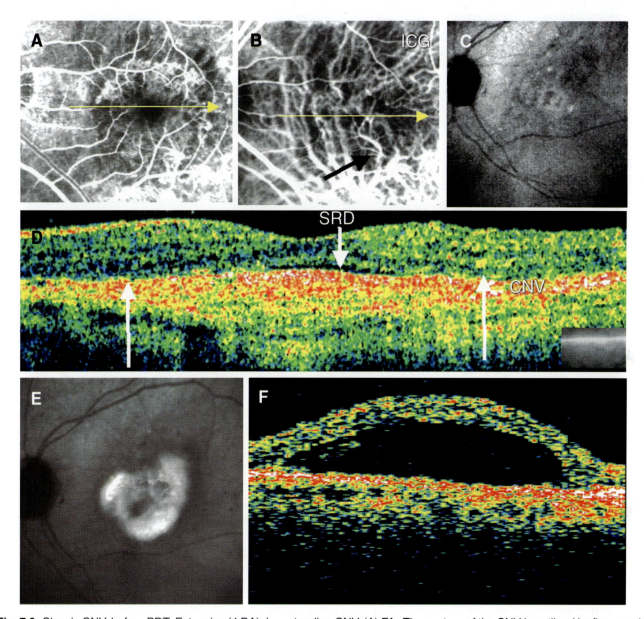

Fig. 7.9: Classic CNV, before PDT: Extensive (4 DA), longstanding CNV. (A) FA : The contour of the CNV is outlined by fluorescein filling. The blocked hypofluorescence of the center is due to xanthophyll pigment. (B, C) ICG-A : Well-delineated CNV, with rapid wash-out and draining vessels at 5 o'clock (black arrow). Late staining. (D) OCT : Hyper-reflective fusiform area (long arrows) anterior to the RPE but separated by a (poorly visible) less reflective area. Note the thin band of overlying serous retinal detachment (small arrow). (E, F) Thirty minutes after PDT, ICG-A and OCT: Massive leakage of ICG at distance.

On SLO ICG, most are converted into a well defined network, filling early and encircled by a hypofluorescent halo. Progressively during the sequence, the fluorescence of the net decreases until the *inversion phase* of ICG where the CNV are barely visible on the background choroidal fluorescence. However, if the amount of fibrosis tissue is more important than the neovascular component, the typical late staining of the plaque will be evident. The association with a RPE elevation (more or less accentuated) is frequent and detectable on SLO ICG-A.

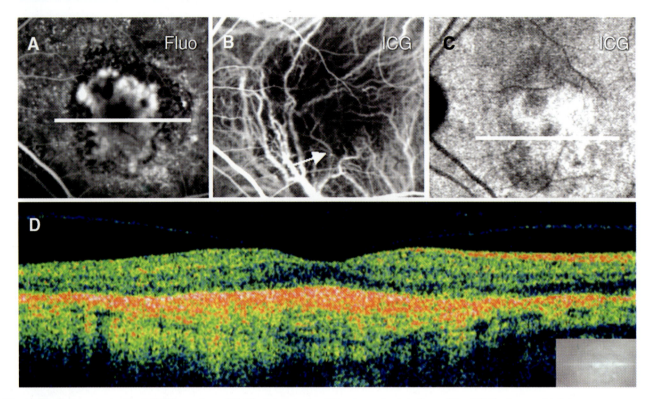

Fig. 7.10: Same case after 3 PDT sessions (A) FA: Progressive fibrosis and retraction of the CNV edges, which become concave at the periphery. Absent or minimal leakage and persistence of the hypofluorescent (hyper-pigmented ?) ring surrounding the CNV edges. (B and C) ICG-A: Practically no filling of the CNV (arrow). Late hyperfluorescent staining of fibrosis. (D) OCT: The fibrosis appears as a fusiform, hyper-reflective area, merged with the retinal pigment epithelium. No sub-retinal fluid accumulation.

On OCT, direct signs of neovascularization are difficult to confirm in this initial stage but can visualize the presence of a hyper-reflective thickened band confounded with the retinal pigment epithelium usually irregular and sometimes fusiform (cigar-like) with shadowing towards the choroid in the corresponding area. In a number of eyes a small and limited elevation of the retinal pigment epithelium might be underlying the hyper-reflectivity of the CNV

The *indirect signs* are less prominent at this early stage. Sub-retinal and/or intra-retinal accumulation of serous fluid with or without intra-retinal cystoid edema confirms the presence of exudation from the CNV. OCT can also demonstrate a limited retinal pigment epithelium detachment, in the vicinity of the hyper-reflective CNV.

During post-treatment follow-up, OCT provides important information about the persistence of active CNV or about the healing processes and eventual development fibrosis. Fibrotic scarring is usually evidenced by the absence of fluid and the presence of a dense, hyper-reflective zone extending posterior towards the choroid often associated to cystic spaces.

Fibrovascular Pigment Epithelial Detachment

The current clinical classification of PED is based on biomicroscopic and stereoscopic analysis as well as on FA, ICG, and OCT. Different types of PED secondary to AMD may be recognized:

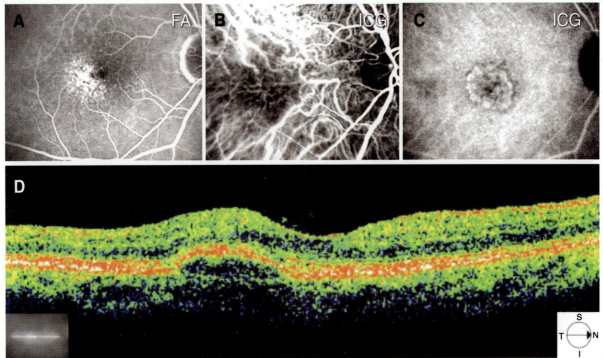

Fig. 7.11: Typical occult CNV. Initial stage. VA: 20/25 (A) FA: Stippled, poorly demarcated hyperfluorescence (arrow) with pinpoints and leakage suggestive of occult CNV. (B and C) SLO ICG-A : A 1.5 DD CNV delineated from the early phase, with late hyperfluorescence and a dark halo. This membrane is centered on the fovea. The occult CNV on FA is "converted" into a well-defined CNV network, entirely localized. (D) OCT : Slight elevation and increase of thickness of the sensory retina and the retinal pigment epithelium with moderate shadowing.

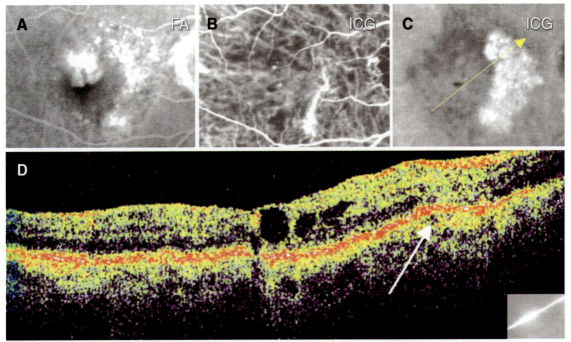

Fig. 7.12: Progression of typical occult CNV. VA : 20/200. (A) FA : Progressive extension of the occult CNV, visible in the nasal area and in the supra-macular area with leakage and cystoid macular edema. (B and C) SLO ICG-A : *In early phase*, neovascular network with central vessel and extensive branches. *In the late phase*, well-demarcated area of hyperfluorescence corresponding to this membrane. (D) OCT : Increased retinal thickness and subfoveal cystic spaces. Note the hyper-reflective area corresponding to the large occult CNV (arrow) in the nasal region.

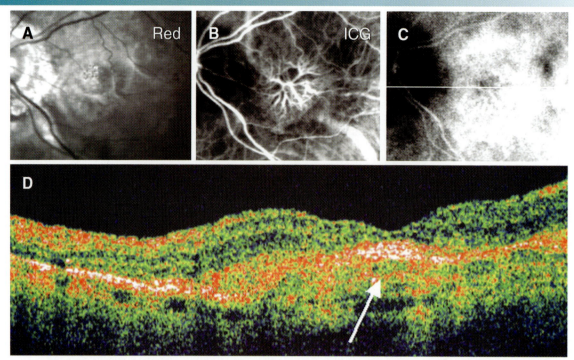

Fig. 7.13: Typical occult CNV. Late stage of the natural course. VA : 20/500 (A) Red-free photograph : Extensive fibrotic lesion with a mature neovascular network. Note the relative atrophy in the central region (B and C) SLO ICG-A : *In the early phase*, rapid filling of the central, large-caliber neovascular network, contrasting with the peripheral vessels of the lesion small and rarefied. *In the late phase*, progressive hyperfluorescent staining of the entire fibrous lesion with minimal late leakage. (D) OCT : Absence of fluid accumulation. A large, hyper-reflective subfoveal zone, corresponding to the fibrous tissue, is obvious in the central zone (arrow). Note the relative thinning of the central sensory retina

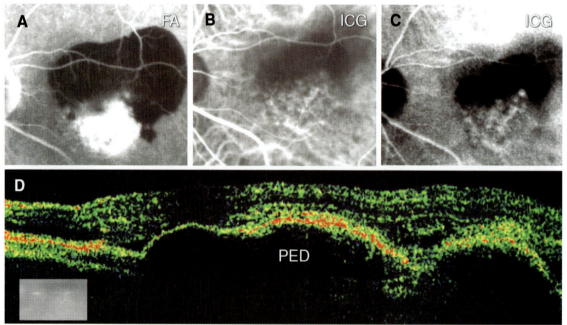

Fig. 7.14: Occult CNV. Occurence of subretinal hematoma. VA: 20/500 (A, B, and C) FA and ICG-A : Sub-retinal hematoma extending in the posterior pole at the superior edge of an irregular hyperfluorescent area suggestive of occult CNV. ICG-A confirms the presence of occult CNV, partialy masked by the thick hematoma. (D) OCT : Hemorrhagic PED with marked shadowing towards the choroid. Note the hyper-reflective central zone corresponding to occult CNV. Alteration and thinning of the retinal pigment epithelium on either side of the central zone.

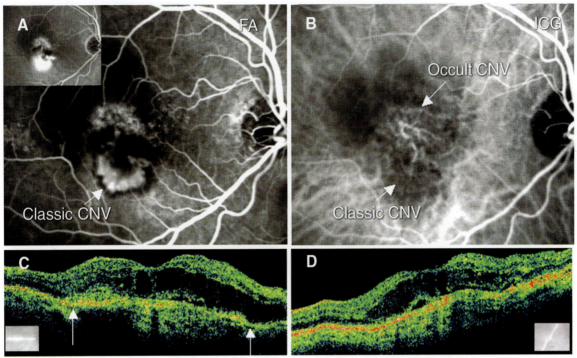

Fig. 7.15: Typical occult CNV: Progression to ingrowth of classic CNV. VA : 20/80 (A) FA : Recent and rapid progression of an active classic CNV (arrow). (B) ICG-A : Well-defined occult CNV network in the upper part of the lesion. Rapid wash-out of the classic component (arrow). (C and D) OCT : Marked exudative reaction with cystoid edema.

- *Avascular serous PED* : extremely rare or transient in AMD (1%) (usually in young adults).
- *Drusenoid PED* : due to progressive confluence of soft drusen. Drusenoid PED usually remains avascular for a long time.
- *Fibro-vascular PED is* a subgroup of occult CNV.
- *Hemorrhagic PED* : complication of typical occult CNV or associated with idiopathic choroidal vasculopathy
- *Serous PED associated with CNV.*

Fibrovacular PED is one of the common forms of exudative AMD, also recognized as type I occult CNV in the Macular Photocoagulation Study classification. It is an advanced form of occult CNV in AMD often associated with typical occult CNV that might preceed its clinical detection. Decrease in vision and guarded prognosis is the main risk of fibrovascular PED.

On fluorescein angiography, an irregular elevation of the retinal pigment epithelium appears as stippled hyperfluorescence, with boundaries that are often poorly demarcated, and fluorescein leakage into the late phase of the angiogram are the characteristic features of fibrovascular PED (Fig. 7.16A).

On ICG, the occult CNV are mostly converted into a lacy network that will progressively invade the entire PED and even extend at distance (Figs 7.16B, C and D).

OCT can distinguish a fibrovascular PED from a serous elevation of the retinal pigment epithelium. The content of the PED is slightly hyper-reflective. The elevated retinal pigment epithelium is highly hyper-reflective possibly due to the different focus plane. A thicker hyper-reflectivity notch appended on the choroidal side of the elevated retinal pigment epithelium might represent CNV (Fig. 7.16E).

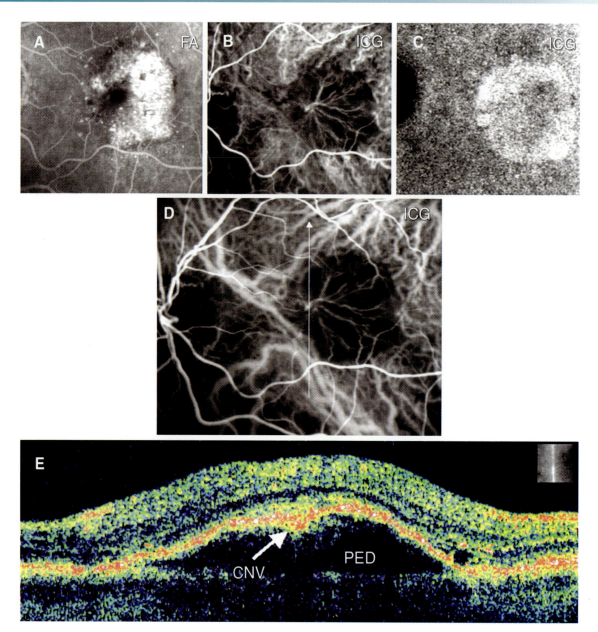

Fig. 7.16: Fibrovascular PED. Medium-sized lesion (2.5 DD). VA: 20/100. (A) FA : Irregular stippled (pinpoints) hyper fluorescence with late leakage predominant in temporal of the macula. (B, C, and D) SLO ICG-A: The CNV is converted into an extensive network with central feeding vessels resolving in multiple branches. This network contrasts against a hypofluorescent round area representing the elevated retinal pigment epithelium. A well-demarcated hyper fluorescent plaque is observed in the very late phase (inversion phase). (E) OCT: The fibro-vascular PED is evidenced on OCT examination, with an associated hyper-reflective zone related to CNV (arrow).

The course of fibrovascular PED is usually one of progressive invasion of the entire PED by the CNV. Overtime the fibrovascular PED may flatten and the associated CNV retract and become fibrotic (Fig. 7.17). Moreover cases appear to be associated with a high risk of retinal pigment epithelium tear. However, these tears are part of the natural history of fibrovascular PED, although they are predictable at least after the first eye involvement.

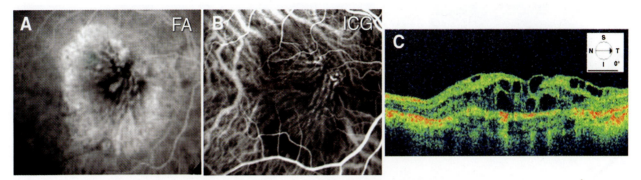

Fig. 7.17: Fibrovascular PED : advanced stage (A) FA : Progressive hyperfluorescence of the PED, predominant at the margins. The PED has an irregular but well-demarcated shape. In the foveal region, a stippled hyperfluorescent area with late leakage is noted (pre-tear stage). (B) SLO ICG-A : The PED is hypofluorescent. In the foveal region, the hyperfluorescence is due to filling of a large network of occult CNV, which is converted by ICG into well-defined CNV that seems to invade the entire PED. (C) OCT : Moderately hyper-reflective and shadow PED. Accentuated increase of thickness of the sensory retina with numerous cystoid spaces

Serous Retinal Pigment Epithelial Detachment and Occult Choroidal Neovascularisation

Occult CNV associated with serous retinal pigment epithelium detachment (frequently termed *"vascularised PED"*) is a severe clinical form of AMD. Exudation originates mainly from CNV (usually occult CNV) and plays a major role in the development of serous PED associated with AMD.

Clinical features reveal elevation of the retinal pigment epithelium that is usually well demarcated and accentuated by a light-reflex. The association with a retinal detachment, more or less accentuated is often detected.

Fluorescein angiography demonstrates the features of PED with early, progressive, uniform, bright hyperfluorescence and late pooling of fluorescein dye into the PED. The CNV may reveal as a more intense hyperfluorescent area. However, CNV may not always be distinguished within the bright hyperfluorescence of PED (Fig. 7.18B). The RPE detachment may be observed with various clinical patterns ; either the CNV is beneath or contiguous or even remote to the retinal pigment epithelium detachment, or the entire PED may be hemorrhagic, masking the CNV (Fig. 7.15). In the later cases, CNV associated with fibrosis can extend into the entire area of the PED with subsequent high risk of eventual retinal pigment epithelium tear.

ICG angiography reveals additional angiographic features of vascularized PED :
- With the traditional fundus camera, the serous component of the PED is seen as a well-demarcated, grayish, isofluorescent area that obscures the underlying choroidal vessels.
- With the SLO, the serous component of the PED remains dark and hypofluorescent throughout the entire angiographic sequence (Figs 7.18C and D). Its shape and contour are well delineated until the very late phase (inversion phase).
- The hyperfluorescence of *chor*oidal neovascularisation is then, seen clearly against the dark background (Fig. 7.18E).

OCT examination provides characteristic imaging of the elevated retinal pigment epithelium in front of an optically empty space without shadowing, regardless of the dimensions and the progressively associated changes during natural history. This technique can distinguish the serous component of the PED from

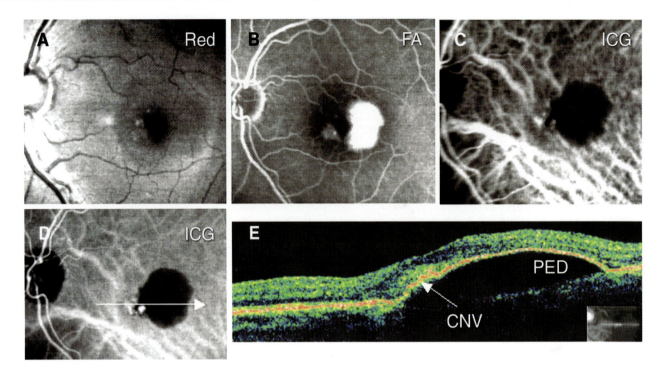

Fig. 7.18: Occult CNV associated with serous PED within a notched area. (A) Red-free photograph: Recent symptomatic, elevated, round, well-defined PED in the macular region. Note the retinal pigment epithelium changes, without hemorrhage, in the nasal juxta-foveal area. (B) FA : Small localized nasal area of hyperfluorescence demonstrating as progressive, uniform pooling of dye. The PED remains well demarcated, with a notch in the nasal region. The vascular network is undetectable (C and D) SLO ICG-A: The serous component of the PED is hypofluorescent and remains very dark in the late phase. The PED has a round, regular shape. In the foveal region, a progressive, hyperfluorescent area is seen in the notch at the PED edge, indicating the presence of (occult) CNV (arrow). (E) OCT: Regular smooth bullous retinal pigment epithelium elevation with an optically empty space posteriorly, without shadowing. Note the hyper-reflective area (arrow) corresponding to the occult CNV

organized fibro-vascular PED. The CNV might be suspected as a hyper-reflective notch attached to the deep face of the elevated retinal pigment epithelium.

The different imaging techniques (FA, SLO ICG-A, and OCT), will distinguish the *various locations* of CNV :

— either *extention* of varying degrees into the PED.

— or secondary to AMD *at the margin* of the PED. The PED has developed adjacent to the CNV (*PED-notch*) (Fig. 7.18)

— or CNV *within the PED*. The so-called "hot spot" is a small and very limited lesion that is usually associated with *chorioretinal anastomosis*. A small juxta-foveal hemorrhage on the border of the FAZ at the end of a retinal vessel may indicate their presence. On FA, its identification is challenging even if not hidden by hemorrhage (Fig. 7.19A and B)

SLO ICG-angiography allows detection of the anastomosis, showing dilated retinal vessels diving deeply towards the choroidal "hot spot" of occult CNV (Fig. 7.19C, D and E). Communication between one or multiple macular retinal vessels (arterial or venous) and the CNV is common and evolving.

On OCT, the elevation of the PED is associated with indirect exudative signs (Fig. 7.19F). The occult CNV can be suspected at the site of thickened retinal pigment epithelium.

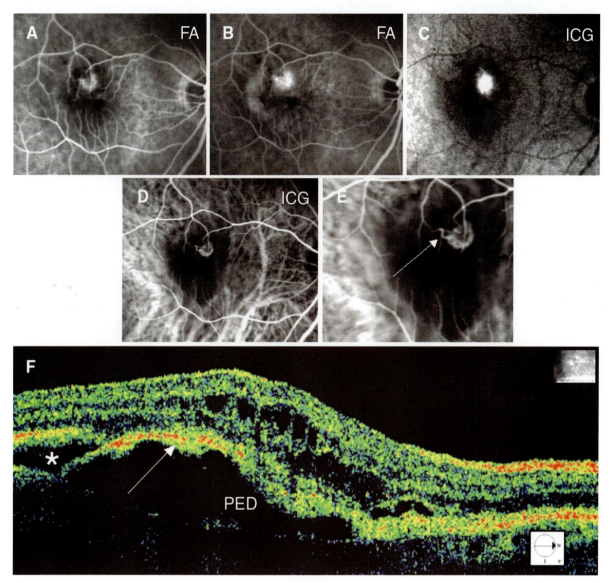

Fig. 7.19: Vascularised PED with chorioretinal anastomosis. VA : 20/50 (A and B) FA: Three-month history of symptoms. Juxtafoveal "hot spot" with lacy pattern of classic CNV and leakage "in contact" with the retinal vessels. (C, D and E) SLO ICG-A : Dilated macular retinal artery and veinules are "diving" into the deep, lacy clearly demonstrated on the enlarged view (E) (arrow); late leakage is seen. (F) OCT: Extensive PED associated with a limited serous retinal detachment (asterix) and intra-retinal fluid accumulation with cystic spaces. Note the irregular, thinned RPE except in the hyper-reflective zone associated with the CNV (arrow)

Natural History

The serous component of vascularized PED can remain relatively stable for a long period; or progressively, the PED may increase in size over time. The presence and rapid accentuation of the irregular shape and aspect constitute the pre-tear stage of PED. Vascularized PED may often present as bilateral, symmetrical lesions appearing at different times. The bilateral nature of the lesions is particularly striking in PED with chorioretinal anastomosis.

Spontaneous retinal pigment epithelial tears may occur. These can be limited or extensive and may be accompanied or preceded by arcuate hemorrhages or sometimes a large or even extensive hematoma (Fig. 7.20).

From the initial stage of typical occult CNV, an associated PED may be detected with SLO ICG and especially with OCT. After a period of apparent stabilization, the lesions extend and deteriorate. and the outcome is usually poor.

The final outcome, whatever the presentation of vascularised PED was, is poor; a *disciform fibro-vascular lesion* or, more rarely, an *atrophic scar* develops, resulting in a large central scotoma.

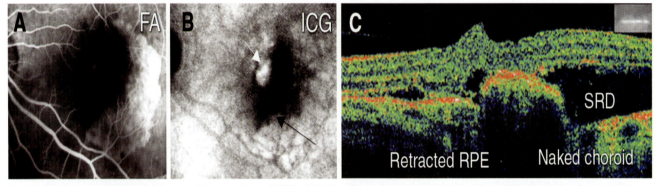

Fig. 7.20: Recent retinal pigment epithelium tear of PED. (A) FA : Early, rapid, and intense hyperfluorescence (transmission or window defect) in the temporal half of the PED, where the retracted and folded retinal pigment epithelium has denuded the underlying choroid. There is no leakage. (B) ICG-A: Abnormal visibility of the large choroidal vessels in the area of the retinal pigment epithelium tear (black arrow). The retracted and folded retinal pigment epithelium is very dark and blocks the underlying fluorescence. The hyperfluorescence in the supero-nasal area (small white arrow) corresponds to the area of CNV in the remaining PED. (C) OCT : Marked hyper-reflectivity of the retracted and folded retinal pigment epithelium in the nasal half. A large, serous retinal detachment is present in the temporal half. The naked choroid induces posterior hyper-reflectivit

CONCLUSION

Classic choroidal neovascularisation, vedette form of exudative age-related macular degeneration has a rapid course to a visual acuity decline. Although well defined on fluorescein angiography classic CNV may be associated with CNV so called occult on fluorescein angiography, either immediately or subsequently. One of the major roles and advantages of ICG angiography is to identify, outline and localize occult CNV.

This imaging system has reclassified the entire group of occult CNV. In addition to the typical occult CNV, the fibrovascular PED, the serous PED, the early occurrence of chorioretinal anastomosis has been recognize and proven. The origin of polypoidal choroidal vasculopathy (PCV) although neovascular is still in debate as retinal or choroidal; similarly the PCV first described as idiopathic can occur secondarily in AMD (Fig. 7.21).

Optical coherance tomography provides a qualitative and quantitative assessment of the various AMD phenotypes. It improves the clinician knowledge in imaging often in typical occult CNV subclinical associated elevation of the retinal pigment epithelium, supporting the natural progression from typical occult CNV to vascularized PED. On the other hand, the evaluation of intra or subretinal fluid, the intraretinal cystoid spaces and the retinal pigment epithelium detachment might identify different AMD subgroups and precisely evaluate the CNV activity.

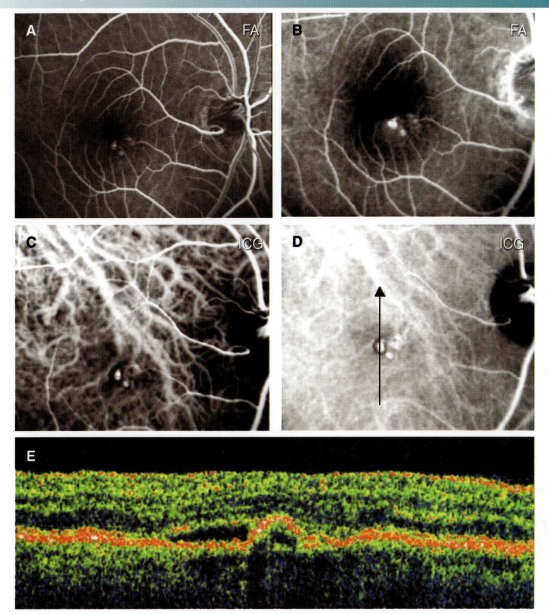

Fig. 7.21: Idiopathic polypoidal choroidal vasculopathy. (A and B) FA: Progressive appearance of a cluster of small, deep ectasiae in the inferior juxtafoveal region with discrete staining of a small, adjacent serous retinal detachment, against which the ectasiae are markedly hyperfluorescent. (C and D) SLO ICG-A: Ectasiae are initially hypofluorescent on ICG, then slowly fill, inducing increased persistent and localized hyperfluorescence. These multiple lesions are relatively clustered, and one of them is surrounded by pigment. (E) OCT : Cross-section through a polypoidal ectasia: a characteristic polypoidal choroidal vasculopathy appearance, with a sharp-edged, dome-liked RPE-Bruch's membrane band elevation, optically empty, with some posterior shadowing. An adjacent serous retinal detachment is observed.

These exudative signs will help to monitor and control all treatment effects. Only precise analysis of the signs and very carefull follow-up with modern imaging can advance our knowledge of this disease and offer the possibility of more effective treatment, as illustrated by the ongoing research.

The results of the various treatment modalities should be improved by judicious use and confrontation of the various modalities. With the advent of ultra high-resolution tomograms with a resolution of axial images of approximately 3 microns and the possibility of 3D reconstruction the classification of AMD will be even more refined.

REFERENCES

1. Coscas G, Coscas F, Zourdani A, Soubrane G. Optical coherence tomography and ARMD. J Fr Ophthalmol 2004;27:7-30.
2. Costa RA, Calucci D, Paccola L, et al. Occult chorioretinal anastomosis in age-related macular degeneration: a prospective study by Optical coherence tomography. Am J Ophthalmol. 2005;140:107-116.
3. Drexler W, Sattmann H, Hermann B, et al. Enhanced visualization of macular pathology with the use of ultrahigh-resolution optical coherence tomography. Arch Ophthalmol. 2003;121:695-706.
4. Hassenstein A, Ruhl R, Richard G. Optical coherence tomography in geographic atrophy—a clinicopathologic correlation. Klin Monatsbl Agenheilkd. 2001;218:503-509.
5. Hee MR, Baumal CR, Puliafito CA, et al. Optical coherence tomography of age-related macular degeneration and choroidal neovascularization. Ophthalmology. 1996;103:1260-1270.
6. Hee MR, Izatt JA, Swanson EA, et al. Optical coherence tomography of the human retina. Arch Ophtalmol 1995;113:325-332.
7. Macular Photocoagulation Study Group. Subfoveal neovascular lesions in age-related macular degeneration. Arch Ophthalmol. 1991;109:1242-1257.
8. McClearly CD, Guier CP, Dunbar MT. Polypoidal choroidal vasculopathy. Optometry. 2004;75:756-770.
9. Puliafito CA, Hee MR, Lin CP et al. Imaging of macular diseases with optical coherence tomography. Ophthalmology .1995;102:217-229.
10. Salinas-Alaman A, Garcia-Layana A, Maldonado MJ, et al. Using optical coherence tomography to monitor photodynamic therapy in age-related macular degeneration. Am J Ophthalmol. 2005;140:23-28.
11. Sato T, Iida T, Hagimura N, Kishi S. Correlation of optical coherence tomography with angiography in retinal pigment epithelial detachment associated with age-related macular degeneration. Retina. 2004;24:910-914.
12. Schuman JS, Puliafito CA, Fujimoto JG. Age-related macular degeneration in optical coherence tomography of ocular diseases, 2nd ed. New York: Slack Incorporated, 2004:243-344.
13. Spraul CW, Lang GE, Lang GK. Value of optical coherence tomography in diagnosis of age-related macular degeneration. Correlation of fluorescein angiography and OCT findings. Klin Monatsbl Augenheilkd. 1998;212:141-148.
14. Treatment of Age-related Macular Degeneration with Photodynamic Therapy (TAP) Study Group. Photodynamic therapy of subfoveal choroidal neovascularization in age-related macular degeneration with verteporfin. One year results of 2 randomised clinical trials – TAP Report 1. Arch Ophthalmol. 1999;117:1329-1345.
15. Treatment of Age-related Macular Degeneration with Photodynamic Therapy (TAP) Study Group. Photodynamic therapy of subfoveal choroidal neovascularization in age-related macular degeneration with verteporfin. Two year results of 2 randomised clinical trials – TAP Report 2. Arch Ophthalmol. 2001;119:198-207.
16. Verteporfin in Photodynamic therapy (VIP) Study Group. Photodynamic therapy of subfoveal choroidal neovascularization in pathological myopia with verteporfin. One year results of a randomised clinical trial – VIP Report Number 1. Ophthalmology. 2001;108:841-852.
17. Verteporfin in Photodynamic therapy (VIP) Study Group. Verteporfin therapy of subfoveal choroidal neovascularization in age-related macular degeneration: two year results of a randomised clinical trial including lesions with occult with no classic choroidal neovascularization – VIP Report Number 2. Am J Ophthalmol. 2001;131:541-560.

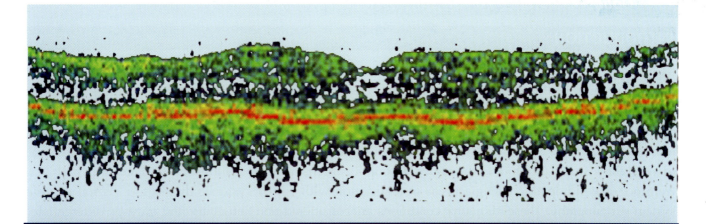

CHAPTER

8

Juxtafoveal Telangiectasis

**Richard Hamilton, Judy E Kim,
Richard F Spaide**

INTRODUCTION

Retinal vascular telangiectasis can occur in the peripheral retina and in the macula. Those entities which occur near the fovea have been designated parafoveal or juxtafoveal telangiectasis, and those which are believed idiopathic have been divided into three groups. Group 1 telangiectasias occur unilaterally in middle aged patients and generally cause minimal decrease in vision and are readily identifiable on clinical examination. Group 2 patients have symmetric bilateral involvement by occult telangiectasias that progress to affect the visual acuity more profoundly. Group 3 patients have central loss of visual acuity in both eyes from occlusive idiopathic telangiectasias in association with varied systemic diseases or central nervous system vasculopathy. These idiopathic conditions are considered non-hereditary and must be differentiated from other secondary causes of telangiectasias including diabetic retinopathy, carotid occlusive disease, branch retinal vein occlusion, radiation retinopathy, Eales disease and sickle cell maculopathy.[1]

Gass and Blodi modified the categorization into three groups with two subgroups each.[2] In group 1A, patients develop mild decrease in visual acuity from 20/25 to 20/40 in one eye secondary to a one to one and a half disc areas of retinal telangiectasias in the temporal half of the macula. These telangiectasias will hyperfluoresce early and leak later. A circinate pattern of hard exudates is generally present and cystoid macular edema may develop. Patients in group 1B complain of metamorphopsia and mild blurring of vision secondary to a small area of capillary telangiectasias encompassing approximately 2 clock hours of the foveolar avascular zone. These telangiectasias will also hyperfluoresce but exhibit minimal leakage.

The most common form of idiopathic juxtafoveal telangiectasis is the group 2A. This form generally progresses to one of five well-described stages. Patients are typically in their fifties or sixties. In the first stage, the patient is asymptomatic and reveals no remarkable findings on biomicroscopy. Angiography reveals hyperfluorescence consistent with minimal capillary dilation and late staining of the temporal fovea (Figs 8.1 and 8.2). In the second stage, the temporal aspect of the macula takes on a grayish discoloration. Development of right angle venules into outer layers of the retina is the hallmark of stage 3 (Fig. 8.3). Stage 4 is characterized by retinal pigment epithelium hyperplasia and migration anteriorly along the right angle venules. Finally, in stage 5, a subretinal choroidal neovascular membrane develops in the areas of retinal pigment epithelium hyperplasia. Half of all group 2A patients will have yellow refractile deposits on the inner surface of the retina and 5% will have a "yellow spot" over the fovea.

Two siblings comprise group 2B. They developed subretinal choroidal neovascular membranes with angiographically demonstrated telangiectasias and graying of the temporal macula but no right angle venules or retinal pigment epithelium hyperplasia.

Patients in groups 3A and 3B develop occlusive juxtafoveal telangiectasias in association with systemic disease and neurological vasculopathy, respectively. In group 3A, the loss of vision is fairly sudden and clinical findings include occlusion of the perifoveal capillaries and central whitening of the macula. Telangiectasias develop as sequelae to the occlusive event and must be differentiated from radiation retinopathy, diabetic retinopathy and sickle cell retinopathy. Patients in this subgroup have varied associated systemic conditions including myeloproliferative disorders, polycythemia and ulcerative colitis. Group 3B patients also suffer from an obliteration of the perifoveal capillaries leading to central visual loss. In these patients, there are often neurological findings including diminished deep tendon reflexes and optic atrophy.

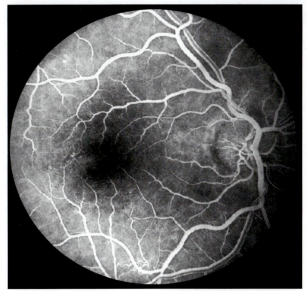

Fig. 8.1: Laminar venous phase revealing multiple small telangiectatic structures in Group 2A patient.

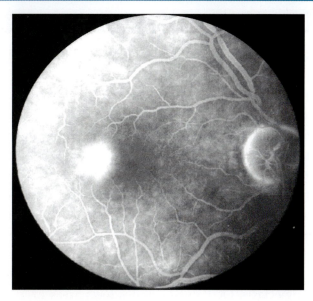

Fig. 8.2: Late leakage at the temporal aspect of the fovea in Group 2A patient.

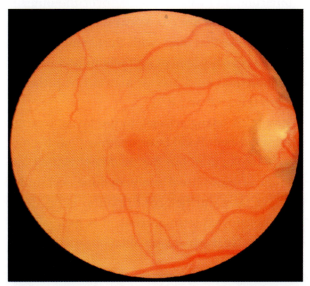

Fig. 8.3: The right eye of a Group 2A patient. Note the right angled venule temporal to the fovea.

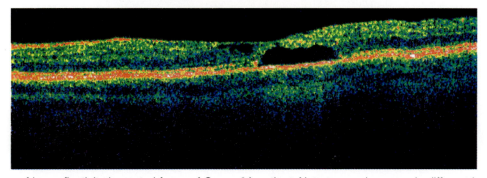

Fig. 8.4: Spaces of low reflectivity in central fovea of Group 2A patient. Note two such spaces in different layers of the retina

OPTICAL COHERENCE TOMOGRAPHY

Optical coherence tomography (OCT) imaging of the central macula has recently been applied to patients with juxtafoveal telangiectasis group 2A.[3] These typically show well demarcated areas of nonreflective clear spaces within the retina at or near the fovea. These spaces can occur at different levels of the retina and are usually elongated (Figs 8.4 and 8.5). They most likely represent the lumens of telangiectactic vessels, being imaged at different "cuts" depending on the OCT scan line orientation. In a sense, what we are imaging is similar to that already described in a diagram form by Gass in his atlas, where he described presumed anatomic changes in the development of acquired juxtafoveal telagiectasis involving the deep retinal plexus.[1] These cavities may represent areas of fluid accumulation.[3] Interestingly, despite significant late leakage noted on fluorescein angiogram, the macula is thickened only minimal to moderate degree (Fig. 8.6). In some cases, there is thinning of the central retina recorded on OCT. Furthermore, there is lack of large cystoid changes seen on OCT images, unlike that of macular edema due to other retinal conditions, such as diabetic retinopathy or vein occlusions. In the eyes with lipid exudates associated with juxtafoveal telangiectasis, OCT demonstrates focal areas of intraretinal high reflectivity.

In stage 4 eyes, there are areas of high reflectivity that correspond to retinal pigment epithelium migration (Fig. 8.7). They block the light reflection and cast a shadow over the outer retinal layers and choroid. In stage 5 eyes, OCT images reveal changes that are consistent with presence of choroidal neovascularisation (CNV). The CNV appears as a highly reflective mass with thickening along the retinal pigment epithelium signal. They are commonly above the retinal pigment epithelium and under the retina, consistent with the type 2 CNVM described by Gass. Subretinal fluid may or may not be present on OCT, despite leakage from CNV seen on fluorescein angiogram (Figs 8.8 and 8.9).

Due to the proximity of the group 2A telangiectasias to the fovea, treatment options have been limited and no firm guidelines have been established. Focal laser treatment has been performed in some cases to the areas of leakage seen on fluorescein angiogram, but the treatment benefit appears to be limited. Although there is a case report on the benefit of intravitreal triamcinolone acetonide injection for macular edema associated with juxtafoveal telangiectasis, further confirmation is needed in the future.[4] For choroidal neovascularisation associated with juxtafoveal telangiectasis, it is generally felt that those lesions closest to the foveal avascular zone should not receive thermal laser ablation so as to avoid a foveal burn and subsequent

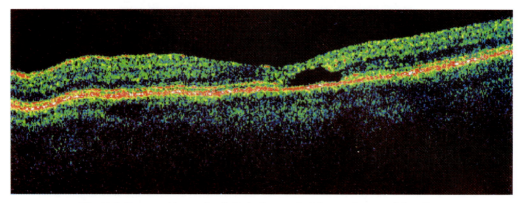

Fig. 8.5: Space of low reflectivity in the central fovea of group 2A patient.

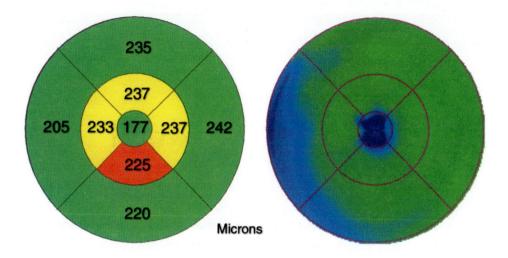

Fig. 8.6: There is a mild increase in thickness of the central 3 mm of the macula, but the central fovea is not thickened.

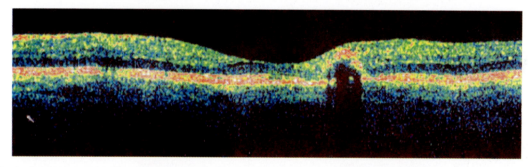

Fig. 8.7: Retinal pigment epithelium migration into the retina is seen as a highly reflective area adjacent to fovea. It blocks the reflections of the tissues below and exhibits shadowing into the choroid. Small slit-like nonreflective cavity is seen at the fovea.

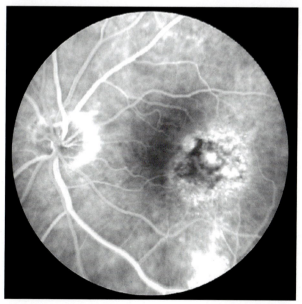

Fig. 8.8: Fluorescein angiogram depicting hyperfluorescence from a choroidal neovascular membrane associated with juxtafoveal telangiectasis.

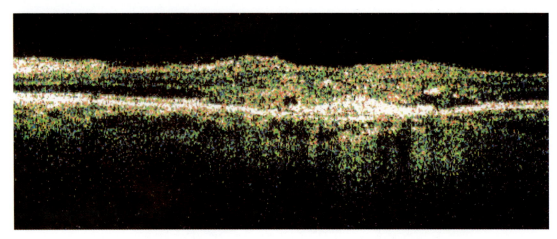

Fig. 8.9: Optical coherence tomography image of the same patient in Figure 8.8 demonstrating the subretinal choroidal neovascular membrane, seen as hyperreflective region between the retina and retinal pigment epithelium.

central scotoma. Recent reports have shown that photodynamic therapy alone or photodynamic therapy combined with intravitreal triamcinolone may be beneficial for treatment of choroidal neovascular membranes secondary to juxtafoveal telangiectasis.[5,6]

In summary, OCT can be a valuable tool in the evaluation and management of patients with juxtafoveal telangiectasis. In these patients, OCT shows intraretinal nonreflective clear cavities which may be present at different layers of the retina. The retina is usually not significantly thickened, although foveal depression may be lacking. Depending on the stage of the disease, various other associated findings may be present.

REFERENCES

1. Gass JDM. Stereoscopic Atlas of Macular Diseases: Diagnosis and Treatment, 4th ed. St Louis. Mosby-Year Book, Inc. 1997:504-513.
2. Gass JDM, Blodi B. Idiopathic juxtafoveal retinal telangiectasis: update of classification and follow-up study. Ophthalmology. 1993;100:1536-1546.
3. Cruz-Villegas V, Puliafito C, Fujimoto J. "Retinal Vascular Diseases". Optical Coherence Tomography of Ocular Diseases, 2nd ed. Thorofare, NJ. SLACK Incorporated, 2004:103-156.
4. Martinez JA. Intravitreal triamcinolone acetonide for bilateral acquired parafoveal telangiectasis. Arch Ophthalmol. 2003;121:1658-1659.
5. Potter MJ, Szabo SM, Chan EY, Morris AH. Photodynamic therapy of subretinal neovascular membrane in type 2A idiopathic juxtafoveal retinal telangiectasis. Am J Ophthalmol. 2002;133:149-151.
6. Smithen LM, Spaide RF. Photodynamic therapy and intravitreal triamcinolone for subretinal neovascularization in bilateral idiopathic juxtafoveal telangiectasias. Am J Ophthalmol. 2004;138: 884-885.

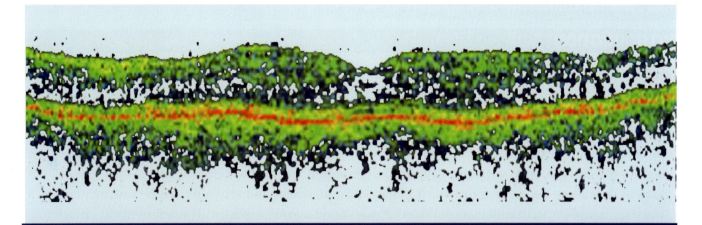

CHAPTER
9

Central Serous Chorioretinopathy

Muna Bhende, Bijoy K Nair

INTRODUCTION

Central serous chorioretinopathy (CSR) [1, 2] is a condition that typically occurs in males around the age of 40 years, and is characterized by neurosensory detachment of the macula.

Presenting symptoms include central visual loss, a sudden decrease in vision which can be corrected with an increased hyperopic correction, metamorphopsia, central scotoma and decreased color saturation. The symptoms are usually self limiting, but can recur in the same or opposite eye in 40-50% of cases. The association with type 'A' personality, systemic hypertension and corticosteroid intake is well known.

It can present as the acute form which is classically unilateral and characterized by one or more focal leaks at the retinal pigment epithelium level on fundus fluorescein angiography. The neurosensory detachment contains clear subretinal fluid, but may be cloudy or have subretinal fibrin in some cases. It is typically self limiting and may not lead to a gross visual deficit after resolution. The chronic form, believed to be due to diffuse retinal pigment epithelium disease occurs in the older age group and is usually bilateral. It presents with diffuse retinal pigment epithelium atrophic changes, varying degrees of subretinal fluid, pigmentary alterations and flask shaped retinal pigment epithelium tracks. It is characterized by diffuse areas of retinal pigment epithelium leakage on fluorescein angiography and areas of focal choroidal hyperpermeability on indocyanine green angiography. This has a relatively poorer visual prognosis due to associated retinal pigment epithelium atrophy and cystoid changes at the fovea.

Theories regarding the pathogenesis of the disease include abnormal ion transport across the retinal pigment epithelium and focal choroidal vascular compromise which results in retinal pigment epithelium dysfunction.

Diagnosis of the disease can be made on slit lamp biomicroscopy, and can be confirmed with fluorescein angiography. Indocyanine green angiography is used in cases of chronic CSR especially as a guide to treatment. Optical coherence tomography (OCT) is used to diagnose, prognosticate and follow the course of the disease and its response to therapy. Multifocal electroretinogram has also been used to demonstrate the diffuse retinal dysfunction, sometimes bilateral, that has been seen to be associated with the disease. Recently, demonstration of fundus autofluorescence[10] has also been used as a tool in diagnosis and prognosis of CSR.

Management options include observation in most cases of typical CSR and focal laser for non resolving cases. Photodynamic therapy[11, 12] and indocyanine green mediated photothrombosis[13] have emerged as recent techniques in the management of chronic CSR.

OPTICAL COHERENCE TOMOGRAPHY

Optical coherance tomography features of central serous chorioretinopathy are as follows:

Acute Central Serous Chorioretinopathy (Figs 9.1 to 9.4)

1. Thickening of the neurosensory layer at the macula with detachment.
2. Presence of retinal pigment epithelial detachment. Isolated small pigment epithelial detachment may be seen in the fellow eyes of patients with CSR.
3. Combination of both. This is seen in active CSR. The pigment epithelial detachment may be small or large and corresponds to the site of leakage on fundus fluorescein angiography.

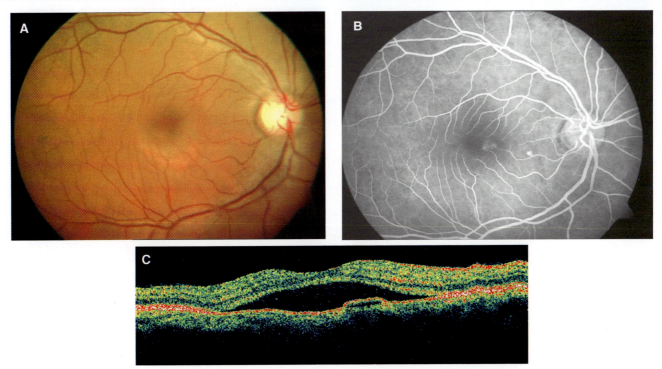

Figs 9.1A to C: Acute CSR. Clinical photograph, fundus fluorescein angiogram and OCT images of the right eye of a young lady with acute CSR. Note the neurosensory detachment at the macula with a small point leak nasal to the fovea. The OCT image – line scan in the horizontal meridian shows a neurosensory elevation of the macula and a small pigment epithelial detachment just nasal to the fovea. This corresponds to the leak on fluorescein angiography.

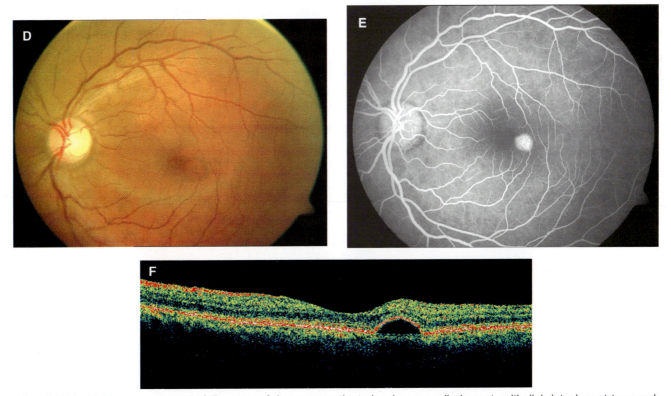

Figs 9.1D to F: The asymptomatic fellow eye of the same patient showing a small pigment epithelial detachment temporal to the fovea. Note the absence of a neurosensory elevation on the OCT.

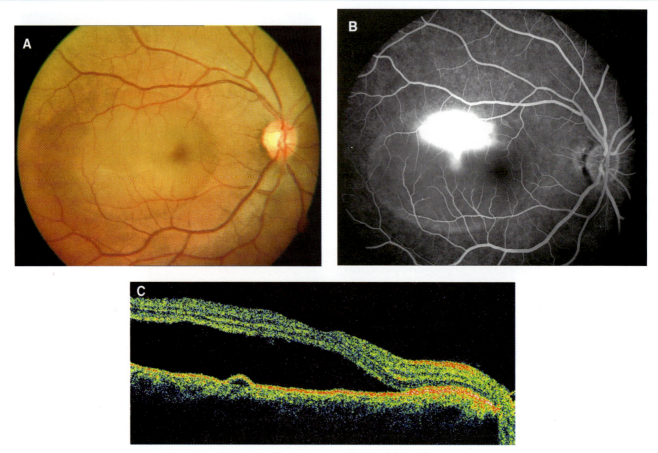

Figs 9.2A to C: Acute CSR .The right eye of a young male with drop in vision of three months duration. The color photograph shows a serous detachment of the macula. Fluorescein angiography shows a classical smoke stack leak of CSR. The OCT image taken in the horizontal meridian through the area of leak on fluorescein angiography shows a large neurosensory elevation with a small elevation of the retinal pigment epithelium corresponding to the site if leak.

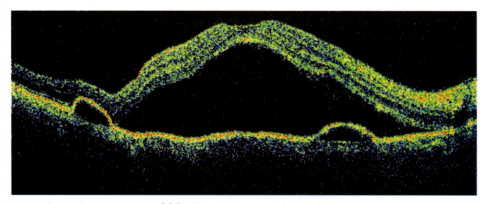

Fig. 9.3: OCT image of a patient with acute CSR showing a highly elevated neurosensory retina at the macula and two small pigment epithelial detachments.

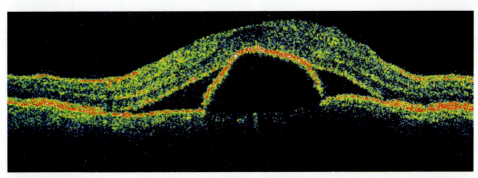

Fig. 9.4: OCT image of a patient with a neurosensory elevation at the macula and a large serous pigment epithelial detachment under the fovea. These large PEDs can sometimes develop into acute tears or rips of the retinal pigment epithelium and cause sudden severe visual loss.

4. Presence of moderately high reflective mass bridging the detached neurosensory retina and retinal pigment epithelium may be seen in eyes with subretinal fibrin.

Chronic Central Serous Chorioretinopathy (Figs 9.5 and 9.6)

1. Presence of foveal atrophy or thinning.
2. Cystoid changes at the fovea.

Associated Findings/Complications

1. Rips of the retinal pigment epithelium.
2. Choroidal neovascularisation.

Role of Optical Coherence Tomography in Central Serous Chorioretinopathy (Figs 9.7 and 9.8)

1. *Diagnosis of the disease*: Optical coherence tomography can aid in the diagnosis of the disease. Detection of neurosensory detachments can be of special use in conditions where fluorescein angiography may be contraindicated but the clinical suspicion is high.
2. *Following the progress of the disease*: The neurosensory thickening as well as elevation is seen to reduce with resolution of the disease either spontaneously, after laser photocoagulation or photodynamic therapy.
3. *Prediction of visual acuity recovery*: Prediction of visual acuity recovery after macular reattachment may be made depending on the optical coherence tomography of the outer plexiform layer.
4. *Explanation of poor visual acuity recovery*: Optical coherence tomography can provide an explanation for poor visual recovery in the presence of apparent resolution — may detect shallow persistent neurosensory detachment at the fovea, foveal atrophy or cystoid changes at the fovea.[3-9]

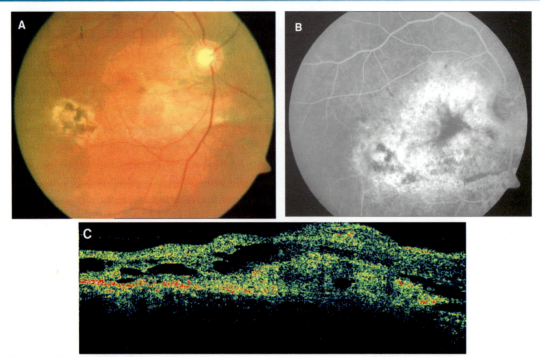

Figs 9.5A to C: Chronic CSR. Color photograph, fluorescein angiography and OCT images of a middle aged male with history of progressive loss of vision over a few years. The color photograph shows a shallow retinal elevation the macula with pigmentary changes and subretinal fibrin. The pigmented lesion temporal to the macula is a photocoagulation scar where laser was done for CSR. Fluorescein angiography shows diffuse mottled hyperfluorescence at the posterior pole along with areas of blocked fluorescence. The OCT image in a horizontal plane shows irregular thickening and elevation of the neurosensory retina with bands and clumps of moderate to high reflectivity in the subretinal space corresponding to the subretinal fibrin.

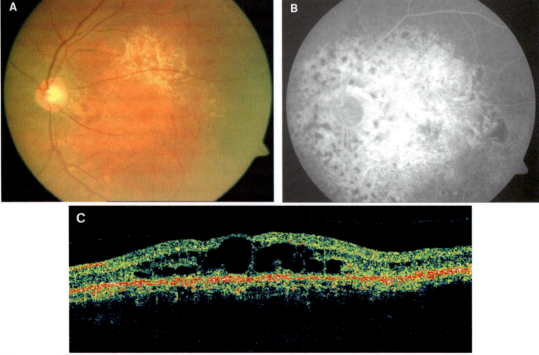

Figs 9.6A to C: Chronic CSR. The left eye of the same patient showing diffuse pigmentary alterations at the macula and corresponding mottled hyperfluorescence on fluorescein angiogram. The OCT image shows large intraretinal cystoid spaces involving the neurosensory retina.

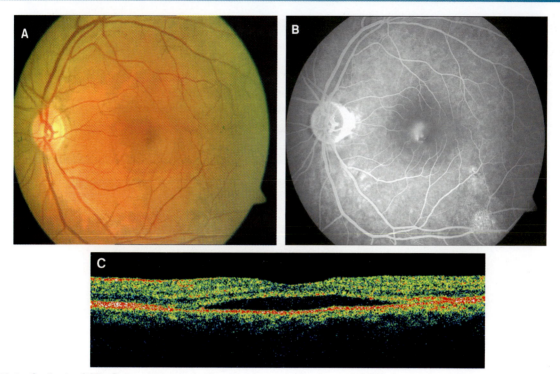

Figs 9.7A to C: Acute CSR. Color photograph, fluorescein angiography and OCT of a young patient with recent loss of vision. Fig. A shows a shallow elevation at the macula. There is a point leak just adjacent to the fovea. The OCT shows a shallow neurosensory elevation involving the fovea.

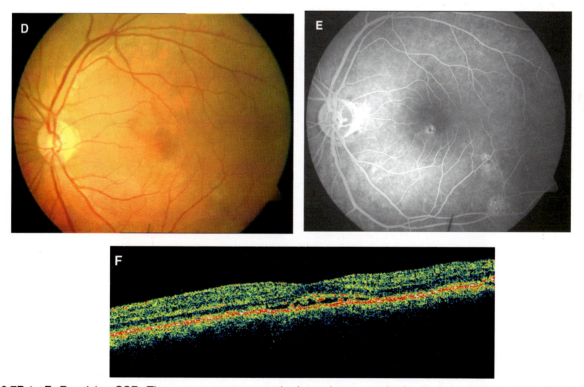

Figs 9.7D to F: Resolving CSR. The same case two months later shows a reduction in the retinal elevation. The fluorescein angiography shows only transmission defects at the macula. The OCT shows a shallow neurosensory elevation with presence of deposits on the outer retinal surface.

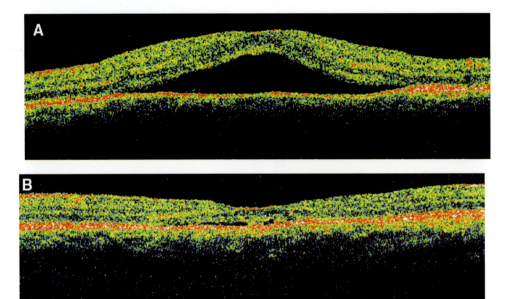

Figs 9.8A and B: OCT images of an eye with acute CSR. Figure A shows a neurosensory elevation of the macula. Figure B shows the same eye 3 months later showing almost total resolution of the detachment with a very small area of neurosensory separation. There are a few deposits on the retinal pigment epithelium layer as well as foveal atrophy.

REFERENCES

1. Gass JDM. Pathogenesis of disciform detachment of the neuroepithelium, II: Idiopathic central serous choroidopathy. Am J Ophthalmol. 1967;63:587-615.
2. Spaide RF, Campeas L, Haas A, et al. Central Serous Chorioretinopathy in younger and older adults. Ophthalmology. 1996;103:2070-2079.
3. Hee MR, Puliafito CA, Wong C, et al. Optical coherence tomography of central serous chorioretinopathy. Am J Ophthalmol. 1995;120:65-74.
4. Wang M, Sander B, Lund-Andersen H, Larsen M. Detection of shallow detachments in central serous chorioretinopathy. Acta Ophthalmol Scand. 1999; 77:402-405.
5. Iida T, Hagimura N, Sato T, Kishi S. Evaluation of central serous chorioretinopathy with optical coherence tomography. Am J Ophthalmol. 2000;129:16-20.
6. Wang MS, Sander B, Larsen M. Retinal atrophy in idiopathic central serous chorioretinopathy. Am J Ophthalmol. 2002; 133:787-793.
7. Iida T, Yannuzzi LA, Spaide RF, et al. Cystoid macular degeneration in chronic central serous chorioretinopathy. Retina. 2003;23:1-7.
8. Montero JA, Ruiz-Moreno JM. Optical coherence tomography characterization of idiopathic central serous chorioretinopathy. Br J Ophthalmol. 2005;89:562-564.
9. Piccolino FC, de la Longrais RR, Ravera G, et al. The foveal photoreceptor layer and visual acuity loss in central serous chorioretinopathy. Am J Ophthalmol. 2005;139:87-99.
10. Spaide RF, Klancnik JM Jr. Fundus auto fluorescence and central serous chorioretinopathy. Ophthalmology. 2005;112:825-833.
11. Taban M, Boyer DS, Thomas EL, Taban M. Chronic central serous chorioretinopathy: photodynamic therapy. Am J Ophthalmol. 2004;137:1073-1080.
12. Cardillo Piccolino F, Eandi CM, Ventre L, et al. Photodynamic therapy for chronic central serous chorioretinopathy. Retina. 2003; 23:752-763.
13. Costa RA, Scapucin L, Moraes NS, et al. Indocyanine green –mediated photothrombosis as a new technique of treatment for persistent central serous chorioretinopathy. Curr Eye Res. 2002; 25:287-297.

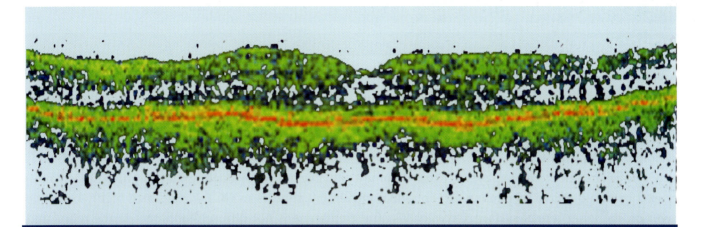

10

Idiopathic
Epiretinal
Membranes

Hiroko Terasaki, Yasuki Ito

INTRODUCTION

An idiopathic epiretinal membrane usually develops after a partial or complete posterior vitreous detachment, and appears as a translucent membrane over the inner retinal surface in the macular area by ophthalmoscopy or biomicroscopy. Contraction of these membranes can result in various retinal pathologies, such as retinal distortion, increased thickness of the macula with or without increased permeability of retinal vessels, and cystoid macular edema.[1]

Optical coherence tomography (OCT) has become a valuable tool for evaluating the morphological changes caused by an epiretinal membrane. An epiretinal membrane appears in OCT images as a highly reflective layer on the inner retinal surface. Occasionally, the membrane is not diffusely adherent to the retina and appears contracted with wrinkling of the retinal surface. More specifically, the morphological changes of the retina detected in the OCT images of eyes with epiretinal membranes are: increased retinal thickness, loss of normal foveal contour, and cystoid macular edema.[2,3] Retinoschisis has not been commonly reported, however, OCT-3 images can capture this condition not only in the inner layer but also in the outer layer of macular retina.

Our studies of correlating focal macular electroretinograms (ERGs) and OCT images in eyes with epiretinal membrane have demonstrated that the mean amplitudes of all components of the focal macular ERGs were significantly smaller than in the normal fellow eyes, with the decrease largest for the oscillatory potentials, followed by the b-waves and then the a-waves.[4] There appears to be a dissociation in the course of reduction of the a- and b-waves.

After removal of the epiretinal membrane by surgery, the mean foveal and parafoveal thicknesses evaluated by OCT are significantly less; however, they are still thicker than the non-affected fellow eyes. With the decrease in macular thickness, the mean amplitudes of the a-waves, b- waves, and the oscillatory potentials become significantly larger; the relative amplitudes (affected eye/fellow eye) was 102% for the a-wave, but still 81% for the b-wave, and 71% for the oscillatory potentials. Only 3 of the 29 eyes studied showed more than a 90% recovery of the amplitudes of all components of the focal macular ERGs. The decrease of the oscillatory potentials after surgery was correlated with increased parafoveal thickness.

INTERESTING CASE EXAMPLES

Case 1

A 62-year-old woman had a 2 months history of metamorphopsia in her left eye. Her best-corrected visual acuity was 20/70 in her left eye. An epiretinal membrane could be seen mainly in the temporal parafoveal area. The foveal retina was slightly pulled toward the temporal epiretinal membrane. The arcade vessels, especially the inferior vessels, are also pulled toward the membrane (Fig. 10.1A). Preoperative OCT image showed macular edema. An epiretinal membrane was observed as a bright yellowish line on the surface of the macular retina. No large cystic space could be seen in the macular edema. The foveal thickness was 532 μm (Fig. 10.1B). Macular thickening was identified at the location corresponding to the epiretinal membrane (Fig. 10.1C). She had a combined surgery of phacoemulsification, intraocular lens implantation, vitrectomy, and epiretinal membrane peeling. Three months after surgery, the epiretinal membrane had been completely removed but slight hemorrhage that occurred during the epiretinal membrane peeling could still be observed. The arcade vessels and fovea were not under tension (Fig. 10.1D). Postoperative OCT showed that epiretinal membrane was not present, however a moderate macular thickening still remained. The foveal thickness was 407μm (Fig. 10.1E). However, macular edema had improved (Fig. 10.1F). Her visual acuity recovered to 20/25 seven months after surgery.

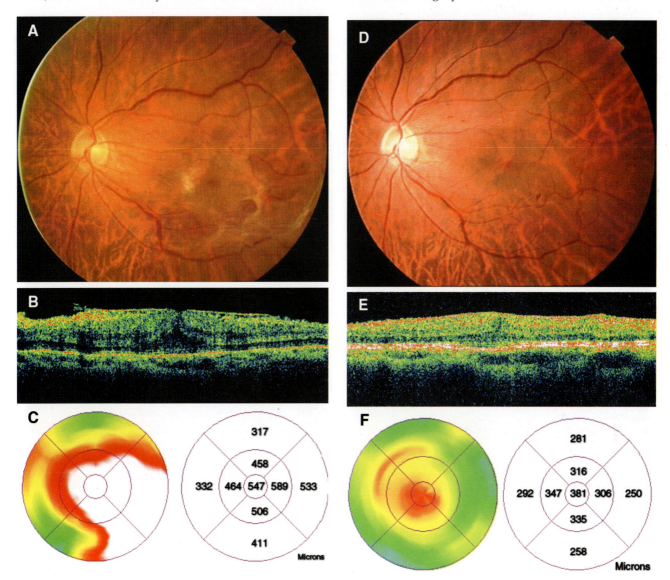

Figs 10.1A to F: (A) Preoperative fundus photograph. An epiretinal membrane can be seen mainly in the temporal parafoveal area. The foveal retina is slightly pulled toward the temporal epiretinal membrane. The arcade vessels, especially the inferior vessels, are also pulled toward the membrane. (B) Preoperative OCT image from a 5 mm vertical scan over the macula. Macular edema can be seen. An epiretinal membrane is observed as a bright yellowish line on the surface of the macular retina. No large cystic space can be seen in the macular edema. The foveal thickness is 532 μm. (C) Preoperative OCT map. Macular thickening is identified at the location corresponding to the epiretinal membrane. The diameters of circles are 1, 3, and 6 mm. (D) Postoperative fundus photograph 3 months after surgery. The epiretinal membrane has been completely removed. Slight hemorrhage that occurred during the epiretinal membrane peeling can still be observed. The arcade vessels and fovea are not under tension. (E) Postoperative OCT map 3 months after surgery. An epiretinal membrane is not present, however a moderate macular thickening still remains. The foveal thickness is 407 μm. (F) Postoperative OCT map 3 months after surgery. Macular edema has improved.

Case 2

An epiretinal membrane was found in the left eye of a 64-year-old woman during a comprehensive medical examination. Her corrected visual acuity was 20/25 in the left eye without metamorphopsia. A cellophane maculopathy could be seen (Fig. 10.2A). Preoperative OCT image showed a small epiretinal membrane. The foveal thickness was 331 µm (Fig. 10.2B). Preoperative OCT map showed macular thickening (Fig. 10.2C). Vitrectomy with epiretinal membrane peeling was performed. Six months after surgery, the epiretinal membrane had been completely removed (Fig. 10.2D). Foveal depression had recovered (Fig. 10.2E). However, mild macular thickening remained (Fig. 10.2F). Her visual acuity recovered to 20/20, six months after surgery.

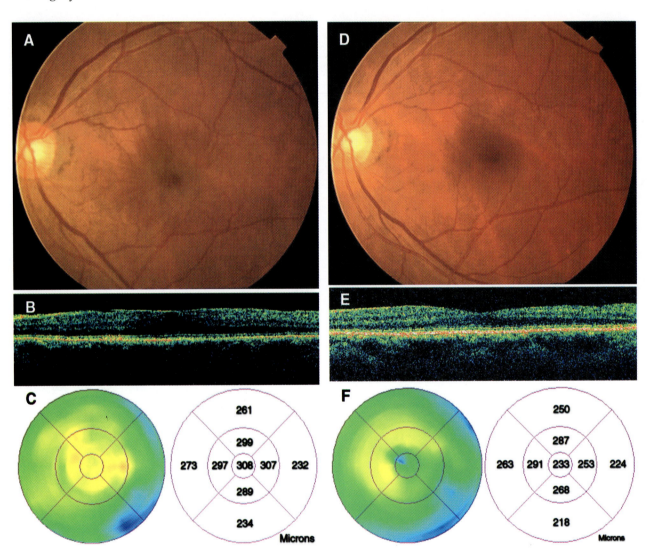

Figs 10.2A to F: A. Preoperative fundus photograph. A cellophane maculopathy can be seen. B. Preoperative OCT image from a 5 mm horizontal scan over the macula. A small epiretinal membrane is seen. The foveal thickness is 331 µm. C. Preoperative OCT map. Macular thickening is present. The diameters of circles are 1, 3, and 6 mm. D. Fundus photograph 6 months after vitrectomy. E. Postoperative OCT image 6 months after surgery. Foveal depression has recovered. The foveal thickness is 224 µm. F. Postoperative OCT map 6 months after surgery. Mild macular thickening is still observed.

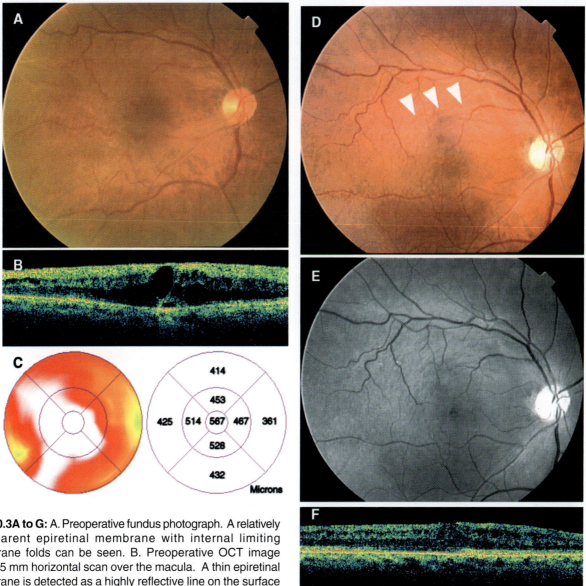

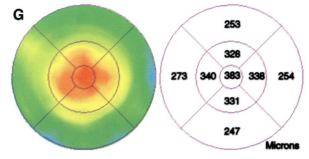

Figs 10.3A to G: A. Preoperative fundus photograph. A relatively transparent epiretinal membrane with internal limiting membrane folds can be seen. B. Preoperative OCT image from a 5 mm horizontal scan over the macula. A thin epiretinal membrane is detected as a highly reflective line on the surface of the retina. Large cystoid space and a small retinal detachment are seen at the fovea. Macular edema especially in the inner nuclear layer and probably the outer plexiform layer is also present. Foveal thickness is 617 μm C. Preoperative OCT map. Macular edema is apparent. The diameters of circles are 1, 3, and 6 mm. D. Postoperative fundus photograph 3 months after surgery. The epiretinal membrane is not present. A dissociated optic nerve fiber layer, which is seen as retinal striae running along the optic nerve fibers in the macular area, is visible especially in the superior macula (arrow head). E. Red-free fundus photograph 3 months after surgery. The dissociated optic nerve fiber layer can be seen more clearly. F. Postoperative OCT image 3months after surgery. An epiretinal membrane is not present but mild macular edema still remains. Foveal thickness is 398 μm. G. Postoperative OCT map 3 months after surgery. Mild macular edema is still present especially in the inner nuclear layer.

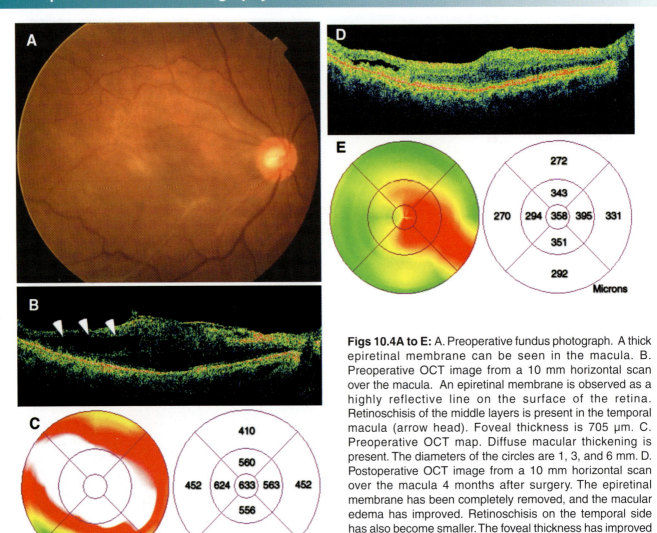

Figs 10.4A to E: A. Preoperative fundus photograph. A thick epiretinal membrane can be seen in the macula. B. Preoperative OCT image from a 10 mm horizontal scan over the macula. An epiretinal membrane is observed as a highly reflective line on the surface of the retina. Retinoschisis of the middle layers is present in the temporal macula (arrow head). Foveal thickness is 705 µm. C. Preoperative OCT map. Diffuse macular thickening is present. The diameters of the circles are 1, 3, and 6 mm. D. Postoperative OCT image from a 10 mm horizontal scan over the macula 4 months after surgery. The epiretinal membrane has been completely removed, and the macular edema has improved. Retinoschisis on the temporal side has also become smaller. The foveal thickness has improved to 456 µm. E. Postoperative OCT map 4 months after surgery. Macular thickening has improved.

Case 3

A 72-year-old man had a 6 months history of visual decrease in his right eye. His best-corrected visual acuity was 20/80 in the right eye. A relatively transparent epiretinal membrane with internal limiting membrane folds was observed (Fig. 10.3A). Preoperative OCT revealed a thin epiretinal membrane, detected as a highly reflective line on the surface of the retina. Large cystoid space and a small retinal detachment were also seen at the fovea. Macular edema especially in the inner nuclear layer and probably the outer plexiform layer was also present. Foveal thickness was 617 µm (Fig. 10.3B). Preoperative OCT map also showed macular edema (Fig. 10.3C). He had a combined surgery of phacoemulsification, intraocular lens implantation, vitrectomy, and epiretinal membrane peeling. Three months after surgery, the epiretinal membrane was not present. A dissociated optic nerve fiber layer, which was seen as retinal striae running along the optic nerve fibers in the macular area, was visible especially in the superior macula (Fig. 10.3D).

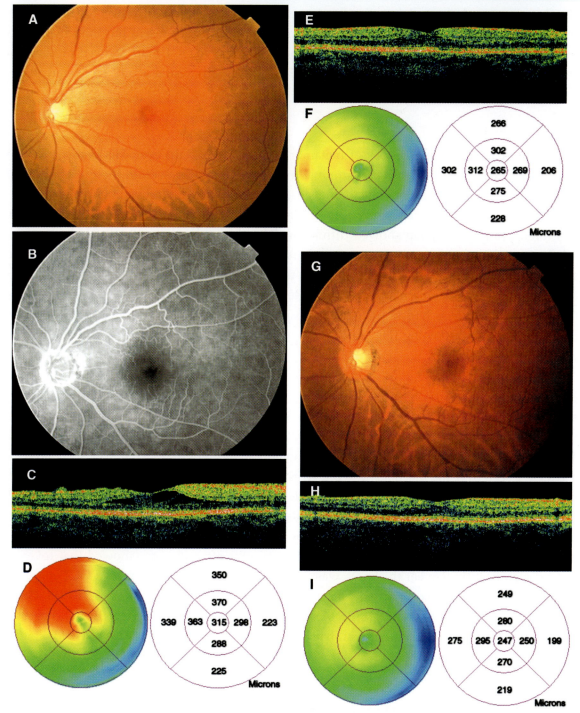

Figs 10.5A to I: A. Preoperative fundus photograph. An epiretinal membrane can be seen mainly in the superonasal parafovea. B. Preoperative fluorescein angiogram. Vessel tortuosity can be observed but no dye leakage is present. C. Preoperative OCT image from a 5 mm vertical scan over the macula. A schisis cavity can be seen noted at the fovea. Foveal thickness is 307 µm. D. Preoperative OCT map. Macular thickening is identified. The diameters of the circles are 1, 3, and 6 mm. E. Postoperative OCT image 2 months after surgery. Foveal schisis has decreased significantly. Foveal thickness is 249 µm. F. Postoperative OCT map 2 months after surgery. Macular edema has improved but mild macular thickening is still present. G. Fundus photograph 5 months after vitrectomy. A macular pseudohole is observed. H. Postoperative OCT image 5 months after surgery. Macular configuration has become almost normal. I. Postoperative OCT map 5 months after surgery. Localized macular thickening is still observed.

Red-free fundus photograph showed dissociated optic nerve fiber layer more clearly (Fig. 10.3E). Postoperative OCT, 3 months after surgery, showed that epiretinal membrane was not present but mild macular edema still remained. Foveal thickness was 398 µm (Fig. 10.3F). Postoperative OCT map, showed presence of mild macular edema especially in the inner nuclear layer (Fig. 10.3G). His visual acuity recovered to 20/50, 6 months after surgery.

Case 4

A 69-year-old man had a 3 month history of metamorphopsia in his right eye. His best-corrected visual acuity was 20/80 in the right eye. A thick epiretinal membrane could be seen in the macula (Fig. 10.4A). Preoperative OCT showed an epiretinal membrane, observed as a highly reflective line on the surface of the retina. Retinoschisis of the middle layers was present in the temporal macula. Foveal thickness was 705 µm (Fig. 10.4B). Preoperative OCT map showed diffuse macular thickening (Fig. 10.4C). He had a combined surgery of phacoemulsification, intraocular lens implantation, vitrectomy, and epiretinal membrane peeling. Postoperative OCT, 4 months after surgery showed that the epiretinal membrane had been completely removed, and the macular edema had improved. Retinoschisis on the temporal side had also become smaller. The foveal thickness had improved to 456 µm (Fig. 10.4D). Postoperative OCT map showed improvement in macular thickening (Fig. 10.4E). His visual acuity recovered to 20/33, four months after surgery.

Case 5

An epiretinal membrane was found in the left eye of a 63-year-old woman during a comprehensive medical examination. Her best-corrected visual acuity was 20/25 in the left eye, although she did not complain of metamorphopsia. An epiretinal membrane can be seen mainly in the superonasal parafoveal area (Fig. 10.5A). Preoperative OCT scan over the macula showed a schisis cavity at the fovea. Foveal thickness was 307 µm (Fig. 10.5B). Preoperative fluorescein angiogram showed tortuosity of vessels however, no dye leakage was present (Fig. 10.5C). On preoperative OCT map, macular thickening was identified (Fig. 10.5D). Vitrectomy with epiretinal membrane peeling was performed. The internal limiting membrane was also peeled during the epiretinal membrane peeling. Postoperative OCT, 2 months after surgery, showed that foveal schisis had decreased significantly. Foveal thickness was 249 µm (Fig. 10.5E). Postoperative OCT map revealed that macular edema had improved but mild macular thickening was still present (Fig. 10.5F). On fundus examination 5 months after vitrectomy, a macular pseudohole was observed (Fig. 10.5G). Postoperative OCT image showed that macular configuration had become almost normal (Fig. 10.5H). Postoperative OCT map showed localized macular thickening. Her visual acuity recovered to 20/20, 5 months after surgery (Fig. 10.5I).

REFERENCES

1. Gass JD. Stereoscopic Atlas of Macular Diseases: Diagnosis and Treatment, 4th edition. St. Louis, Mosby. 1997:938-951.
2. Mavrofrides EC, Rogers AH, Truong S, et al. Vitreoretinal interface disorders. In: ….. Optical Coherence Tomography of Ccular Diseases, Second Edition. Thorofare, Slack. 2004:57-77.
3. McDonald HR, Johnson RN, Ai E, Schatz H. Macular epiretinal membrane. In: Ryan SJ (ed.). Retina. St. Louis, Mosby. 2001: 2531-2546.
4. Niwa T, Terasaki H, Kondo M, et al. Function and morphology of macula before and after removal of idiopathic epiretinal membrane. Invest Ophthalmol Vis Sci. 2003 ;44:1652-1656.

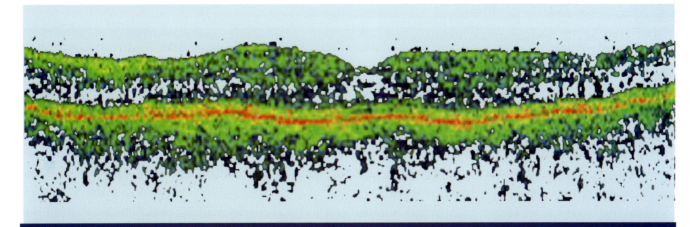

11

Secondary Epiretinal Membrane, Macular Pseudoholes, and Vitreomacular Traction Syndrome

Keisuke Mori

INTRODUCTION

The pathogenesis of epiretinal membrane may differ depending on the clinical setting in which they are found. Idiopathic epiretinal membrane occurs unassociated with other ocular disorders. In contrast, secondary epiretinal membranes are associated with a number of other ocular disorders, including limited form of proliferative vitreoretinopathy, retinal vascular diseases, intraocular inflammatory disorders, ocular trauma, all types of ocular surgeries and other diseases with blood retinal barrier breakdown.[14] Epiretinal membranes of differing pathogenesis have different characteristics. Among the features that may vary are etiology, morphology, prognosis and treatment response.

Epiretinal membranes occasionally induce retinal distortion that creates macular pseudoholes. Continuous contraction of epiretinal membranes may induce appearance of pseudohole to change from round or oval to slit-like, but usually vision decrease is limited.[5] Visual prognosis of eyes with macular pseudoholes is generally good since foveal structure is unaffected. Optical coherence tomography provides useful information for understanding the pathology of macular pseudoholes.

Macula is one of the regions of physiological vitreoretinal adhesions, which plays a key role in vitreomacular traction in an idiopathic macular hole development. In cases with incomplete posterior vitreous detachment persistent vitreomacular traction results in morphological distortion of macula, termed vitreomacular traction syndrome.[6,7] Vitreoretinal attachment in vitreomacular traction syndrome may vary from a broad area around the optic nerve and macula to narrow foveal zone with vitreous strands attachment.[6] Macular distortion induced persistent macular traction results in cystoid macular edema associated with central vision decrease and metamorphopsia.

Therapeutic intervention for these three clinical categories is vitreous surgery releasing retinal traction by removal of epiretinal membrane and posterior vitreous cortex. Optical coherence tomography (OCT) provides useful information of surgical response.

OPTICAL COHERENCE TOMOGRAPHY

Optical coherence tomography demonstrates epiretinal membranes as thin, highly reflective bands anterior to the retina. Wilkins and associates [8] identified morphologic characteristics of epiretinal membranes that allowed their separation into two distinct groups; those with focal points of attachment to the retina and those with global adherence to the retina. Based on the reports by Wilkins and associates[8] and Mori and associates[9] the majority of epiretinal membranes (approximately 70%) are globally adherent to the retina. The remaining eyes have focally adherent epiretinal membranes. Occasionally OCT can not distinguish between the epiretinal membrane and the anterior surface of the retina if the epiretinal membrane is globally adherent to the retina. Discriminating features were a difference in contrast between the epiretinal membrane (higher reflectivity) and the retina (lower reflectivity) and the appearance of a membrane tuft or edge contiguous with the retinal surface.[8,9] When correlated to clinical pathogenesis, secondary epiretinal membranes are more likely to be characterized by focal retinal adhesion than are idiopathic epiretinal membranes. Idiopathic epiretinal membranes tend to be globally adherent. The majority of eyes with macular pseudoholes are associated with globally adherent membranes.

An OCT image of fovea with secondary epiretinal membrane typically demonstrates diffuse thickening with loss of foveal pit. In idiopathic epiretinal membranes mean central macular thickness measured with

OCT correlates with visual acuity.[8] Vision in eyes with secondary epiretinal membranes may be affected additionally by associated diseases. Optical coherence tomography provides beneficial information in monitoring surgical removal of epiretinal membrane and decrease of intraretinal edema after vitreous surgery. The foveal pit reappears occasionally in successful cases. However, preoperative and postoperative mean macular thickness do not correlate with postoperative vision, thus indicating that preoperative macular thickness is not predictive of postoperative visual outcome.[10] Macular electrophysiological function measured by multifocal electroretinogram after epiretinal membrane removal may correlate residual macular thickening.[11]

Optical coherence tomography is beneficial in distinguishing macular pseudoholes from ophthalmoscopically similar-appearing lesions such as macular holes, macular lamellar holes, and macular cysts. Typical OCT configuration of macular pseudohole is the contour of the foveal pit, a thickening of the macular edges, a steeper foveal pit contour and the presence of normally reflective retinal tissue at the base of the pseudohole.[8,10]

Vitreoretinal attachment in vitreomacular traction syndrome may vary from a broad area around the optic nerve and macula to narrow foveal zone with a perifoveal vitreous detachment and focal adhesion to the fovea. Optical coherence tomography enables us to understand vitreomacular tractional force due to membrane adherent to macula with attachment of the posterior hyaloid, inducing significant retinal elevation and edema. Optical coherence tomography is also useful in demonstrating anatomic response after surgery for vitreomacular traction syndrome.[12]

INTERESTING CASE EXAMPLES

Case 1. Secondary Epiretinal Membrane Associated with Chronic Retinal Angitis

A 68-year-old male had a 6-month history of mild blurred vision and metamorphopsia. His right vision was 20/20. Fundus examination revealed perifoveal epiretinal membrane (Fig. 11.1A). Fluorescein angiography showed moderate intraretinal leakage in the macula and peripheral fundus. Capillary occlusion was also delineated in the temporal peripheral retina (Fig. 11.1B). Vertical OCT scan showed that the epiretinal membrane was delineated as a highly reflective band and was globally adherent to the retina without apparent retinal distortion. The foveal depression was moderately decreased with mild fluid accumulation (Fig. 11.1C).

Case 2. Secondary Epiretinal Membrane Associated with Chronic Retinal Vasculitis

A 56-year-old female had a 2-year history of chronic retinal vasculitis similar to case 1. Fundus examination demonstrated thick macular edema associated with the advanced secondary epiretinal membrane (Fig. 11.2A). A horizontal OCT scan delineated partially adherent epiretinal membrane to the retinal surface. Optical coherence tomography depicted increased retinal thickness and spaces of reduced optical reflectivity consistent with intraretinal cystic fluid accumulation (Fig. 11.2B).

Case 3. Macular Pseudohole with Idiopathic Epiretinal Membrane

A 61-year-old male had a 24-month history of mild metamorphopsia. His right eye vision was 20/20. Fundus examination demonstrated an oval macular pseudohole surrounded by idiopathic epiretinal membrane

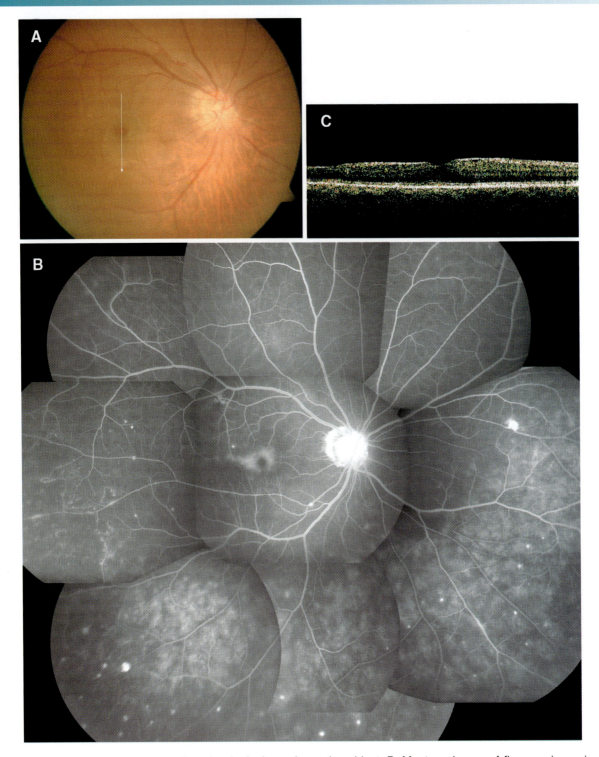

Fig. 11.1: A. Fundus photograph. Perifoveal epiretinal membrane is evident. B. Montage image of fluorescein angiography shows moderate intraretinal leakage in the macula and peripheral fundus. Capillary occlusion is also delineated in the temporal peripheral retina. C. A vertical OCT scan. The epiretinal membrane is delineated as a highly reflective band and is globally adherent to the retina without apparent retinal distortion. The foveal depression is moderately decreased with mild fluid accumulation.

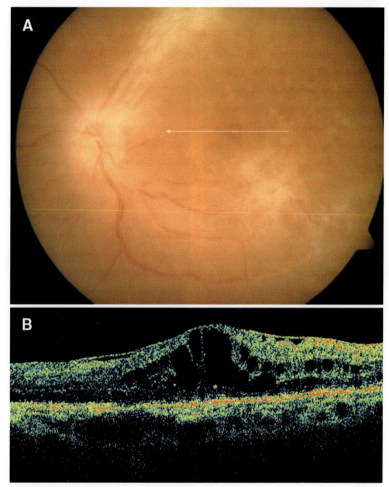

Fig. 11.2: A. Fundus photograph demonstrates thick macular edema associated with the advanced secondary epiretinal membrane. B. A horizontal OCT scan delineates partially adherent epiretinal membrane to the retinal surface. Optical coherence tomography depicts increased retinal thickness and spaces of reduced optical reflectivity consistent with intraretinal cystic fluid accumulation.

(Fig. 11.3A). A horizontal OCT scan showed deep and steep foveal pit with lamellation and thinning at the base of the fovea. Epiretinal membrane was globally adherent to the inner surface of the retina and difficult to distinguish from sensory retina (Fig. 11.3B). His vision and symptoms were stable during the 12-month follow-up.

Case 4. Macular Pseudohole with Focally Adherent Epiretinal Membrane

A 59-year-old female had a 5-month history of mild metamorphopsia. Her right eye vision was 20/20. Fundus examination showed macular pseudohole surrounded by retinal striae and dense epiretinal membrane superior to fovea (Fig. 11.4A). An OCT scan delineated the epiretinal membrane as a highly reflective band focally adherent to the inner retinal surface superior to fovea. The foveal pit encountered was wide and steep with thin fovea at the base, representing macular pseudohole (Fig. 11.4B).

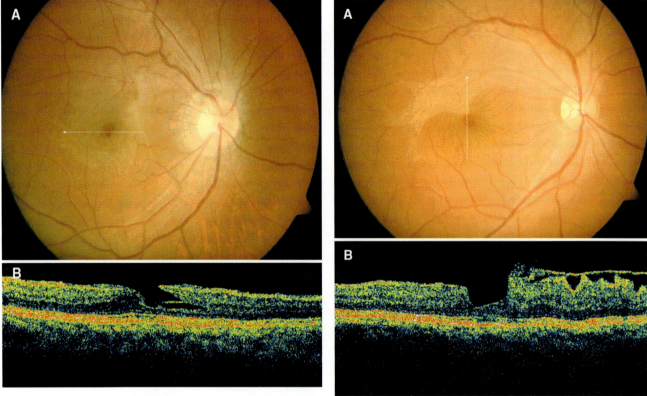

Fig. 11.3: A. Fundus photograph demonstrates an oval macular pseudohole surrounded by idiopathic epiretinal membrane. B. A horizontal OCT scan shows deep and steep foveal pit with lamellation and thinning at the base of the fovea. Epiretinal membrane is globally adherent to the inner surface of the retina and difficult to distinguish from sensory retina.

Fig. 11.4: A. Fundus photograph shows macular pseudohole surrounded by retinal striae and dense epiretinal membrane superior to fovea. B. An OCT scan delineates the epiretinal membrane as a highly reflective band focally adherent to the inner retinal surface superior to fovea. The foveal pit encountered is wide and steep with thin fovea at the base, representing macular pseudohole.

Case 5. Vitreomacular Traction Syndrome with Branch Retinal Vein Occlusion

A 72-year-old female had a 10-month history of branch retinal vein occlusion. Biomicroscopic fundus examination revealed vitreomacular traction syndrome. Her right vision was 20/400. Pars plana vitrectomy with membrane peeling was performed. Her vision improved moderately to 20/200 one month after vitreous surgery. Fundus examination before surgery demonstrated advanced branch retinal vein occlusion with glistening epiretinal fibrosis (Fig. 11.5A). Fluorescein angiograms of early (Fig. 11.5B) and late (Fig. 11.5C) phases demonstrated capillary occlusion and intensive vascular leakage. Horizontal (Fig. 11.5D) and vertical (Fig. 11.5E) cross-sectional OCT images showed dense membrane adherent to macula with attachment of the posterior hyaloid. The vitreomacular tractional force induces significant retinal elevation and edema. Fundus photograph one-month after vitreous surgery is shown in Figure 11.5F. A vertical OCT scan demonstrated release of macular traction, resolution of macular edema, relative increase of intraretinal exudation and significant reduction of retinal thickness (Fig. 11.5G).

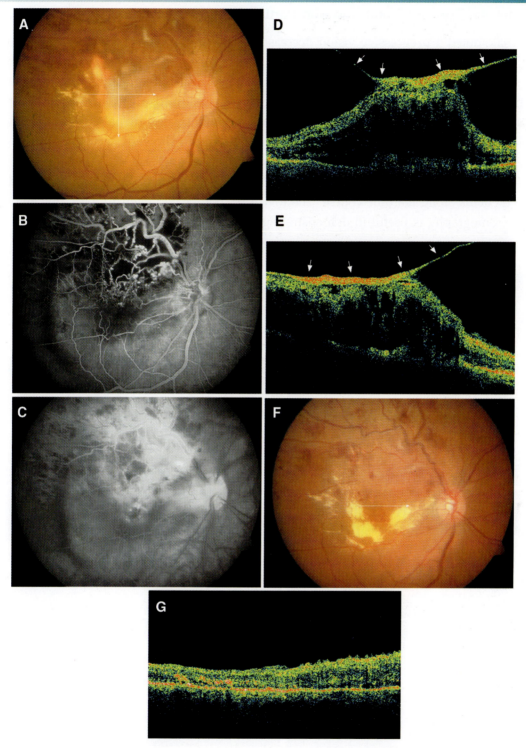

Fig. 11.5: **A.** Fundus photograph before surgery demonstrates advanced branch retinal vein occlusion with glistening epiretinal fibrosis. Fluorescein angiograms of early (B) and late (C) phases demonstrate capillary occlusion and intensive vascular leakage. Horizontal (D) and vertical (E) cross-sectional OCT images show dense membrane adherent to macula with attachment of the posterior hyaloid (arrows). The vitreomacular tractional force induces significant retinal elevation and edema. F. Fundus photograph one-month after vitreous surgery. G. A vertical OCT scan demonstrates release of macular traction, resolution of macular edema, relative increase of intraretinal exudation and significant reduction of retinal thickness.

Case 6. Vitreomacular Traction Syndrome with Partial Vitreous Detachment

A 57-year-old female noted a progressive vision decrease and metamorphopsia. Her right eye vision was 20/50. Biomicroscopic fundus examination revealed partial posterior vitreous detachment in the nasal quadrants and vitreoretinal traction in the posterior pole. The cortical vitreous and epiretinal membrane were removed by vitreous surgery and vitreomacular traction was released. Her visual acuity improved to 20/25 six month after vitreous surgery. Fundus examination demonstrated retinal edema and folds with thick glistening epiretinal membrane (Fig. 11.6A). A vertical OCT scan showed macular edema associated with thick epiretinal membrane partially adherent to the retinal surface (Fig. 11.6B). Vertical OCT scans 4 days (Fig. 11.6C), 10 days (Fig. 11.6D), 28 days (Fig. 11.6E) and 6 month (Fig. 11.6F) after surgery delineate recovery of retinal edema along the time course. The foveal pit reappeared even 10 days after the surgery. Optical coherence tomography is useful in demonstrating anatomic response after surgery.

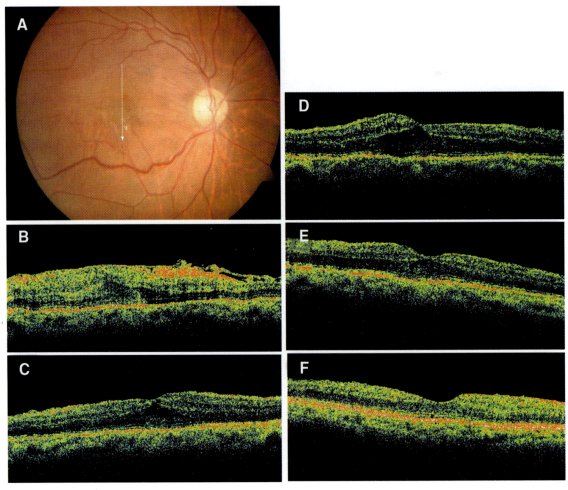

Fig. 11.6: A. Fundus photograph demonstrates retinal edema and folds with thick glistening epiretinal membrane. B. A vertical OCT scan shows macular edema associated with thick epiretinal membrane partially adherent to the retinal surface. Vertical OCT scans 4 days (C), 10 days (D), 28 days (E) and 6 month (F) after surgery delineate recovery of retinal edema along the time course. The foveal pit reappeared even 10 days after the surgery. OCT is useful in demonstrating anatomic response after surgery.

REFERENCES

1. Mcdonald HR, Schatz H, Johnson RN. Introduction to epiretinal membrane. In: Ryan S (ed.) Retina. St. Louis, Mosby. 1994:1819-1825.
2. Tannenbaum, HL, Schepens CL, Elzeneiny I, Freeman HM. Macular pucker following retinal detachment surgery. Arch Ophthalmol. 1970; 83: 286-293.
3. Wise GN. Congenital preretinal macular fibrosis. Am J Ophthalmol. 1975;79:363-365.
4. Lobes LA Jr, Burton TC. The incidence of macular pucker after retinal detachment surgery. Am J Ophthalmol. 1978;85:72-77.
5. Gass JDM. Stereoscopic Atlas of Macular Diseases: Diagnosis and Treatment. St. Louis, Mosby. 1987.
6. Smiddy WE, Michels RG, Glaser BM, de Bustos S. Vitrectomy for macular traction caused by incomplete vitreous separation. Arch Ophthalmol. 1988;106:624-628.
7. Margherio RR, Trese MT, Margherio AR, Cartright K. Surgical management of vitreomacluar traction syndromes. Ophthalmology. 1989; 96: 1437-1445.
8. Wilkins JR, Puliafito CA, Hee MR, et al. Characterization of epiretinal membrane using optical coherence tomography. Ophthalmology. 1996; 103:2142-2151.
9. Mori K, Gehlbach PL, Sano A, et al. Comparison of epiretinal membranes of differing pathogenesis using optical coherence tomography. Retina. 2004;24:57-62.
10. Massin P, Allouch C, Haouchine B, et al. Optical coherence tomography of idiopathic macular epiretinal membranes before and after surgery. Am J Ophthalmol. 2000;130:732-739.
11. Niwa T, Terasaki H, Kondo M, et al. Function and morphology of macula before and after removal of idiopathic epiretinal membrane. Invest Ophthalmol Vis Sci. 2003;44:1652-1656.
12. Carpineto P, Ciancaglini M, Aharrh-Gnama A, et al. Optical coherence tomography imaging of surgical resolution of bilateral vitreomacular traction syndrome related to incomplete posterior vitreoschisis: a case report. Eur J Ophthalmol. 2004;14:438-441.

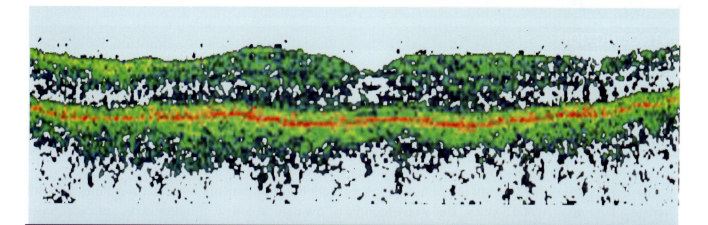

12

Idiopathic Macular Hole

Michael S Ip, Marni Grage Feldmann

INTRODUCTION

Idiopathic macular holes represent a retinal defect involving the fovea. There is a marked predilection for macular holes occurring in women in the 6th to 7th decade with an incidence of approximately three per 1,000.[1,2] Most macular holes are idiopathic, however up to 9% are traumatic and some may be associated with chronic cystoid macular edema. Symptoms of macular holes include decreased visual acuity, central scotoma, and metamorphopsia. Retinal detachments secondary to macular holes are rare; occurring predominantly in highly myopic eyes in the setting of trauma.

The Eye Disease Case Control Study had long-term follow-up of patients with macular holes with an average follow-up time of 4.5 years. This study found that the natural course of full-thickness macular holes is to progress in size. Only 8% showed spontaneous resolution and of these patients, one-third had improvement in visual acuity. Forty-five percent of patients will have a loss of at least two Snellen lines of visual acuity; 28% will lose three lines. Vision loss typically stabilizes around 20/200 to 20/400. The rate of macular hole formation in the fellow eye without evidence of posterior vitreous detachment is 4.6% within three years, 6.5% within four to five years, and 7.1% within six or more years of follow-up. If the fellow eye has already had a posterior vitreous detachment, the risk is nearly zero percent.[2]

Clinical features of full-thickness macular holes include a circular defect in the region of the fovea with a surrounding cuff of subretinal fluid and retinal edema. Ancillary tests that may be used to as an adjunct to the clinical examination in the diagnosis of macular holes include the Watzke-Allen test, the laser aiming beam test, fluorescein angiography, and optical coherence tomography (OCT). The Watzke-Allen test is positive for macular hole when a narrow, vertical slit light beam is projected over the fovea and the patient notes a break or thinning of the beam. The laser aiming beam test is positive for macular hole when a 50 µm beam is projected within the hole and the patient cannot detect the light because of the lack of retinal tissue at the macular hole. Fluorescein angiography reveals window defects secondary to the absence of xanthophyll pigment and retinal tissue within the hole. The window defect may be particularly prominent because of partial blockage of choroidal fluorescence around the hole secondary to surrounding subretinal fluid. Optical coherence tomography which is described in further detail below is used to demonstrate the full-thickness foveal defect.

OPTICAL COHERENCE TOMOGRAPHY

Optical coherence tomography is a medical imaging technology that has improved the understanding of the pathophysiology and anatomy of idiopathic macular holes well as well as their management.

Pathogenesis of Macular Holes

The proposed pathophysiology for formation of macular hole has undergone revision throughout this century. In the 1920s, Lister proposed that macular holes develop from anteroposterior traction from vitreous bands adherent to the foveola.[3] In the late 1960s, Jaffe supported the concept of anteroposterior vitreomacular traction as a contributing factor to macular hole formation.[4] It has also been proposed that tractional forces created during the process of posterior vitreous detachment may lead to development of macular holes.[5,6]

In the 1980s, Gass proposed that macular holes developed as a result of tangential traction of the vitreous cortex at the foveolar edges; and that foveal dehiscence was followed by centripetal retraction of retinal elements. In his hypothesis, the posterior hyaloid face of the vitreous remained attached to the foveola and surrounding macular region in the initial stages of hole formation.[7,8,9] This hypothesis was generated using only biomicroscopy.

The pathogenesis of macular hole formation, as described above, can be paralleled by optical coherence tomography with minor modification. Optical coherence tomography is able to demonstrate changes in the vitreomacular interface not visible with biomicroscopy (Figs 12.1 and 12.2). For example, OCT can demonstrate adherence of the vitreous to the fovea which has previously been described in histologic studies.[10,11] On OCT images, most early stage macular holes have been found to have a separation of the posterior perifoveal vitreous from the retina. A convexity of the posterior hyaloid face has been demonstrated with perifoveal separation and continued attachment at the foveola, disc and peripheral to the foveal region.[12, 13] This creates a convex trampolining or tenting effect, which causes a combination of anteroposterior and tangential traction (oblique traction), resulting in macular hole formation. This force is concentrated on the foveola, particularly during eye movement. Posterior vitreous detachment starting in the perifoveal region has been confirmed by anatomical studies,[14] ultrasonography, and biomicroscopy.[15, 16]

Anatomy / Staging

In 1988, Gass published a staging classification for macular holes, based on biomicroscopy. He speculated that Muller cells in the fovea or retina could migrate through the internal limiting membrane to form a prefoveolar vitreoglial membrane, which could then contract, causing a focal contraction of prefoveolar vitreous cortex. This could cause tangential traction on the retina resulting in a foveolar detachment which appears as a yellow spot on biomicroscopy (Fig. 12.1). This is described as a Stage 1A macular hole. This yellow spot changes to a yellow ring, Stage 1B, with lateral spread of photoreceptors and xanthophyll from centrifugal retraction (Fig. 12.3). Stage 1B holes were subsequently divided into occult and impending holes when Gass published a reappraisal of the biomicroscopic classification of stages of macular hole development in 1995.[8] Occult holes have a separation between retinal elements that is not present in impending holes and the surface of occult holes are bridged by internal limiting membrane, Muller cells, and contracted prefoveolar vitreous cortex. When an eccentric tear occurs in these bridging elements, the hole may enlarge forming a Stage 2 hole which by definition is less than 400 microns in width (Fig. 12.4). At this stage, the contracted vitreous cortex could separate from the surface of the hole, forming a pseudooperculum. The 1995 classification stated that this prefoveal condensation, the pseudooperculum, was usually not composed of retinal tissue. A Stage 3 hole is larger than or equal to 400 microns in diameter and was associated with a prefoveal condensation (Fig. 12.5) without a posterior vitreous detachment. A Stage 4 hole was defined as a full thickness macular hole associated with a complete posterior vitreous detachment (Fig. 12.6). In the initial three stages, the posterior hyaloid face is attached except at the vitreofoveolar interface in Stage 3 and some Stage 2 holes.

Optical coherence tomography images provide excellent visualization of the earliest stages of macular hole formation and demonstrate the anatomy more clearly than biomicroscopy. The OCT images show that the initial traction on the macula, as described by Gass, is concentrated at the foveola, but with earlier separation of the vitreous from the fovea. In 1999, Gaudric and associates used OCT to demonstrate perifoveal posterior vitreous detachment in patients with early macular holes.[17] In 2001, Haouchine and associates demonstrated the same finding of perifoveal posterior vitreous detachment surrounding a focal area of vitreofoveal adhesion in pre-macular hole lesions.[18]

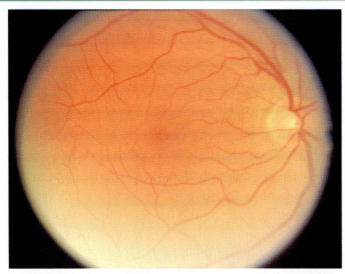

Fig. 12.1: Stage 1A macular hole, yellow spot is noted.

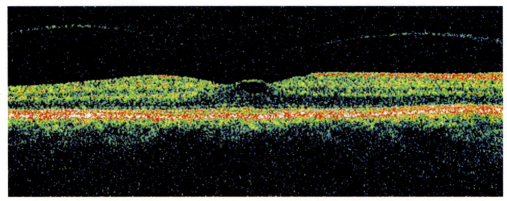

Fig. 12.2: Stage 1A macular hole OCT highlighting perifoveal posterior vitreous detachment with continued foveolar adherence and obliquely oriented tractional forces which are not evident on photographs. Retinal tissue remains at the base of the pseudocyst.

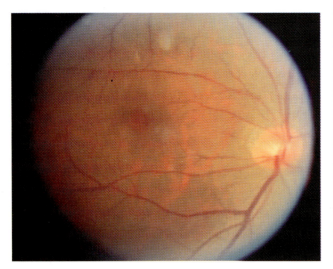

Fig. 12.3: Stage 1B macular hole, yellow ring develops.

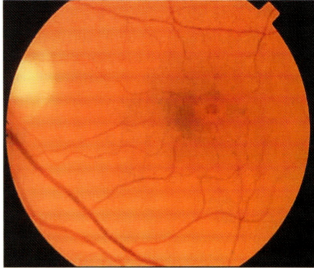

Fig. 12.4: Stage 2 full thickness macular hole with diameter < 400 µm.

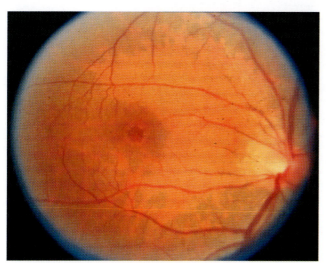

Fig. 12.5: Stage 3 full thickness macular hole with diameter=< 400 µm.

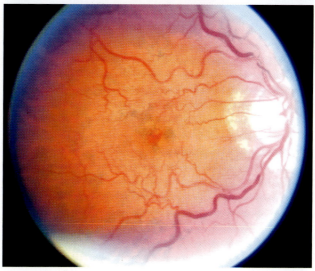

Fig. 12.6: Stage 4 full thickness macular hole with complete posterior vitreous detachment.

Given that OCT is able to demonstrate anatomical changes that are not visible biomicroscopically, the staging of macular holes with OCT differs from that originally proposed by Gass. Optical coherence tomography has allowed the proposal of a new staging scheme while maintaining certain conventions to allow this staging system to supplement, rather than replace, the biomicroscopic staging (Fig. 12.7).[19] This convention is important for allowing comparison of previously published reports and future studies.

Optical coherence tomography of Stage 1 holes reveals foveal splitting rather than foveolar detachment (Fig. 12.2). On OCT images, a pseudocyst is formed and may be observed prior to a yellow spot being visible with biomicroscopy. Optical coherence tomography has shown retinal tissue at the base of the pseudocyst in Stage 1A and B holes.[20] Optical coherence tomography has documented the progression to a Stage 1B hole as this pseudocyst enlarges and extends to the retinal pigment epithelium. In addition to being imaged with OCT, these pseudocysts have also been described with biomicroscopic examination and confirmed with both scanning laser ophthalmoscopy as well as retinal thickness analysis.[21,22]

In distinction to biomicroscopic staging, OCT demonstrates perifoveal posterior vitreous detachment with continued adhesion at the foveola in the early stages of macular hole formation. This finding has been confirmed with ultrasonography patients with Stage 1 or 2 macular holes (without opercula).[9]

Full-thickness Stage 2 macular holes, less than 400 microns in diameter, result from partial or complete unroofing of the pseudocyst present in a Stage 1B holes (Fig. 12.8). In this stage, the posterior hyaloid face may remain attached to the roof of the pseudocyst or it may result in operculation which remains contiguous with the posterior hyaloid face. These two different forms of Stage 2 holes (OCT staging) are easily differentiated with OCT imaging. This distinction is important as they may have a different natural course and/or respond differently to intervention. To this effect, the classification of Stage 2 holes has been subdivided: Stage 2A has continued attachment of the flap to the retina and Stage 2B is operculated (Fig. 12.8 and 12.9). This new classification maintains the convention set forth by the Gass classification scheme of Stage 2 holes being less than 400 microns and Stage 3 being greater than in or equal to 400 microns in diameter. This is important as the conventional method has been utilized in several publications on the

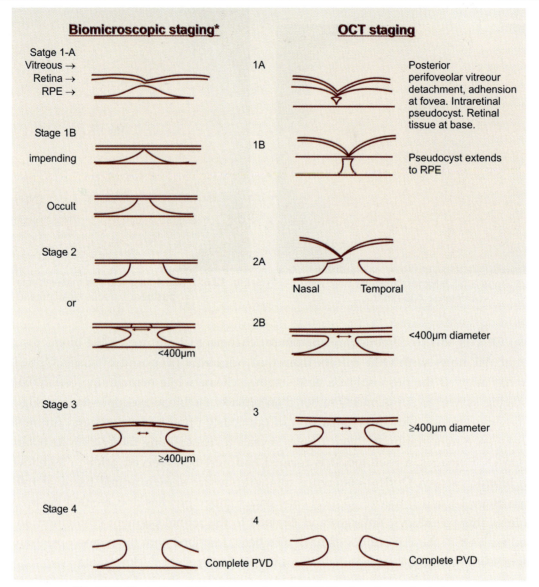

Fig. 12.7: Illustration of biomicroscopic and OCT Staging of macular holes.

Biomicroscopic staging *(Gass, Am J Ophthalmol. 1995)*
Stage 1A: Yellow spot, foveal dehiscence, posterior hyaloid attached to IL Minternal limiting membrane
Stage 1B: Yellow ring, lateral spread of photoreceptors
Stage 2: Full thickness macular hole, can opener tear or pseudooperculumpseudo operculum, ≥ 400 μm diameter
Stage 3: Full thickness macular hole, pseudooperculum = ≥400 μm diameter
Stage 4: Full thickness macular hole with complete posterior vitreous detachment

OCT Staging
Stage 1A: Partial thickness pseudocyst with perifoveal posterior vitreous detachment
Stage 1B: Full thickness pseudocyst with roof
Stage 2A: Full thickness macular hole with partial opening of the roof, focal vitreous attachment to flap
Stage 2B: Full thickness operculated macular hole, traction to retina released
Stage 3: Full thickness operculated macular hole, traction released, ≥ 400 μm diameter
Stage 4: Full thickness macular hole with complete posterior vitreous detachment, vitreous face may or may not be evident on OCT

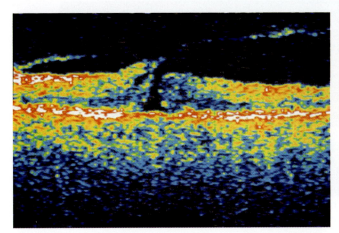

Fig. 12.8: Optical coherence tomography of Stage 2A macular hole – the roof of the pseudocyst has been torn open and continues to have traction exerted by the vitreous attachment.

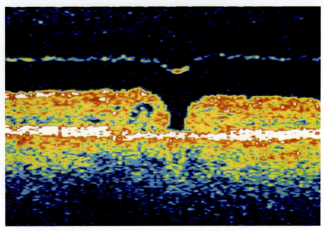

Fig. 12.9: Optical coherence tomography of Stage 2B macular hole – the roof of the pseudocyst has completely separated from the retina. Full thickness macular hole with diameter < 400 µm.

natural course and surgical intervention utilizing biomicroscopy and OCT for follow-up. It is important to note that former papers on OCT findings in macular holes have referred to the hole with the attached flap as Stage 2 and the operculated hole as Stage 3.

Stage 2 holes (OCT staging) may have posterior hyaloid which remains adherent the incompletely detached roof of the pseudocyst. This tissue has the same reflectivity on OCT as retinal tissue and in continuous with the retina prior to separation. Ezra and associates[23] suggested that this tissue may indeed be retinal tissue. This has now been confirmed though immunohistochemical studies. Up to two-thirds of intra-operative specimens consist of cone photoreceptors, glial cells, and internal limiting membrane rather than a vitreous condensation.

On OCT, a Stage 3 hole (Fig. 12.10) appears to have thickening of the retina with intraretinal cystoid spaces. In contrast to the Gass classification where the posterior hyaloid is attached in the perifoveal region, OCT reveals that in many cases the retinal traction has been released as the posterior perifoveal hyaloid face is completely separated and can be visualized anterior to the hole. The posterior hyaloid may or may not be visualized on OCT images of Stage 4 holes (Fig. 12.11) depending on whether it has moved too far anteriorly for imaging. A complete posterior vitreous detachment can be confirmed with biomicroscopy and ultrasonography when the vitreous face is not imaged on OCT.

In summary, the significant differences in the Gass' biomicroscopic and the OCT classification of macular hole stages are:

1. The finding of obliquely oriented focal foveolar attachment of the posterior hyaloid face with surrounding vitreomacular separation demonstrated on OCT in distinction to the tangential traction proposed by Gass.

2. Formation of a pseudocyst with retinal tissue at the base of Stage 1A holes versus the foveolar dehiscence proposed by Gass as an initial event in macular hole formation, and 3) Subdivision of Stage 2 holes into two distinct anatomical appearances, which may respond differently to intervention.[19]

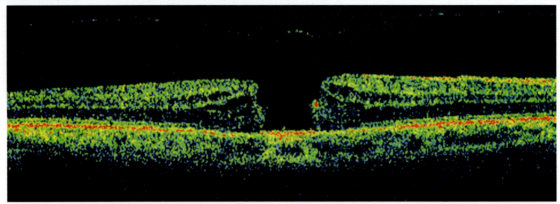

Fig. 12.10: Optical coherence tomography of Stage 3 macular hole – the retinal elements have separated to = ≥ 400 µm apart and the retina has thickened. An operculum/pseudooperculum is attached to the visible posterior hyaloid face.

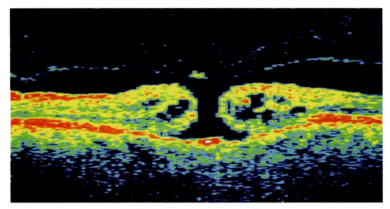

Fig. 12.11: Optical coherence tomography of Stage 4 macular hole – note that the posterior hyaloid face is detached off the surface of the retina. The posterior hyaloid face may no longer be visible on OCT if it has moved too far anteriorly.

Treatment Implications

Optical coherence tomography has improved both our understanding of the pathogenesis and staging of macular holes. Preoperative OCT can assist in the staging of macular holes and is useful in discussing surgical prognosis with patients. In addition, the images obtained with OCT can be used to enhance patient education in obtaining informed consent for surgery and in demonstrating the results of surgical intervention.

Natural Course

Optical coherence tomography is an excellent modality for imaging pre-macular hole lesions and their potential progression to full thickness macular holes. The Vitrectomy for Prevention of Macular Hole Study Group reported that over a two-year period, 14 of 35 patients (40%) with a pre-macular hole lesion who were randomized to observation progressed to a full-thickness macular hole.[24] Optical coherence tomography has been useful to document that, in macular holes that resolve spontaneously, the foveolar adhesion observed in Stage 1A and 1B holes is released with resultant settling of the pseudocyst. In patients who progress to a full thickness macular hole, there is continued traction on the foveolar retina which creates either an operculum or a can-opener tear with secondary flap formation. Lewis et al demonstrated that if an individual has a macular hole in one eye, the risk for developing a macular hole in the contralateral eye is 13% at 48 months.[25] Optical coherence tomography may be helpful in identifying those patients who have already developed a central hyaloid detachment and would subsequently be at reduced risk of developing a macular hole versus those who have an attachment and are at continued risk.

Optical coherence tomography can also provide information concerning the risk of developing a macular hole within an individual eye because OCT delineates the anatomy in more detail than biomicroscopy. For example, Gaudric and associates demonstrated in a study of 61 fellow eyes that although biomicroscopy demonstrated six patients with a posterior vitreous detachment and 55 with an attached posterior hyaloid, the OCT examination found that 26 of these 55 had perifoveal hyaloid detachment with continued adherence at the fovea and 19 had central hyaloid detachment.[17] These 19 would therefore be much less likely to develop a macular hole.

DIFFERENTIAL DIAGNOSIS

The diagnosis of macular hole in some cases is difficult. Many entities can mimic macular hole on biomicroscopic examination. For example, the yellow spot seen on biomicroscopy in a Stage 1A macular hole may appear to be central serous retinopathy. Similarly, a full thickness Stage 2 or Stage 3 macular hole may appear to be an epiretinal membrane with pseudohole. OCT can usually help distinguish these entities and is an important ancillary test to biomicroscopy in these situations. Distinguishing these lesions apart is important because the natural course and treatment of these lesions are different. The differential diagnosis includes central serous retinopathy, epiretinal membrane with pseudohole, lamellar hole, solar retinopathy, cystoid macular edema, and drusen.[12, 13, 26]

PATIENT EDUCATION

Patient education regarding the presence and management of macular hole is enhanced by the ability to use OCT to demonstrate the discontinuity of retinal architecture on a cross-sectional image of the retina. It is also helpful when explaining the purpose and mechanism of surgical repair as the tractional element of macular hole formation can often be visualized in earlier stage holes. The enhanced patient education offered by OCT may help improve compliance with prone positioning required in the postoperative period.

Optical coherence tomography may also be utilized to monitor for enlargement of the macular hole or change in architecture if an individual elects to proceed with observation rather than surgical repair. This knowledge will assist the patient in making future decisions. The postoperative OCT confirmation of hole closure can also be compared with preoperative OCT for the patient's benefit (see case examples 1 and 2). It is helpful to demonstrate anatomical closure considering that visual improvement is a prolonged process with functional improvement often lagging behind anatomical success.

MANAGEMENT

Kelly and Wendel reported on a series of patients in 1991 where they showed that it was possible to surgically close macular holes and improve the visual acuity in many of the patients studied.[27] Currently, success rates for macular hole closure range from 88% to 97%.[28,29] Recently, attention has been directed at the use of indocyanine green (ICG) in macular hole surgery. Indocyanine green may be a useful surgical adjuvant as ICG facilitates visualization of the internal limiting membrane during surgical peeling. Slaughter and Lee found that macular hole closure rate was 97% with ICG and 91% without ICG, although this difference was not statistically different. However, in another study here was a statistically significant improvement in visual acuity in patients who underwent peeling of the internal limiting membrane compared with those that did not have the internal limiting membrane removed.[30]

de Bustros and associates demonstrated that Stage 1 holes may be observed since approximately 60% of Stage 1 macular holes may resolve spontaneously.[24] In contrast, Stage 2 holes are much more likely to progress with enlargement and further decrease in visual acuity; Hikichi and associates reported progressive hole enlargement in 84% of Stage 2 holes observed over 3 years, with 81% of these eyes losing 2 or more lines of vision.[30]

The current standard of care is to offer surgical repair for Stage 2 or larger holes. Optical coherence tomography is helpful to distinguish between stage 1 and 2 holes as treatment options are clearly different. The anatomical and visual outcome of macular hole surgery is better for macular holes of more recent onset and of an earlier stage and therefore it is helpful to identify full thickness macular holes as soon as they develop.[31]

Measurements of macular hole diameter with OCT have been correlated with surgical results. A study by Ip and associates [32] confirmed earlier studies demonstrating increased closure rates with Stage 2 versus Stage 3 and 4 holes.[16,28,33] In 40 patients, 22 of 24 eyes with a hole diameter of less than 400 microns closed with one operation (92%) whereas only 9 of 16 eyes with macular hole diameter greater than or equal to 400 microns achieved hole closure with one surgery (56%, p=0.02). Late reopening of the macular hole after anatomical closure was seen only in holes which measured greater than 400 microns, in 3 of the 31 eyes. Based on this, it was concluded that the preoperative hole diameter on OCT was predictive of the immediate postoperative closure rate and the rate of late reopening. Ullrich and associates have supported that preoperative hole size is a prognostic factor for hole closure and vision outcome and indicated that the best correlation with the biomicroscopic appearance was the diameter of the hole measured at its narrowest point on OCT.[34]

Successfully repaired macular holes have been subdivided by Imai and associates into three patterns based on OCT configuration: the U-type with normal foveal contour, the V-type with steep foveal contour and the W-type with a foveal defect of the neurosensory retina. Theses patterns have also be shown to correlate with postoperative visual acuity (U>V>W).[35]

As described above, OCT allows for subdivision of Stage 2 macular holes into those with an elevated flap of retinal tissue with continued adherence of the posterior vitreous face and those in which an operculum or pseduo-operculum has already formed which may have implications for treatment. Patients who continue to have an adhesion may benefit from more limited surgical intervention than those who have already had a spontaneous resolution of traction but yet continue to have an open macular hole. Spaide described successful hole closure with minimal vitrectomy and dissection of this adhesion followed by fluid gas exchange in patients who have continued adhesion, the OCT Stage 2A appearance.[36] Chan and associates and Costa and associates have used OCT to demonstrate a gas injection induced separation of vitreofoveolar adhesion that resulted in closure of a Stage 2A macular hole.[37,38] Peeling of the internal limiting membrane during the standard surgical procedure may improve macular hole closure rates.[39,40] Based on OCT findings, it is possible that this may be of greater necessity in patients who have a OCT Stage 2B hole or larger rather than in patients with Stage 2A holes in which more limited surgery is likely to be successful.

Visualization of the retinal structures through intraocular gas or silicone oil with OCT is possible. Kasuga and associates has demonstrated OCT confirmation of macular hole closure with surgery has been reported within 24 hours in four of seven eyes through gas.[41] Although early anatomical hole closure on OCT does not necessarily indicate complete healing, such evaluations may eventually assist investigators in determining the optimum length of time for prone positioning in the postoperative period. Optical coherence tomography images of closed macular holes confirm the centripetal repositioning of photoreceptors in successful surgery and mimic the histopathologic appearance of closed holes.[42]

INTERESTING CASE EXAMPLES

Case 1. Cystoid macular edema developing into a full-thickness macular hole.

Seventy-three-year-old man presented with blurry vision and floaters in his left eye three weeks prior to presentation. Visual acuity was 20/400 in affected eye. He was found to have an extremely elevated central macula with cystic changes and a very early epiretinal membrane in the left eye. The cystic macular edema was confirmed with OCT and fluorescein angiography (Figs 12.12A to C). He was treated with prednisolone acetate 1% QID and ketorolac QID. On follow-up 6 weeks later, visual acuity improved to 20/100, but he developed a large cyst in the left macula which had a clinical appearance suggestive of a macular hole. However, OCT was consistent with a large macular cyst, not a macular hole (Figs 12.12 D and E). He then underwent subtenon injection of 40 mg of trimcinolone and continued the prednisolone acetate and ketorolac, both QID. The patient continued these medications and the cystoid macular edema remained stable. Approximately four months later, he developed a full-thickness macular hole which was successfully repaired [Figs 12.12F and G (pre op) and Figure 12.12H and I (post op)].

Case 2. Risk of vitreoretinal interface abnormalities (i.e. stage 1 macular holes) in fellow eyes of patients with full-thickness macular holes.

Seventy-six-year-old man presented with an "oval ball" in his central vision, left eye, for one week without metamorphopsia. Visual acuity was 20/40 in each eye. Optical coherence tomography documented a stage 2 macular hole in the left eye (Figs 12.13 A and B). An OCT was also performed in the patient's asymptomatic right eye and a Stage 1 macular hole was documented (Figs 12.13C and D). The patient underwent macular hole repair in the left eye. On follow-up one month later, the macular hole was closed OS (Fig. 12.13E); however the patient's right eye then progressed to a full-thickness macular hole which was subsequently repaired. This case demonstrates the utility of OCT to document fellow eye changes which occurs with a relatively high frequency in patients with macular holes.

Case 3. Macular holes can be repaired with silicone oil without use of face-down positioning.

Seventy six year-old man presented with complaints of "images jumping around" in the right eye. Past ocular history is significant for cryotherapy for a retinal tear in his right eye, cataract extraction, both eyes, and an epiretinal membrane peel in the right eye 2 years prior to presentation. Visual acuity in the affected

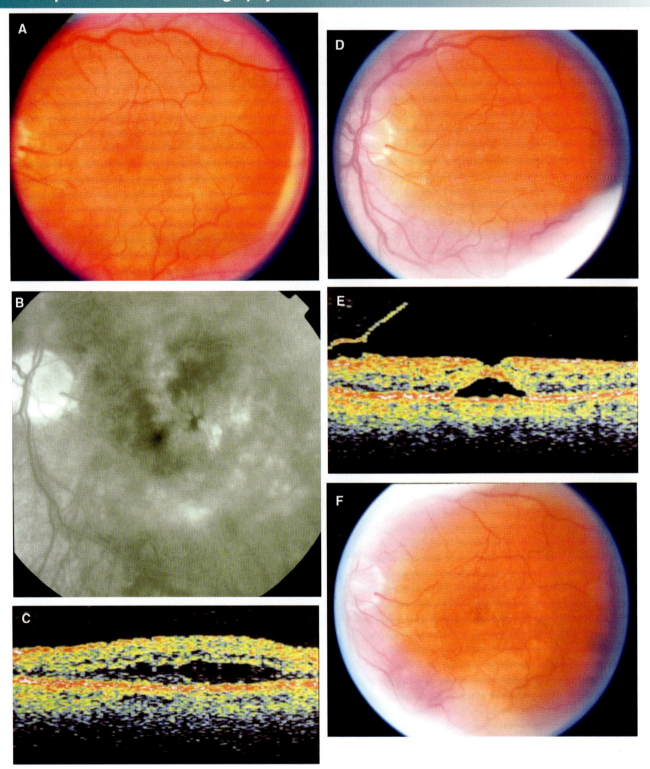

Figs 12.12A to F: A. Fundus photograph of cystic macular edema of the left eye, B. Late fluorescein angiogram revealing hyperfluorescent cystic spaces, C. Optical coherence tomography revealing cystic macular edema, D. Fundus photograph of large macular cyst with appearance suggestive of a full-thickness macular hole, E. Optical coherence tomography confirming large macular cyst, not full-thickness macular hole, F. Fundus photograph of full-thickness macular hole.

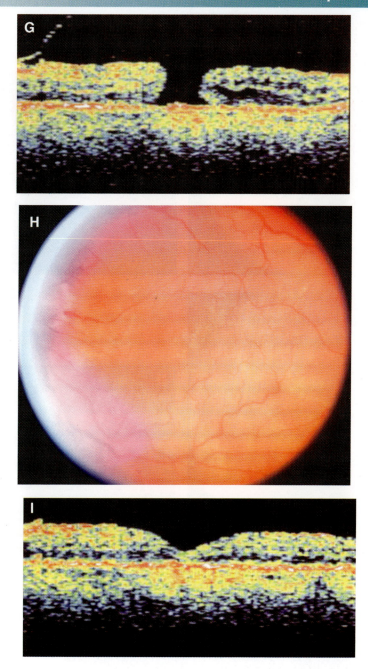

Figs 12.12G to I: G. Optical coherence tomography of full-thickness macular hole, H. Fundus photograph of closed macular hole, I. Optical coherence tomography confirming macular hole closure after repair OS.

eye was 20/40. At presentation the patient was found to have a large epiretinal membrane with pseudohole in the right eye and subsequently underwent epiretinal membrane peel. On follow-up three months following repair, his visual acuity improved to 20/30 and he continued to appear to clinically have a macular hole, but OCT revealed a pseudo-hole due to regrowth of the epiretinal membrane (Figs 12.14 A and B). On subsequent follow-up visits, his vision dropped to 20/80 due to development of a macular hole and he elected to have repeat macular hole repair with placement of silicone oil. The macular hole was successfully closed using

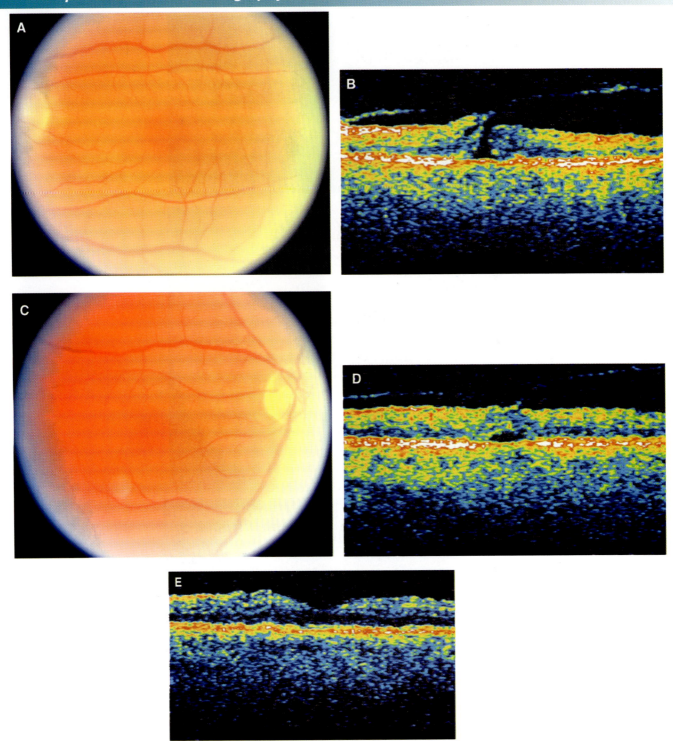

Figs 12.13A to E: A. Fundus photograph of Stage II macular hole OS, B. Optical coherence tomography of Stage II macular hole OS, C. Fundus photograph of stage I macular hole OD, D. Optical coherence tomography Stage I macular hole OD, E. Optical coherence tomography confirming macular hole closure after repair OS.

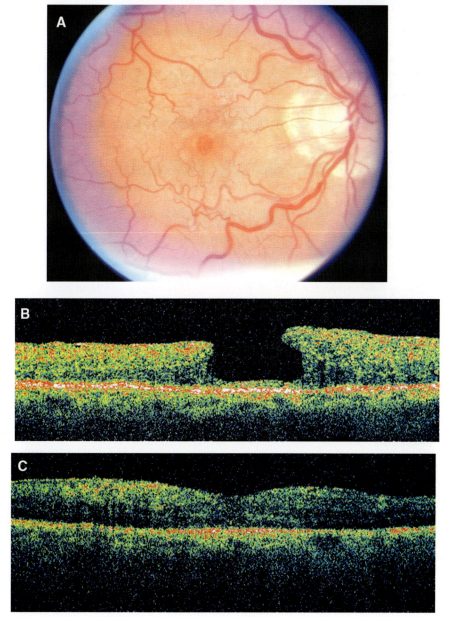

Figs 12.14A to C: A. Fundus photograph of pseudohole, B. Optical coherence tomography of pseudohole, C. Optical coherence tomography under silicone oil confirming macular hole closure.

silicone oil without any postoperative positioning (Fig. 12.14C). The OCT image was taken when the eye was filled with silicone oil, demonstrating the ability to perform OCT in eyes filled with silicone oil.

REFERENCES

1. Aaberg TM, Blair CJ, Gass JDM. Macular holes. Ophthalmology. 1970; 69:555-562.
2. Chew EY, Sperduto RD, Hiller R, et al. The eye diseases case-control study. Clinical course of macular holes. Arch Ophthalmol. 1999; 117:242-246.
3. Lister W. Holes in the retina and their clinical significance. Br J Ophthalmol. 1924;8:1-20.

4. Jaffe NS. Vitreous traction at the posterior pole of the fundus due to alterations in the vitreous posterior. Trans Am Acad Ophthalmol Otolaryng. 1967;71:642-652.
5. Reese AB, Jones IS, Cooper WC. Macular changes secondary to vitreous traction. Am J Ophthalmol 1967;64:544-549.
6. McDonnell PJ, Fine SL, Hills AI. Clinical features of idiopathic macular cysts and holes. Am J Ophthalmol 1982; 93:777-786.
7. Gass JDM. Idiopathic senile macular hole: its early stages and pathogenesis. Arch Ophthalmol. 1988;106:629-639.
8. Gass JDM. Reappraisal of biomicroscopic classification of stages of development of a macular hole. Am J Ophthalmol. 1995;-119:752-759.
9. Johnson MW, Van Newkirk MR, Meyer KA. Perifoveal vitreous detachment is the primary pathogenic event in idiopathic macular hole formation. Arch Ophthalmol. 2001;119:215-222.
10. Grignolo A. Fibrous components of the vitreous body. Arch Ophthalmol. 1952;47:760-774.
11. Eisner G. Clinical anatomy of the vitreous. In: Jakobiec FA; (ed.)=Ocular Anatomy, Embryology, and Teratology. Philadelphia,, PA: Harper & Row Publishers.;-1982:413-417.
12. Hee MR, Puliafito CA, Wong C, et al. Optical coherence tomography of macular holes. Ophthalmology. 1995; 102:748-756.
13. Puliafito, CA, Hee MR, Lin CP, et al. Imaging of macular diseases with optical coherence tomography. Ophthalmology. 1995; 102:217-219.
14. Foos RY. Vitreoretinal juncture; topographical variations. Invest Ophthalmol. 1972; 11:801-808.
15. Kakehashi A, Schepens CL, Trempe CL. Vitreomacular observations, II: data on the pathogenesis of idiopathic macular breaks. Graefes Arch Clin Exp Ophthalmol. 1996;234:425-433.
16. Kim JW, Freeman WR, Azen SP, et al. for the Vitrectomy for Macular Hole Study Group. Prospective randomized trial of vitrectomy or observation for stage 2 macular holes. Am J Ophthalmol 1996; 121:605-614.
17. Gaudric A, Haouchine B, Massin P, et al. Macular hole formation: new data provided by optical coherence tomography. Arch Ophthalmol. 1999; 117:744-751.
18. Haouchine B, Massin P, Gaudric A. Foveal pseudocyst as the first step in macular hole formation: a prospective study by optical coherence tomography. Ophthalmology. 2001;108:15-22.
19. Altaweel, M and Ip, M. Macular hole: improved understanding of pathogenesis, staging, and management based on optical coherence tomography. Semin Ophthalmol. 2002;18:58-66.
20. Azzolini C, Patelli F, Brancato R. Correlation between optical coherence tomography data and biomicroscopic interpretation of idiopathic macular hole. Am J Ophthalmol 2001;132:348-355.
21. Tolentino FI, Schepens CL, Freeman HM. Vitreoretinal Disorders: Diagnosis and Management, Philadelphia, PA: WB Saunders Co.; 1976:400-412.
22. Asrani S, Zeimer R, Goldberg M, et al. Serial optical sectioning of macular holes at different stages of development. Ophthalmology. 1998; 105:66-77.
23. Ezra E, Fariss RN, Possin DE, et al. Immunocytochemical characterization of macular hole opercula. Arch Ophthalmol. 2001; 119:223-231.
24. de Bustros S, The Vitrectomy for Prevention of Macular Hole Study Group. Vitrectomy for prevention of macular holes: results of a randomized multicenter clinical trial. Ophthalmology. 1994;101:1055-1060.
25. Lewis MI, Cohen SM, Smiddy WE, et al. Bilaterality of idiopathic macular holes. Graefes Arch Clin Exp Ophthalmol. 1996; 234:241-245.
26. Smiddy WE, Gass JDM. Masquerades of macular holes. Ophthalmic Surg. 1995; 26:16-24.
27. Kelly NE, Wendel RT. Vitreous surgery for idiopathic macular holes: Results of a pilot study. Arch Ophthalmol. 1991;109:654-659.
28. Ryan EH Jr, Gilbert HD. Results of surgical treatment of recent-onset full-thickness idiopathic macular hole. Arch Ophthalmol. 1994;112:1545-1553.
29. Slaughter K, Lee I. Macular hole surgery with and without indocyanine green assistance. Eye. 2004;18:376-378.
30. Hikichi T, Yoshida A, Akiba J, et al. Natural outcomes of stage 1, 2, 3, and 4 idiopathic macular holes. Br J Ophthalmol. 1995;79:517-520.
31. Kang HK, Chang AA, Beaumont PE. The macular hole: report of an Australian surgical series and meta-analysis of the literature. Clin Exp Ophthalmol. 2000;28:298-308.
32. Ip MS, Baker BJ, Duker JS, et al. Anatomical outcomes of surgery for idiopathic macular hole as determined by optical coherence tomography. Arch Ophthalmol. 2002;120:29-35.
33. Freeman WR, Azen SP, Kim JW, et al. For the Vitrectomy for Treatment of Macular Hole Study Group. Vitrectomy for the treatment of full-thickness stage 3 or 4 macular holes: results of a multicentered randomized clinical trial. Arch Ophthalmol. 1997;115:11-21.
34. Ullrich S, Haritoglou C, Gass C, et al. Macular hole size as a prognostic factor in macular hole surgery. Br J Ophthalmol 2002, 86:390-393.
35. Imai M, Iijima H, Gotoh T, et al. Optical coherence tomography of successfully repaired idiopathic macular holes. Am J Ophthalmol. 1999;128:621-627.
36. Spaide RF. Macular hole repair with minimal vitrectomy. Retina 2002,22:183-186.
37. Costa RA, Cardillo JA, Morales PH, et al. Optical coherence tomography evaluation of idiopathic macular hole treatment by gas-assisted posterior vitreous detachment. Am J Ophthalmol 2001;132:264-266.
38. Chan CK, Wessels IF, Friedrichsen EJ. Treatment of idiopathic macular holes by induced posterior vitreous detachment. Ophthalmology. 1995; 102:757-767.
39. Smiddy WE, Feuer W, Cordahl G. Internal limiting membrane peeling in macular hole surgery. Ophthalmology. 2001;108:1471-1478.
40. Brooks HL Jr. Macular hole surgery with and without internal limiting membrane peeling. Ophthalmology. 2000;107:1939-1949.
41. Kasuga Y, Arai J, Akimoto M, et al. Optical coherence tomography to confirm early closure of macular holes. Am J Ophthalmol. 2000;-130:675-676.
42. Madreperla SA, Geiger GL, Funata M, et al. Clinicopathologic correlation of a macular hole treated by cortical vitreous peeling and gas tamponade. Ophthalmology. 1994;101:682-686.

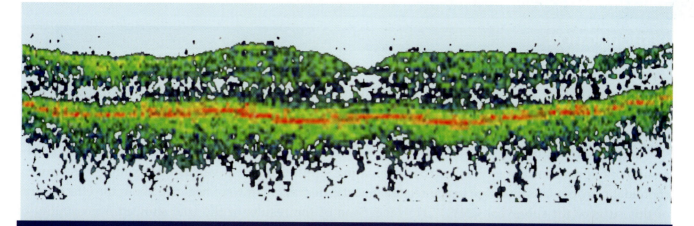

CHAPTER
13

Surgery for Choroidal Neovascular Membrane

Hirokazu Sakaguchi, Masahito Ohji,
Motohiro Kamei, Yasuo Tano

INTRODUCTION

Choroidal neovascular membrane (CNV) caused by several diseases such as age-related macular degeneration (AMD) or myopia is the major cause of legal blindness in developed countries. Various treatments have been attempted, including photocoagulation, photodynamic therapy, surgical removal of CNV, and macular translocation. [1-21] Anti-VEGF aptamer treatment has been also recently approved.

Surgical removal of subfoveal CNV might be effective for classic or predominantly classic CNV. The results of Submacular Surgery Trial (SST) evaluating surgical removal versus observation of subfoveal choroidal neovascularisation due to age-related macular degeneration were negative about the effectiveness of this surgery for subfoveal CNV. [2-4] However, one of the results of the trial showed a possibility of improvement of vision by surgical removal of CNV associated with ocular histoplasmosis. [5]

Macular translocation, in which the fovea is rotated and relocated onto healthier retinal pigment epithelium following creation of an artificial total retinal detachment and 360-degree retinotomy, was first reported by Machemer and Steinhorst in 1993. [6] After the report, several modified surgical techniques, including translocation surgery with partial retinotomy, limited translocation without retinotomy, translocation with scleral out pouching, and translocation with 360-degree retinotomy combined with extraocular muscle surgery have been reported. [7-17] Macular translocation is different from other options in that the goal of this surgery is to improve visual acuity.

In this chapter, we describe the morphological changes of macular structure detected by optical coherence tomography (OCT) after surgical removal of CNV, macular translocation with 360-degree retinotomy or limited macular translocation.

OPTICAL COHERENCE TOMOGRAPHY

The macula in eyes with CNV is characterized by serous retinal detachment, subretinal hemorrhage, macular edema, or serous, hemorrhagic, or fibrovascular pigment epithelial detachment (PED). Therefore, OCT shows the morphological images consistent with the characteristics of these changes. [22-24] The details of OCT images of CNV is described in other chapter, but is briefly described here: Classic CNV is seen as a well-defined, high reflective lesion on retinal pigment epithelium and choriocapillaris. Occult CNV, with fibrovascular PED, presents as a mildly backscattering region below the elevation of the reflective band (retinal pigment epithelium), although retinal pigment epithelium reflectivity may not be found due to CNV. Serous retinal detachment shows as the elevation of reflective structure consistent with the retina and the optically clear space below the retina. Serous PED shows an elevation of the highly reflective band (retinal pigment epithelium) and shadowing of the reflections returning from the deeper choroid. Subretinal hemorrhage shows as bright backscatter corresponding to the accumulation of blood and significant attenuation of the choroidal reflection. Hemorrhagic PED shows as the elevation of the reflective band (retinal pigment epithelium) and bright backscatter corresponding to the accumulation of blood. Macular edema presents as diffuse increase in retinal thickness and reduction in retinal reflectivity. Cystoid space which is corresponding to cystoid macular edema may be found at the macula.

Although surgical removal of subfoveal CNV may not be effective, [2-4] surgical removal of juxtafoveal CNV could achieve a better visual outcome. OCT shows the elevation of retinal reflection and the hyper reflective area below the retina at the macula, which is consistent with CNV resulting from AMD. After the surgery, the elevation of the retina reflection at the macula decreases and the retinal reflective thickness may be reduced because of the reduction of macular edema.

Macular translocation with 360-degree retinotomy and limited macular translocation may be effective for cases with either type of CNV, classic or occult CNV. The fovea is relocated on healthier retinal pigment epithelium after macular translocation, either in macular translocation with 360-degree retinotomy or limited macular translocation. Therefore, in OCT images, the nearly normal retinal reflection is onto normal retinal pigment epithelium reflective band without the reflective lesion representing CNV or PED after the surgeries. The elevation of the reflection before the surgeries due to CNV, PED, or serous retinal detachment, may be bearing down on the almost normal retinal pigment epithelium reflection. Macular translocation with 360-degree retinotomy can achieve a large movement of the fovea and the CNV may not be seen on the same image of OCT including the fovea. On the other hand, the fovea is moved less than 1 disc diameter after limited macular translocation. Therefore, OCT usually detects CNV or other lesions at the same image of OCT including the fovea after the surgery.

After these surgeries, foveal contour may be recovered. Some cases that show cystoid macular edema detected by fluorescein angiography may not show cystoid space in OCT images postoperatively.[25] The newly located macula, or the macula after the CNV removal, may have slight macular edema or subretinal fluid and OCT is effective to detect them as the hyporeflective space. In the follow-up period, enlargement of CNV involving the new fovea may develop after limited translocation. Recurrence of CNV also may be observed in the eyes in which CNV is removed during the surgeries. Optical coherence tomography is also useful to monitor them.

INTERESTING CASE EXAMPLES

Case 1: Surgical Removal of Choroidal Neovascular Membrane

A 76-year-old woman presented with a central gray spot in her left eye for two months prior to examination. She noticed enlargement of this spot over the past two weeks. Her visual acuity in this eye was 10/200 at the first visit. Fundus examination revealed an elevated subretinal lesion superior to the fovea with a small subretinal hemorrhage (Fig. 13.1A). Fluorescein angiography showed a hyperfluorescent lesion at the juxtafoveal area which showed vigorous leakage in the later phases consistent with classic CNV and hyperfluorescence at the area superior temporal to the fovea caused by retinal pigment epithelium damage (Fig. 13.1B).

A vertical OCT image showed a hyper-reflective region including fovea under the retinal reflectivity. Discrepancy between fluorescein angiography and OCT regarding area of CNV could be seen in some cases. The retinal pigment epithelium reflectivity was not clearly shown under CNV. The thickness of the CNV was 650 μm. The fovea had macular edema and the thickness of the fovea was approximately 300 μm (Fig. 13.1C).

The removal of CNV combined with cataract surgery was performed. Fundus examination 6 months after the surgery showed an atrophic area where CNV had existed (Fig. 13.1D). Fluorescein angiography exhibited a window defect at the area of the preexisting CNV which have been probably caused from the damage of the retinal pigment epithelium when the CNV was removed (Fig. 13.1E). The visual acuity improved to 20/100.

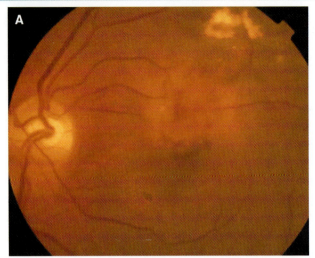

Fig. 13.1A: Case 1. 67-year-old woman with age-related macular degeneration. Fundus photograph of a classic CNV. An elevated subretinal lesion superior to the fovea with a small subretinal hemorrhage is revealed.

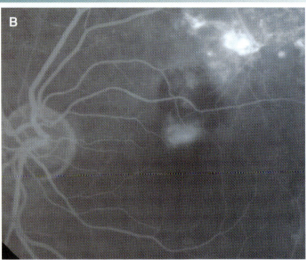

Fig. 13.1B: Fluorescein angiography of the same case. Early fluorescein angiogram shows a hyperfluorescent lesion at the juxtafoveal area which leaked more in the later phases consistent with classic CNV.

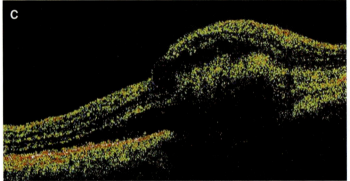

Fig. 13.1C: A vertical OCT image. A hyper-reflective region under the retinal reflectivity which is corresponding to the CNV is detected. Interestingly, the CNV located under the fovea in the OCT image while it located juxtafoveally in fluorescein angiography. The retinal pigment epithelium reflectivity is not clearly shown. The thickness of the CNV is 650 μm. The fovea has reduced intraretinal optical reflectivity which is caused from retinal edema and the thickness of the fovea is 300 μm.

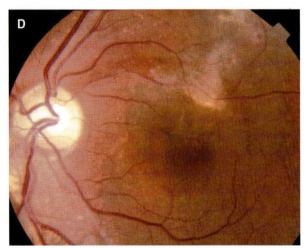

Fig. 13.1D: Fundus photograph 6 months after surgical removal of CNV combined with cataract surgery. An atrophic area where CNV existed is shown.

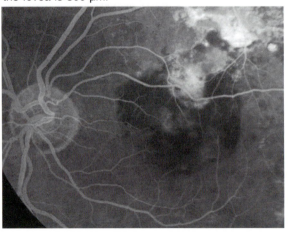

Fig. 13.1E: Fluorescein angiography at early phase exhibits a window defect at the location of the CNV which have been probably caused from the damage of the retinal pigment epithelium when the CNV was removed.

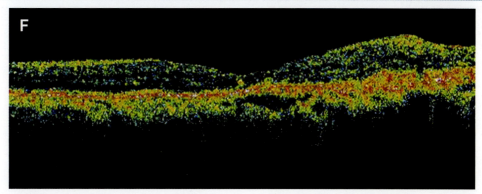

Fig. 13.1F: A vertical OCT image. OCT reveals no CNV reflection and the clearly reduced elevation of the retina. The thickness of the retinal reflectivity reduces to 110 μm and the foveal decompression is recovered. Reflectivity of retinal pigment epithelium-choroid complex at area where CNV existed is increased. This high reflectivity is probably caused by scar formation.

An OCT revealed no CNV reflection and the clearly reduced elevation of the retina. The thickness of the retina reduced to 110 μm and the foveal contour was recovered. Reflectivity of retinal pigment epithelium-choroid complex at area where CNV existed was increased. This high reflectivity was probably caused by scar formation (Fig. 13.1F)

Case 2: Macular Translocation with 360-degree Retinotomy

A 55-year-old woman was referred for evaluation of CNV due to high myopia in her right eye. Her visual acuity was 20/100 at the first visit. Fundus examination revealed a subretinal round gray lesion with subretinal hemorrhage at the fovea (Fig. 13.2A). The early angiographic image revealed a well-defined area of hyperfluorescence. There was diffuse leakage in the late angiographic image (Fig. 13.2B). A vertical OCT image showed an elevation of the retinal reflectivity and hyper reflective lesion under the retina which was corresponding to a CNV. The thickness of the CNV was approximately 330 μm and the thickness of the slightly swollen fovea was 360 μm (Fig. 13.2C).

Macular translocation with 360-degree retinotomy was performed and CNV was removed during the surgery. The fundus photograph 12 months after the surgery showed the rotation of the retina by approximately 40 degree (Fig. 13.2D). The visual acuity was improved to 20/40. A vertical OCT image showed no elevation of the retinal reflectivity. The foveal contour was recovered and the thickness of the retina was reduced to 200 μm. The reflectivity of the retinal pigment epithelium and choroid under the new fovea was normal (Fig. 13.2E).

Case 3: Limited Macular Translocation

A 49-year-old woman was referred for evaluation of idiopathic CNV in her right eye. Her visual acuity was 20/100 at the first visit. Slit-lamp biomicroscopy showed a subretinal well-defined yellowish lesion at the fovea and subretinal hemorrhage (Fig. 13.3A). Fluorescein angiography showed early hyperfluorescence and late leakage and blockage of fluorescein angiography by subretinal hemorrhage (Fig. 13.3B). This was a classic CNV. A vertical OCT image showed a hyper-reflective region which is corresponding to the CNV under the retinal reflectivity at the subfoveal area. The thickness of the CNV was 170 μm. The thickness of the foveal reflectivity including edema was 370 μm (Fig. 13.3C).

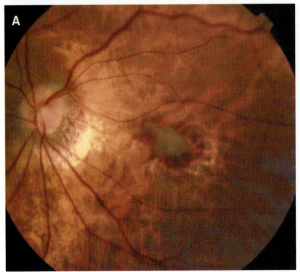

Fig. 13.2A: Fundus photograph in the right eye of Case 2. A round gray lesion with subretinal hemorrhage at the fovea is revealed.

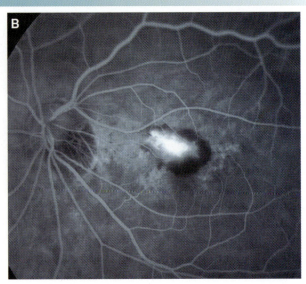

Fig. 13.2B: Early phase fluorescein angiography. The early angiographic image reveals a well-defined area of hyperfluorescence.

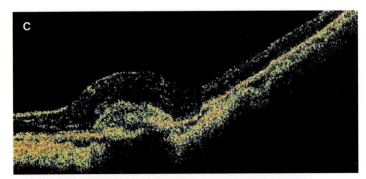

Fig. 13.2C: A vertical OCT image. Optical coherence tomography shows an elevation of the retinal reflectivity and hyper-reflective lesion under the retina which is corresponding to a CNV. The thickness of the CNV is approximately 330 µm and the thickness of the swollen fovea is 360 µm.

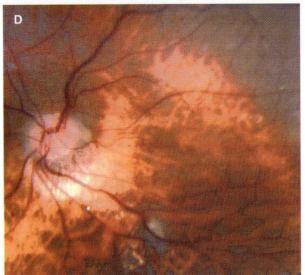

Fig. 13.2D: Fundus photograph 12 months shows the rotation of the retina by approximately 40 degree after macular translocation with 360-degree retinotomy.

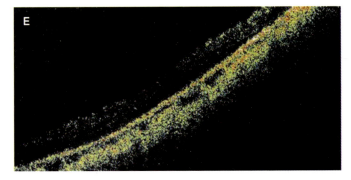

Fig. 13.2E: A vertical OCT image. Optical coherence tomography shows no elevation of the retinal reflectivity. The decompression of the fovea is recovered and the thickness of the retina is reduced to 200 µm. The reflectivity of the retinal pigment epithelium and choroid under the new fovea is normal.

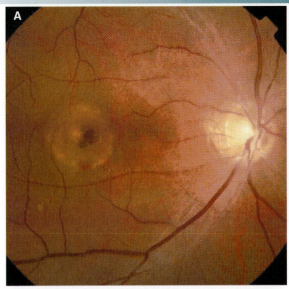

Fig. 13.3A: Fundus examination shows a well-defined round yellowish lesion at the fovea and subretinal hemorrhage.

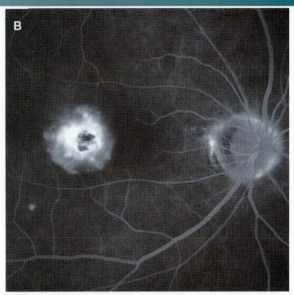

Fig. 13.3B: Fluorescein angiography. Fluorescein angiogram shows early hyperfluorescence and late staining. This is a classic CNV.

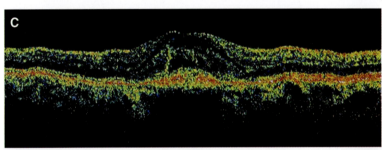

Fig. 13.3C: A vertical OCT image. It shows a hyper-reflective region which is corresponding to the CNV under the retinal reflectivity. The thickness of the CNV is 170 μm. The retina is swollen and its thickness is measured 370 μm.

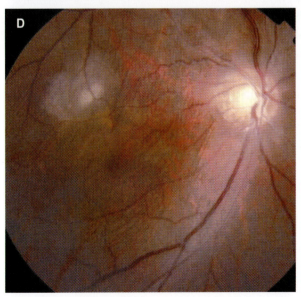

Fig. 13.3D: Fundus photograph 3 months after limited macular translocation. It reveals that the fovea is slightly moved to the area inferiorly to the CNV.

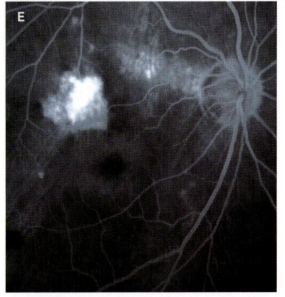

Fig. 13.3E: Fluorescein angiography. Fluorescein angiogram also shows the movement of the fovea inferiorly to the CNV.

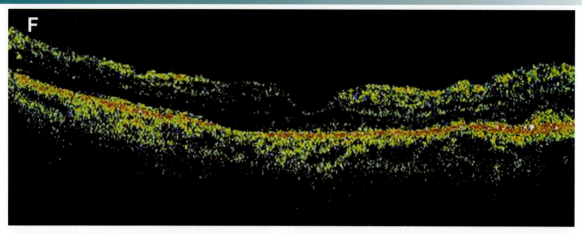

Fig. 13.3F: A vertical OCT image after the surgery. OCT shows a hyper-reflective region which is corresponding to the CNV under the retinal reflectivity. The location of the fovea is moved toward inferiorly to the one measured preoperatively. The thickness of the foveal reflectivity is reduced to 125 µm, and there is an obvious foveal contour.

Limited macular translocation was performed. A fundus photograph (Fig. 13.3D) and fluorescein angiography (Fig. 13.3E) at 6 months after the surgery, revealed that the fovea moved inferiorly to the CNV. The visual acuity was maintained at 20/100. A vertical OCT image showed a hyper-reflective region which was corresponding to the CNV under the retinal reflectivity superior to the fovea (arrow, Fig 3F). The location of the fovea was moved toward inferiorly (toward left side, Fig. 13.3F). The contour of fovea recovered and the foveal thickness was reduced to 125 µm (Fig. 13.3F).

Case 4: Limited Macular Translocation with Choroidal Neovascular Membrane Removal

A 70-year-old woman was referred for evaluation of CNV in her right eye. Her visual acuity was 20/150 at the first visit. Slit-lamp biomicroscopy showed a subfoveal well-defined round yellowish lesion at the fovea (Fig. 13.4A). An early angiographic image showed a well-defined small round hyperfluorescence and fluorescein leakage was evident in a late angiographic image (Fig. 13.4B).

A vertical OCT image showed a hyper reflective region of CNV under the retinal reflectivity of the fovea. The thickness of the CNV was 290 µm and the thickness of the fovea was 90 µm. No cystic space was detected (Fig. 13.4C).

Limited macular translocation was performed and CNV was removed during surgery. The fundus photograph showed the movement of the fovea inferiorly and area from where the CNV was removed became atrophic after the surgery (Fig. 13.4D). Fluorescein angiogram also revealed that the fovea was moved inferiorly (Fig. 13.4E). Fluorescein leakage was found at area where CNV remained. The visual acuity was improved to 20/100. A vertical OCT image showed the movement of the fovea on the normal retinal pigment epithelium and the elevation of the retina was reduced. No CNV reflection was detected. Foveal contour was recovered and the foveal thickness reduced to 161 µm (Fig. 13.4F).

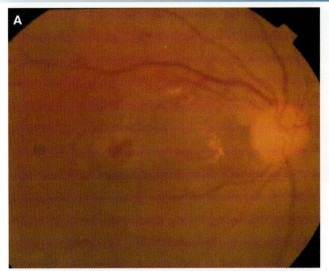

Fig. 13.4A: Fundus photograph of a CNV in Case 4. Slit-lamp biomicroscopy shows a subretinal well-defined round yellowish lesion at the fovea.

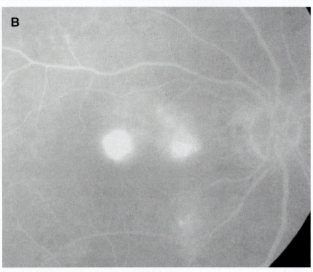

Fig. 13.4B: Fluorescein angiography at the late phase. An early angiographic image shows a well-defined small round hyperfluorescence and leakage is evident in a late angiographic image.

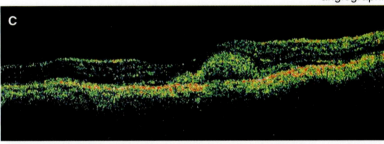

Fig. 13.4C: A vertical OCT image. Optical coherence tomography shows a hyper-reflective region which is corresponding to the CNV under the retinal reflectivity. The thickness of the CNV is 290 μm and the thickness of the fovea is 90 μm. No cystic space is detected.

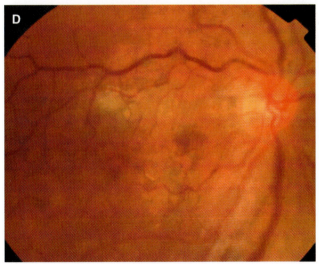

Fig. 13.4D: At 6 months after the limited macular translocation combined with CNV removal, the fundus photograph shows the movement of the fovea inferiorly and area from where the CNV was removed became atrophic.

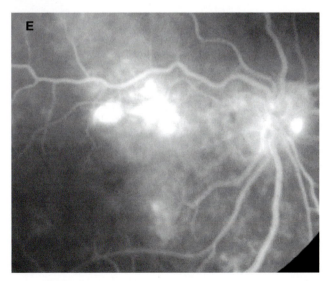

Fig. 13.4E: Fluorescein angiogram also reveals that the fovea is moved inferiorly. Fluorescein leakage is found at area where CNV remained.

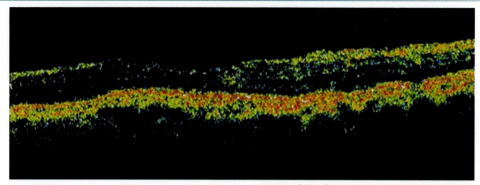

Fig. 13.4F: A vertical OCT image shows the movement of the fovea above the normal RPE and the elevation of the retinal reflectivity is reduced. A hyper-reflective region, which is corresponding to the CNV, under the retinal reflectivity is detected. Foveal contour has recovered and the foveal thickness of the fovea has recovered to 161 μm.

REFERENCES

1. Macular Photocoagulation Study Group. Laser photocoagulation of subfoveal neovascular lesions in age-related macular degeneration. Results of a randomized clinical trial. Arch Ophthalmol. 1991;109:1220-1231.
2. Hawkins BS, Bressler NM, Miskala PH, et al. Submacular Surgery Trials (SST) Research Group. Surgery for subfoveal choroidal neovascularization in age-related macular degeneration: ophthalmic findings: SST Report No. 11. Ophthalmology. 2004; 111:1967-1980.
3. Bressler NM, Bressler SB, Childs AL, et al. Submacular Surgery Trials (SST) Research Group. Surgery for hemorrhagic choroidal neovascular lesions of age-related macular degeneration: ophthalmic findings: SST report no. 13. Ophthalmology. 2004; 111:1993-2006.
4. Brindeau C, Glacet-Bernard A, Coscas F, et al. Surgical removal of subfoveal choroidal neovascularization: visual outcome and prognostic value of fluorescein angiography and optical coherence tomography. Eur J Ophthalmol 2001; 11:287-95.
5. Hawkins BS, Bressler NM, Bressler SB, et al; Submacular Surgery Trials Research Group. Surgical removal vs observation for subfoveal choroidal neovascularization, either associated with the ocular histoplasmosis syndrome or idiopathic: I. Ophthalmic findings from a randomized clinical trial: Submacular Surgery Trials (SST) Group H Trial: SST Report No. 9. Arch Ophthalmol 2004; 122:1597-1611.
6. Machemer R, Steinhorst UH. Retinal separation, retinotomy, and macular relocation: II. A surgical approach for age-related macular degeneration? Graefes Arch Clin Exp Ophthalmol. 1993; 231:635-41.
7. Ninomiya Y, Lewis JM, Hasegawa T, Tano Y. Retinotomy and foveal translocation for surgical management of subfoveal choroidal neovascular membranes. Am J Ophthalmol. 1996; 122:613-621.
8. Fujikado T, Ohji M, Hayashi A, et al. Anatomic and functional recovery of the fovea after foveal translocation surgery without large retinotomy and simultaneous excision of a neovascular membrane. Am J Ophthalmol. 1998; 126:839-842.
9. Wolf S, Lappas A, Weinberger AW, Kirchhof B. Macular translocation for surgical management of subfoveal choroidal neovascularizations in patients with AMD: first results. Graefes Arch Clin Exp Ophthalmol. 1999; 237:51-57.
10. Eckardt C, Eckardt U, Conrad HG. Macular rotation with and without counter-rotation of the globe in patients with age-related macular degeneration. Graefes Arch Clin Exp Ophthalmol. 1999;237:313-325.
11. Cekic O, Ohji M, Hayashi A, et al. Foveal translocation surgery in age-related macular degeneration. Lancet. 1999; 354(9175):340.
12. Lewis H, Kaiser PK, Lewis S, Estafanous M. Macular translocation for subfoveal choroidal neovascularization in age-related macular degeneration: a prospective study. Am J Ophthalmol. 1999; 128:135-146.
13. de Juan E Jr, Vander JF. Effective macular translocation without scleral imbrication. Am J Ophthalmol. 1999;128:380-382.
14. Lewis H. Macular translocation with chorioscleral outfolding: a pilot clinical study. Am J Ophthalmol. 2001;132:156-163.
15. Ohji M, Fujikado T, Kusaka S, et al. Comparison of three techniques of foveal translocation in patients with subfoveal choroidal neovascularization resulting from age-related macular degeneration. Am J Ophthalmol. 2001;132:888-896.
16. Tano Y. Pathologic myopia: where are we now. Am J Ophthalmol. 2002;134:645-60.
17. Kamei M, Tano Y, Yasuhara T, et al. Macular translocation with chorioscleral outfolding: 2-year results. Am J Ophthalmol. 2004; 138:574-581.
18. Treatment of age-related macular degeneration with photodynamic therapy (TAP) Study Group. Photodynamic therapy of subfoveal choroidal neovascularization in age-related macular degeneration with verteporfin: one-year results of 2 randomized clinical trials—TAP report 1. Arch Ophthalmol 1999;117:1329-1345.
19. Treatment of age-related macular degeneration with photodynamic therapy (TAP) Study Group. Photodynamic therapy of subfoveal choroidal neovascularization in age-related macular degeneration with verteporfin: two-year results of 2 randomized clinical trials—TAP report 2. Arch Ophthalmol 2001;119:198-207.
20. Treatment of age-related macular degeneration with photodynamic therapy (TAP) Study Group. Verteporfin therapy of subfoveal choroidal neovascularization in age-related macular degeneration with verteporfin: additional information regarding baseline lesion composition's impact on vision outcomes—TAP report No. 3. Arch Ophthalmol 2002;120:1443-1454.
21. Verteporfin In Photodynamic Therapy Study Group. Verteporfin therapy of subfoveal choroidal neovascularization in age-related macular degeneration: two-year results of a randomized clinical trial including lesions with occult with no classic choroidal neovascularization-Verteporfin in photodynamic therapy report 2. Am J Ophthalmol. 2001;131:541-560.

22. Hee MR, Baumal CR, Puliafito CA, et al. Optical coherence tomography of age-related macular degeneration and choroidal neovascularization. Ophthalmology. 1996;103:1260-1270.
23. Puliafito CA, Hee MR, Schuman JS, et al. Macular degeneration. In: Puliafito CA, Hee MR, Schuman JS, Fujimoto JG, eds. Optical coherence tomography of ocular diseases. New Jersey, SLACK incorporated. 1996: 187-246.
24. Giovannini A, Amato G, Mariotti C, Scassellati-Sforzolini B. Optical coherence tomography in the assessment of retinal pigment epithelial tear. Retina 2000;20:37-40.
25. Terasaki H, Ishikawa K, Suzuki T, et al. Morphologic and angiographic assessment of the macula after macular translocation surgery with 360-degree retinotomy. Am J Ophthalmol 2003;110: 2403-2408.

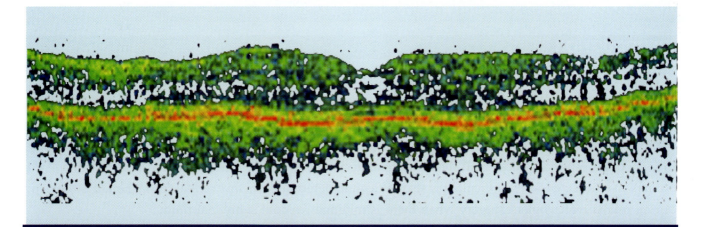

CHAPTER

14

Macula after Retinal Detachment Surgery

Takayuki Baba

INTRODUCTION

In rhegmatogenous retinal detachment, the neurosensory retina is separated from the retinal pigment epithelium. When the retinal detachment involves the macula, severe visual impairment occurs. Treatment for retinal detachment consists of closing the retinal breaks and reattaching the detached retina. Fundus examination with indirect binocular ophthalmoscopy is essential before and after retinal detachment surgery. In some cases, especially those with shallow retinal detachment, the diagnosis of retinal detachment and the estimation of its extension is difficult. It is also difficult to determine whether retinal reattachment is achieved during retinal reattachment surgery when there is minimal residual subretinal fluid. [1-3]

OPTICAL COHERENCE TOMOGRAPHY

Anatomy

With optical coherence tomography (OCT), the normal neurosensory retina is observed as a continuous layer of highly-reflective retinal pigment epithelium. The inner layer of the neurosensory retina is highly-reflective and the outer layer has low-reflectivity. The outer layer, which includes photoreceptor cells, is observed as a dark-colored layer in a false-color representation scale, but not black, which indicates almost no optical reflectivity.

Pathogenesis

In retinal detachment, there is an accumulation of subretinal fluid between the neurosensory retina and retinal pigment epithelium. This pathology was determined from experimental retinal detachment in an animal model.[4] Histopathologic study of retinal detachment is not applicable to in vivo studies, especially in acute retinal detachment cases. Thus, OCT is a highly advantageous technique for in vivo studies. With OCT, subretinal fluid is observed as a low- to non-reflective layer between two highly-reflective layers,[5] the neurosensory retina and the retinal pigment epithelium (Figs 14.1B and 14.7B). Each border of the subretinal fluid is so distinct that differential diagnosis from retinal edema is relatively easy. This OCT finding of subretinal fluid is sometimes called 'optically clear space'.

The detached neurosensory retina has specific characteristics.[6] The OCT findings of detached neurosensory retina are normal (40%), intraretinal separation (28%, Fig. 14.1B), and intraretinal separation with an undulated outer layer (32%). Patients with intraretinal separation and undulation have poor visual acuity. Hagimura and associates [6] reported that patients with a highly detached retina also had severely impaired vision. Intraretinal separation is rapidly resolved after successful retinal reattachment surgery (Fig. 14.1D).

Treatment

The main surgical procedure to repair retinal detachment is scleral buckling and vitrectomy, depending on the case specifics and the surgeon's experience. Optical coherence tomography is useful to disclose a slight elevation of the neurosensory retina in cases with very shallow retinal detachment. It is sometimes difficult

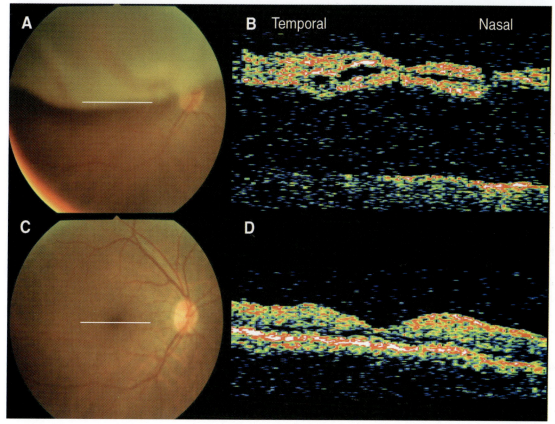

Fig. 14.1: The right eye of a 58-year-old man with macula-off rhegmatogenous retinal detachment. Preoperative visual acuity was 0.3 with a refractive error of -1 diopters. A. Preoperative fundus photograph. B. Preoperative OCT image. Retinal elevation and intraretinal separation around the fovea were observed. C. Postoperative fundus photograph. Two weeks after scleral buckling, the macula was completely reattached and visual acuity was 0.6. D. OCT image 2 weeks after operation. The neurosensory retina was completely reattached and the intraretinal clear space observed preoperatively had disappeared.

to diagnose shallow retinal detachment in a highly myopic eye with severe macular atrophy because of the low contrast between the detached retina and the retinal pigment epithelium. For the same reason, it is difficult to detect retinal detachment of ocular albinism and sunset-fundus after Vogt-Koyanagi-Harada disease (Fig. 14.2). In such cases, shallow retinal detachment can be detected clearly with OCT.

Monitoring

In cases of macula-off rhegmatogenous retinal detachment, the macula is as observed with ophthalmoscopy to be flat after successful retinal reattachment surgery. Pre- and postoperative OCT provides useful information in rhegmatogenous retinal detachment cases. Soon after surgery, some macula-off retinal detachment cases have a completely reattached macula with no subretinal fluid detected with OCT (Fig. 14.3).

On the other hand, OCT can detect even a small amount of residual subretinal fluid, which is difficult to determine using ophthalmoscopy postoperatively (Fig. 14.4D). In our experience, acute macula-off rhegmatogenous retinal detachment has a favorable postoperative visual recovery, even if there is residual

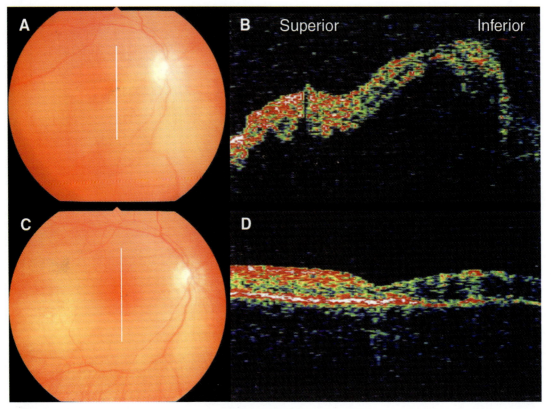

Fig. 14.2: The left eye of a 45-year-old woman with macula-off rhegmatogenous retinal detachment originating from a peripheral tractional tear. In the peripheral retina, Dalen-Fuchs spots were scattered. Preoperative visual acuity was hand movement. The duration of macula-off retinal detachment was estimated to 5 days. A. Preoperative fundus photograph. Due to the bright fundus ("sunset-like fundus") after Vogt-Koyanagi-Harada disease, whether retinal detachment involved the macula or not was unclear. B. Preoperative OCT image. The retinal detachment involved the macula. Because of poor fixation, an OCT scan was performed under a fundus monitor. There was so much subretinal fluid that the retinal pigment epithelium was not observed with OCT. C. Fundus photograph 2 weeks after scleral buckling. Visual acuity recovered to 0.2. D. OCT image 2 weeks after operation. No subretinal clear space was observed. The OCT signal inferior to the fovea was decreased due to the small pupil size and vitreous opacity.

subretinal fluid at the macula. In our patients, there was less than 1 week between acknowledgment of central visual loss and retinal reattachment surgery; a longer duration of macula-off retinal detachment might influence the degenerative changes of the neurosensory retina and result in a poor visual prognosis. Whether this accumulation of residual subretinal fluid influences postoperative visual recovery is not clear, [1-3] therefore follow-up examination with OCT is important. Residual subretinal fluid can take over 1 year to be absorbed completely after successful scleral buckling surgery (Fig. 14.4F).

Rarely, after successful retinal detachment surgery with no postoperative subfoveal fluid confirmed by OCT, a very small amount of subfoveal fluid accumulation occurs during the postoperative period (Fig. 14.5F). In this case, there was no subjective visual acuity loss or decreased vision. The reason for the subfoveal fluid recurrence is unknown. The migration of subretinal fluid in the peripheral retina might contribute to this phenomenon.

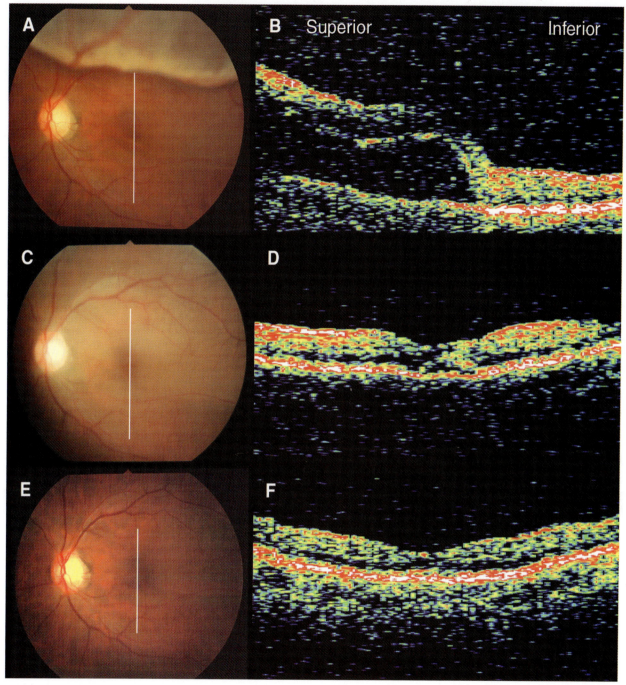

Fig. 14.3: The left eye of a 49-year-old man with macula-off rhegmatogenous retinal detachment. Preoperative visual acuity was 0.08 with a refractive error of −10 diopters. The duration of macula-off retinal detachment was 3 days. A. Preoperative fundus photograph. B. Preoperative OCT image. The retinal detachment involved the macula. C. Fundus photograph 3 months after scleral buckling. Visual acuity was 1.0. D. OCT image 3 months after surgery. No subretinal clear space was observed and foveal configuration was almost normal. E. Fundus photograph 1 year after operation. Visual acuity was 0.8. F. OCT image 1 year after the operation. No subretinal fluid was observed.

Apart from rhegmatogenous retinal detachment involving the macula, subretinal fluid at the macula is postoperatively detected in some cases of retinal detachment with a preoperatively spared macula. Theodossiadis and associates[7] reported that subretinal fluid in a preoperatively uninvolved macula is also sometimes observed after successful scleral buckling and some cases with postoperative accumulation of subfoveal fluid had decreased visual acuity that did not return to the preoperative level. They mentioned that the location of the postoperative subfoveal fluid moved since the original retinal detachment.

A macular pucker sometimes appears several weeks to months after retinal reattachment surgery. As its severity varies, the proliferation and subsequent contraction of thick epiretinal membrane causes visual impairment with metamorphopsia. The OCT findings of a macular pucker is a thickened neurosensory retina with a highly-reflective innermost layer corresponding to the epiretinal membrane (Fig. 14.6D). The foveal pit is sometimes not observed. The thickness of the neurosensory retina can be reduced and foveal configuration becomes almost normal after membrane peeling.

Cystoid macular edema occurs after retinal reattachment surgery. Macular detachment, increased duration of macular detachment, cryotherapy, and pseudophakia are suspected risk factors of cystoid macular edema.[8] The OCT image of cystoid macular edema after retinal detachment surgery is characterized by increased retinal thickness and multiple small intraretinal clear spaces (Fig. 14.7E). The OCT image of an intraretinal cyst is similar to that of cystoid macular edema of diabetic maculopathy or uveitis.[9]

Relevant Study

Subclinical subfoveal fluid is often detected with OCT after scleral procedures in macula-off rhegmatogenous retinal detachment. After vitrectomy with fluid-gas exchange in such retinal detachment cases, complete foveal reattachment can be confirmed with OCT. It is reported to be achieved faster after vitrectomy than after scleral buckling.[10]

INTERESTING CASE EXAMPLE

Macular Hole Retinal Detachment in High Myopia

A case of retinal detachment due to a macular hole in a highly myopic eye is presented.[11] A 65-year-old Japanese woman presented with visual disturbances and metamorphopsia in her left eye. Her visual acuity was 0.02 in the left eye with a refractive error of –12 diopters. A one-quarter disc diameter macular hole was observed in the posterior staphyloma (Fig. 14.8). Optical coherence tomography disclosed retinal detachment due to a macular hole (Fig. 14.8B). The patient underwent retinal reattachment surgery using a macular silicone explant.[12] The OCT image 3 days after surgery revealed a macular hole on the protrusion of the buckle and decreased subretinal fluid (Fig. 14.8D). There was some subretinal fluid for several months. The OCT image 6 months after surgery revealed retinal reattachment around the macular hole with minimal subretinal fluid surrounding the protrusion of the buckle (Fig. 14.8F). Though the macular hole itself was not closed, visual acuity improved to 0.2.

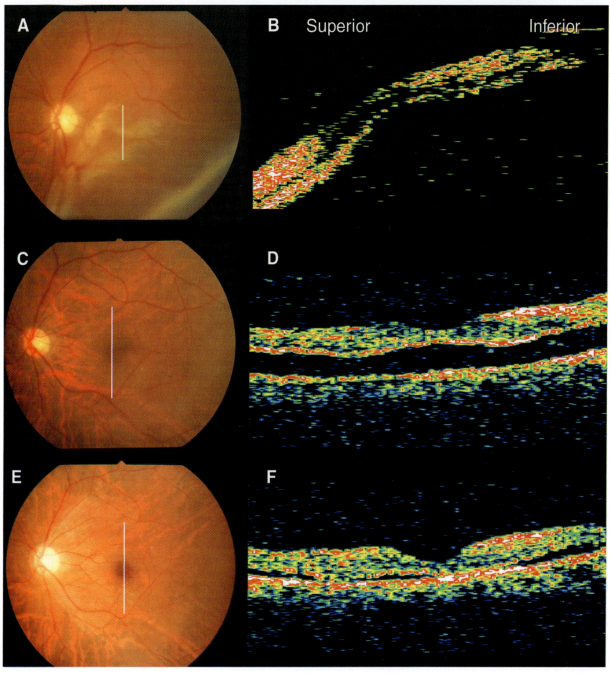

Fig. 14.4: The left eye of a 44-year-old man with macula-off rhegmatogenous retinal detachment. Preoperative visual acuity was 0.05 with a refractive error of −7 diopters. The duration of macula-off retinal detachment was 4 days. A. Preoperative fundus photograph. B. Preoperative OCT image. The retinal detachment involved the macula. There was too much subretinal fluid to observe either the neurosensory retina or the retinal pigment epithelium. C. Fundus photograph 3 months after scleral buckling. The macula was ophthalmoscopically reattached. Visual acuity was 0.3. D. OCT image 3 months after surgery. Thin subretinal clear space was observed. E. Fundus photograph 1 year after surgery. Visual acuity was 0.9. F. OCT image 1 year after surgery. The subretinal clear space was diminished with very limited subretinal fluid.

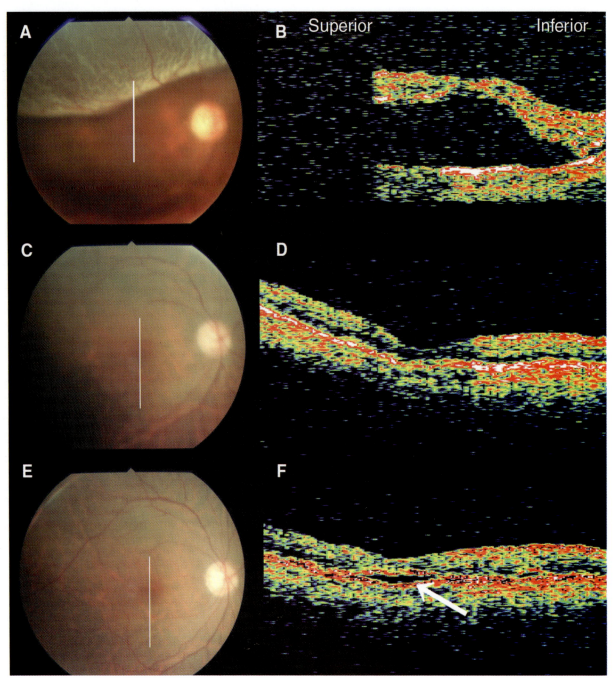

Fig. 14.5: The right eye of a 56-year-old man with macula-off rhegmatogenous retinal detachment. Preoperative visual acuity was 0.01 with a refractive error of –9 diopters. The duration of macula-off retinal detachment was 2 days. A. Preoperative fundus photograph. B. Preoperative OCT image. The retinal detachment involves the macula. The retinal detachment was so bullous that the detached neurosensory retina superior to the macula was out of range. C. Fundus photograph 1 month after scleral buckling. The macula was reattached and visual acuity was 0.7. D. OCT image 1 month after operation. The subretinal clear space observed preoperatively had disappeared. Foveal configuration was almost normal. E. Fundus photograph 3 months after operation. No subretinal fluid was observed ophthalmoscopically and visual acuity was 0.7. F. OCT image 3 months after operation. A very limited subretinal clear space emerged at the subfovea (arrow).

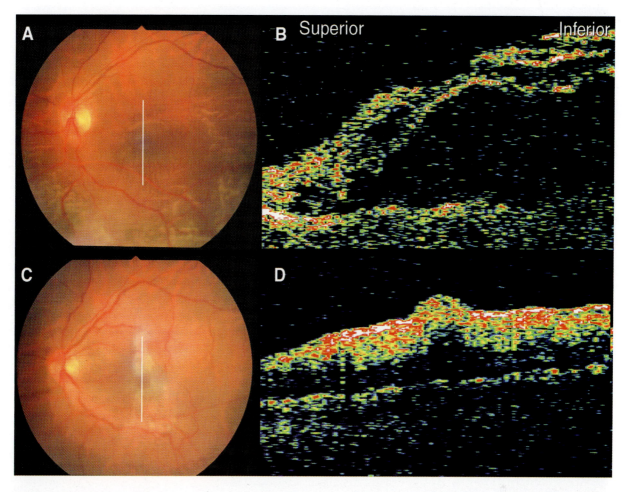

Fig. 14.6: The right eye of a 53-year-old man with a macula-off rhegmatogenous retinal detachment. Preoperative visual acuity was 0.1 with a refractive error of −4 diopters. A. Preoperative fundus photograph. B. Preoperative OCT image. The foveal retina was elevated due to inferior retinal detachment. C. Postoperative fundus photograph. Two months after scleral buckling, apparent epiretinal membrane ("macular pucker") occurred and visual acuity was 0.1. D. OCT image 2 months after operation. The neurosensory retina was thickened and the foveal pit disappeared. The innermost layer of the neurosensory retina was highly-reflective and the fovea protruded conversely to a normal configuration.

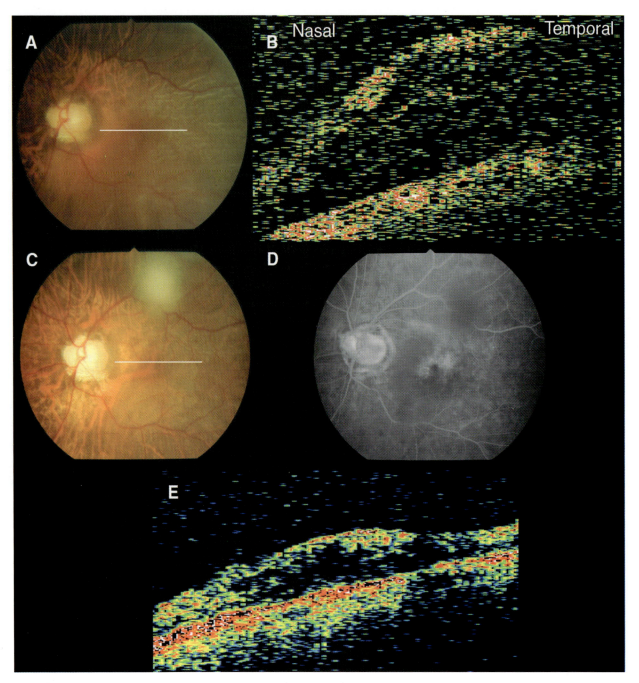

Fig. 14.7: The left eye of a 63-year-old man with macula-off rhegmatogenous retinal detachment. Preoperative visual acuity was 0.1 with a refractive error of –5 diopters. A. Preoperative fundus photograph. B. Preoperative OCT image. Though the OCT image was difficult to obtain due to vitreous hemorrhage, foveal retinal elevation was demonstrated. C. Postoperative fundus photograph. Six months after scleral buckling, macular edema occurred and the visual acuity was 0.3. D. Fluorescein fundus angiography. Cystoid macular edema was observed at the late stage of angiography. E. OCT image 6 months after operation. The neurosensory retina was thickened and multiple small intraretinal cysts were observed.

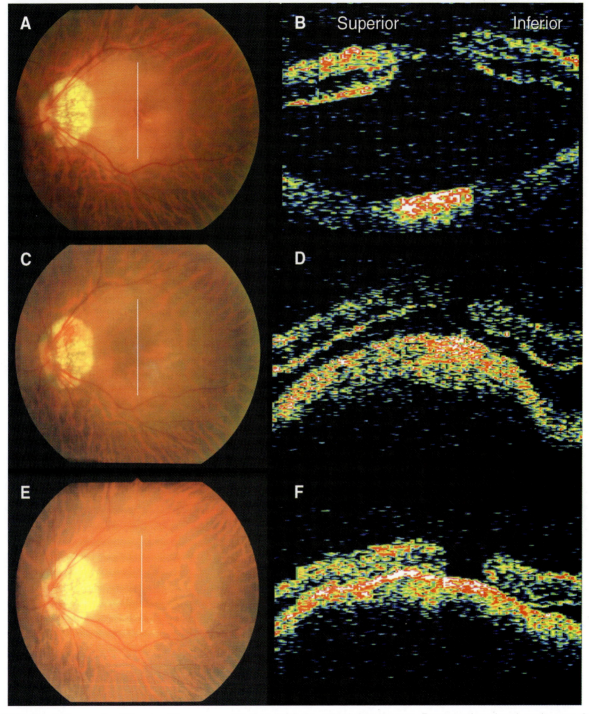

Fig. 14.8: The left eye of a 65-year-old woman with macular hole retinal detachment. Preoperative visual acuity was 0.02 with a refractive error of −12D. A. Preoperative fundus photograph, showing a macular hole accompanied by a limited retinal detachment in the posterior staphyloma. B. Preoperative OCT image. A macular hole and a retinal detachment were observed. C. Fundus photograph 3 days after macular buckling. D. OCT image of the macular hole 3 days after macular buckling. The macular hole on the protrusion of the buckle and decreased subretinal fluid was observed, and the visual acuity was 0.04. E. Fundus photograph 6 months after surgery. F. OCT image 6 months after surgery. The thin layer of clear space observed just after surgery disappeared around the macular hole and visual acuity was improved to 0.2.

REFERENCES

1. Hagimura N, Iida T, Suto K, Kishi S. Persistent foveal retinal detachment after successful rhegmatogenous retinal detachment surgery. Am J Ophthalmol. 2002;133:516-520.
2. Wolfensberger TJ, Gonvers M. Optical coherence tomography in the evaluation of incomplete visual acuity recovery after macula-off retinal detachments. Graefe's Arch Clin Exp Ophthalmol. 2002;240: 85-89.
3. Baba T, Hirose A, Moriyama M, Mochizuki M. Tomographic image and visual recovery of acute macula-off rhegmatogenous retinal detachment. Graefe's Arch Clin Exp Ophthalmol. 2004;242: 576-581.
4. Machemer R. Experimental retinal detachment in the owl monkey. II. Histology of retina and pigment epithelium. Am J Ophthalmol 1968; 66: 396-410.
5. Ip MS, Garza-Karren C, Duker JS, et al. Differentiation of degenerative retinoschisis from retinal detachment using optical coherence tomography. Ophthalmology. 1999;106:600-605.
6. Hagimura N, Suto K, Iida T, Kishi S. Optical coherence tomography of the neurosensory retina in rhegmatogenous retinal detachment. Am J Ophthalmol 2000;129:186-190.
7. Theodossiadis PG, Georgalas IG, Emfietzoglou J, et al. Optical coherence tomography findings in the macula after treatment of rhegmatogenous retinal detachments with spared macula preoperatively. Retina 2003;23:69-75.
8. Sabates NR, Sabates FN, Sabates R, et al. Macular changes after retinal detachment surgery. Am J Ophthalmol. 1989;108:22-29.
9. Antcliff RJ, Stanford MR, Chauhan DS, et al. Comparison between optical coherence tomography and fundus fluorescein angiography for the detection of cystoid macular edema in patients with uveitis. Ophthalmology 2000;107:593-559.
10. Wolfensberger TJ. Foveal reattachment after macula-off retinal detachment occurs faster after vitrectomy than after buckle surgery. Ophthalmology. 2004;111:1340-1343.
11. Baba T, Hirose A, Kawazoe Y, Mochizuki M. Optical coherence tomography for retinal detachment with a macular hole in a highly myopic eye. Ophthalmic Surg Lasers Imaging 2003;34:483-483.
12. Ando F. Use of a special macular explant in surgery for retinal detachment with macular hole. Jpn J Ophthalmol 1980;24:29-34.

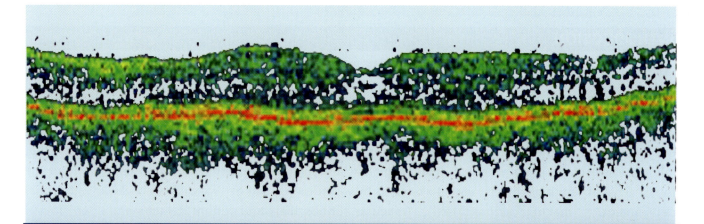

CHAPTER

15

Myopic Foveoschisis

Yasushi Ikuno, Yasuo Tano

INTRODUCTION

Myopic foveoschisis was first reported as a macular detachment without a retinal hole specific to high myopia almost 50 years ago.[1] Myopic foveoschisis was diagnosed as a retinal detachment but not as retinoschisis using a conventional observational system available at that time. Recent improvements in instrumentation including development of optical coherence tomography (OCT) demonstrate more precisely the architecture of the posterior retina in myopic foveoschisis. Using OCT, investigators reported that myopic foveoschisis is not a retinal detachment but a foveal detachment with retinoschisis around the fovea.[2] Several terms have been used to refer to this condition, such as "foveal retinoschisis and retinal detachment",[2] "macular retinoschisis",[3] "macular retinoschisis and retinal detachment",[4] or" foveal detachment and retinoschisis"[5] ; however, in this chapter we use the phrase "myopic foveoschisis," as we have done in previously published studies.[6-9]

OPTICAL COHERENCE TOMOGRAPHY

Anatomy of Myopic Foveoschisis

Myopic foveoschisis is specific to high myopia, which generally is defined as a refractive error greater than –8.0 diopters. The chief complaints at presentation include visual loss, metamorphopsia, relative central scotoma, or all of these; however, some patients can be asymptomatic. The incidence of myopic foveoschisis has been reported to be 10% of highly myopic patients with posterior staphyloma.[10] Optical coherence tomography is an essential tool for diagnosing myopic foveoschisis, because establishing this diagnosis is often difficult when only a conventional slit lamp-based examination is performed.

There are several subtypes of myopic foveoschisis based on retinal morphology including the presence of either a foveal detachment, a lamellar hole, or a macular hole (Fig. 15.1).[3,9] Spontaneous resolution, probably resulting from posterior vitreous detachment may occur;[11] however we believe that this is very rare.

Pathogenesis

The mechanism by which myopic foveoschisis develops is still controversial. At first, vitreous traction on the retina was thought to be a primary cause[2]; however, ultrastructural study of internal limiting membranes excised during vitrectomy performed to treat myopic foveoschisis showed cell migration into the inner retinal surface and consequent development of proliferative tissue.[7] This finding suggests that the tractional force of the epiretinal membrane may cause myopic foveoschisis. Recent studies using OCT have provided more information and indicated that different subtypes of myopic foveoschisis may have processes specific to their development. For instance, local posterior vitreous detachment at the posterior retina as well as a preretinal strand between the edge of the macular hole and the posterior vitreous surface often are observed in myopic foveoschisis in which a macular hole develops.[8] This indicates that a macular hole associated with myopic foveoschisis may develop as the result of posterior vitreous detachment, which generates antero-posterior traction and consequent retinal tearing at the fovea.

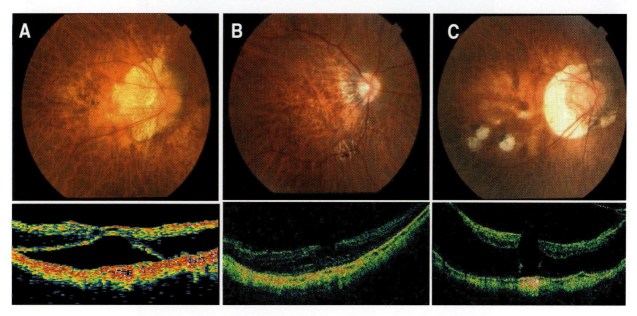

Fig. 15.1: Myopic foveoschisis has several morphologic subtypes. A. The type accompanied by foveal detachment typically presents with a foveal detachment and retinoschisis of the surrounding retina. B. Myopic foveoschisis accompanied by a lamellar hole. C. Myopic foveoschisis accompanied by a macular hole.

Another possible mechanism is retinal vascular traction on the retina.[9] Using OCT, we observed eyes after vitrectomy performed to treat myopic foveoschisis and found that retinal microfolds formed gradually after the surgery. The incidence of microfold development was approximately 60% by 6 months postoperatively. These microfolds are oriented horizontally; however, conventional biomicroscopic examination failed to detect the microfolds because they are so small. Only OCT can detect them (Fig. 15.2). OCT-ophthalmoscope identifies the precise location of the microfolds and shows that they coincide with the retinal arterioles (Fig. 15.3). The microfolds seem to be generated by inward traction of the vessels due to axial length elongation, and intraoperative internal limiting membrane peeling might have disclosed the potent tractional force of these vessels. Further investigation showed that the microfolds were present even in patients with high myopia who did not undergo surgery; the incidence was reported to be 3%.[12] Thus, myopic foveoschisis might be a multifactorial disease.

Does Optical Coherence Tomography Guide Treatment and Is It Useful to Monitor Results?

Vitrectomy, including removal of the vitreous cortex, internal limiting membrane peeling, and gas tamponade, is a useful treatment to achieve foveal reattachment and consequent visual improvement if the fovea is detached.[5,6] After surgery; OCT typically shows that foveal detachment gradually resolves over time. Foveal detachment completely resolves soon after surgery in some cases; however, other cases can take longer than 6 months to resolve, probably depending on the viscosity of the subretinal or intraretinal fluid (Fig. 15.4). Although there is a risk of macular hole formation even after surgery, 80% to 90% of patients have improved visual acuity. The surgery usually results in stabilization of the fixation point in scanning laser ophthalmoscope microperimetry, indicating that retinal function has improved.

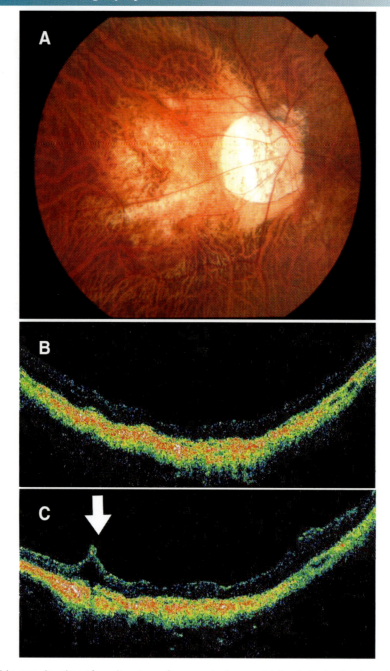

Fig. 15.2: Retinal microfolds can develop after vitrectomy for myopic foveoschisis. A. Color fundus photograph shows atrophic changes due to high myopia and a flattened retina after surgery. B. Horizontal and C. vertical OCT scan shows microfold (arrow) formation inferior to the fovea.

There is a risk that a macular hole may enlarge after surgery in cases in which the hole is small (early hole). We examined two patients who presented with enlargement of the macular hole and progressive retinal detachment after vitrectomy for myopic foveoschisis and early macular hole.[13] These detachments can be treated with additional long-term gas tamponade or another vitrectomy. The visual acuity improved in one patient, but remained unchanged in the other, suggesting that visual outcome might not be favorable

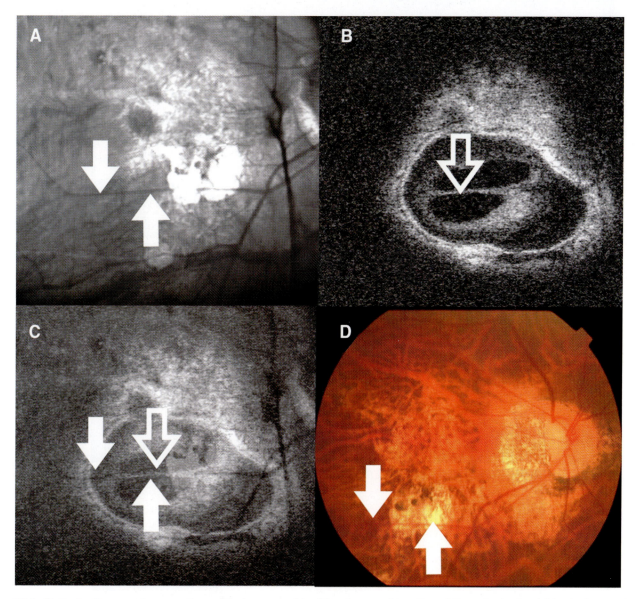

Fig. 15.3: Optical coherence tomography-ophthalmoscopy identifies the exact location of the retinal microfolds. A. A scanning laser ophthalmoscope (SLO) image and B. A C-scan image showing linear retinal microfolds. C. The C-scan image was overlaid onto SLO image that pinpoints the location on the retina. D. The retinal microfolds coincide exactly with the retinal arterioles. Closed arrows in A, C, and D indicate retinal arteriole and open arrows in B and C retinal microfold.

after vitrectomy for myopic foveoschisis with an early macular hole. From this experience, we always take maximum care to detect small macular holes before vitrectomy, since this is very important factor predictive of the visual acuity.

INTERESTING CASE EXAMPLE

A 72-year-old man presented with visual loss in the right eye of 2 years duration. Optical coherence tomography and fundus examination disclosed the presence of myopic foveoschisis as well as atrophy

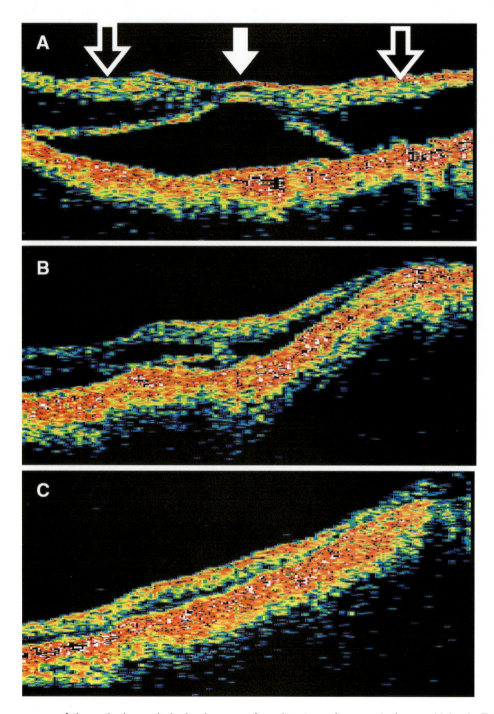

Fig. 15.4: Time course of the retinal morphologic changes after vitrectomy for myopic foveoschisis. A. Foveal detachment (closed arrow) and retinoschisis surrounding the retina (open arrows) are observed preoperatively. B. One month after vitrectomy that included removal of the vitreous cortex, internal limiting membrane peeling, and gas tamponade, the amount of subretinal fluid has decreased; however, the foveal detachment remains. C Six months postoperatively, respectively, the retinal detachment has decreased further, and finally the retina is reattached completely.

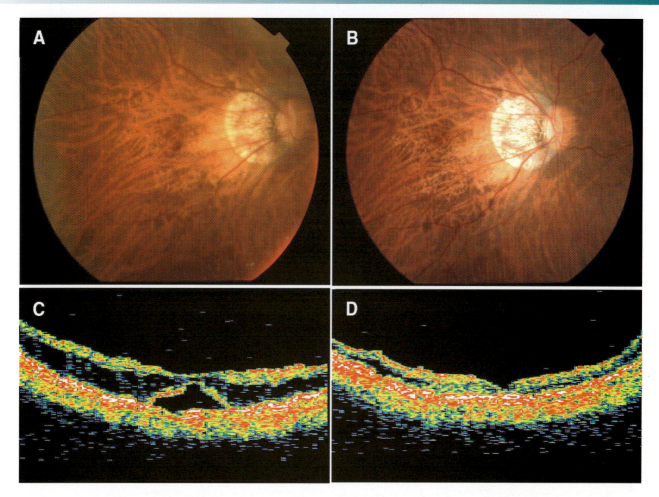

Fig. 15.5: Preoperative fundus appearance of patients who underwent vitrectomy for myopic foveoschisis. A. Color fundus photograph shows almost normal fundus, except for myopic atrophy. B. However, OCT shows apparent foveal detachment and retinoschisis. Fundus appearance, 6 months after surgery. C. The color fundus image has not changed from preoperatively. D However, the OCT image shows complete resolution of the foveal detachment and consequent visual improvement.

associated with high myopia (Figs 15.5A and B). The best-corrected visual acuity at the time was 0.06. The patient underwent vitrectomy including triamcinolone acetonide-assisted removal of the vitreous cortex, internal limiting membrane peeling, and gas tamponade. One month after surgery, the fovea began to reattach toward the pigment epithelium and the fovea was reattached completely 6 months after. His visual acuity improved to 0.2 (Figs 15.5C and D).

REFERENCES

1. Phillips CI. Retinal detachment at the posterior pole. Br J Ophthalmol. 1958;42:749-753.
2. Takano M, Kishi S. Foveal retinoschisis and retinal detachment in severely myopic eyes with posterior staphyloma. Am J Ophthalmol. 1999; 128:472-476.
3. Benhamou N, Massin P, Haouchine B, et al. Macular retinoschisis in highly myopic eyes. Am J Ophthalmol. 2002;133:794-800.
4. Kanda S, Uemura A, Sakamoto Y, Kita H. Vitrectomy with internal limiting membrane peeling for macular retinoschisis and retinal detachment without macular hole in highly myopic eyes. Am J Ophthalmol. 2003;136:177-180.

5. Kobayashi H, Kishi S. Vitreous surgery for highly myopic eyes with foveal detachment and retinoschisis. Ophthalmology. 2003;110:1702-1707.
6. Ikuno Y, Sayanagi K, Ohji M, et al. Vitrectomy and internal limiting membrane peeling for myopic foveoschisis. Am J Ophthalmol. 2004;137:719-724.
7. Bando H, Ikuno Y, Choi JS, et al. Ultra structure of internal limiting membrane in myopic foveoschisis. Am J Ophthalmol. 2005;139:197-199.
8. Matsumura N, Ikuno Y, Tano Y. Posterior vitreous detachment and macular hole formation in myopic foveoschisis. Am J Ophthalmol. 2004; 138:1071-1073.
9. Ikuno Y, Gomi F, Tano Y. Potent retinal arteriolar traction as a possible cause of myopic foveoschisis. Am J Ophthalmol. 2005, in press.
10. Baba T, Ohno-Matsui K, Futagami S, et al. Prevalence and characteristics of foveal retinal detachment without macular hole in high myopia. Am J Ophthalmol. 2003;135:338-342.
11. Polito A, Lanzetta P, Del Borrello M, Bandello F. Spontaneous resolution of a shallow detachment of the macula in a highly myopic eye. Am J Ophthalmol. 2003;135:546-547.
12. Sayanagi K, Ikuno Y, Gomi F, Tano Y. Retinal vascular microfolds in highly myopic eyes. Am J Ophthalmol. 2005, in press.
13. Ikuno Y, Tano Y. Early macular holes with retinoschisis in highly myopic eyes. Am J Ophthalmol. 2003;136:741-744.

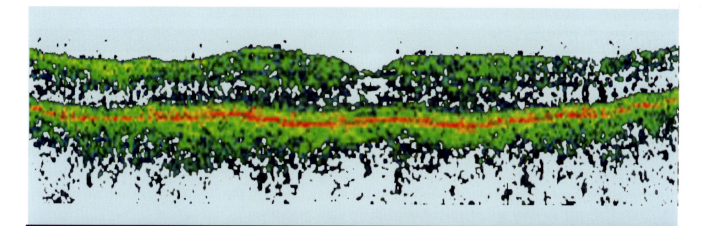

Congenital X-Linked Retinoschisis

Kimberly A Drenser, Michael T Trese

INTRODUCTION

Congenital X-linked retinoschisis is a vitreoretinopathy that is primarily inherited in an X-linked recessive pattern. It is typically bilateral and is the most common cause of juvenile macular degeneration in males. Congenital X-linked retinoschisis affects one in 5,000 to 25,000 live births worldwide and occurs in a broad population, without demonstrating ethnic predisposition[1]. Mothers are asymptomatic obligate carriers, with normal retinal findings on examination. Most patients present between the ages of 5 and 10 years with difficulties in school, but may present in infancy with nystagmus or strabismus. The clinical course is variable with severity ranging from moderate effect on visual acuity (20/50 to the 20/100 range) to legal blindness (20/200 to 20/400) to very severe affectation with no light perception.[2]

The vitreoretinopathy is due to expression of an aberrant retinoschisin protein.[3-5] This protein appears to play an important role in the structural and functional integrity of the retina. Clinically, patients present with a wide array of retinal pathology. The hallmark for the disease is splitting, or schisis, of the retinal layers.[2] Prior to the use of optical coherence tomography (OCT) retinal splitting was thought to occur predominately in the nerve fiber layer, with some splitting occurring in the ganglion cell layer and the internal limiting membrane. Optical coherence tomography analysis has shown that retinal splitting occurs in all layers of the retina, but appears to most commonly occur in the outer plexiform layer.[6,7] Schisis in the fovea, the area of the retina responsible for detailed visual acuity, is seen in all cases and is responsible for the loss of normal vision testing. Retinal splitting can occur, however, in any part of the retina and presents as a bullous or flat schisis cavity. Until the development of OCT, this flat or lamellar schisis was often missed. Lamellar schisis has not been appreciated until recently and it is now understood that this finding may be responsible for vision significantly worse than initial examination may reveal. The advent of OCT analysis, in combination with ophthalmoscopic exam, aids in the accurate diagnosis of congenital X-linked retinoschisis and determining the extent of affected retina.[6,8,9] Based on these findings a new classification system has been developed which better represents the spectrum of this disease.[7] This classification system is shown in Table 16.1.

Table 16.1: Retinoschisis classification system.			
Type	*Foveal schisis*	*Lamellar schisis*	*Peripheral schisis*
Foveal	+	–	–
Foveal-lamellar	+	+	–
Complex	+	+	+
Foveal-peripheral	+	–	+

Electrophysiology has traditionally aided in making the diagnosis of congenital X-linked retinoschisis. The electroretinogram (ERG) typically shows normal a-wave amplitude and reduced b-wave amplitude. This has been attributed to the schisis cavity within the retina causing a delay in electrical impulse conductance.[10] Optical coherence tomography findings demonstrating lamellar schisis explain the finding that ERG dysfunction is found throughout the retina even when clinical evaluation reveals foveal pathology only (Foveal-lamellar, see below). This is supported by the finding that both focal ERG and full-field ERG yield similar results.[11] Foveal congenital X-linked retinoschisis, with only foveal schisis, explains the occasional eye which has a normal ERG.

The importance of a functioning retinoschisin protein in the visual pathway has recently been demonstrated in a mouse model. A mouse retinoschisin (RS1) knockout mouse model displays an electronegative ERG waveform that is characteristic of human retinoschisis disease. This model supports the belief that retinoschisin plays an essential role in maintaining not only the structural integrity of the retina but also maintains normal electrical conductance throughout the retina. Introduction of a wild-type retinoschisin protein in the adult RS1 knock out mouse restored the normal ERG configuration.[4]

Retinoschisin is a secreted protein of 224 amino acids and appears to play a role in cell-cell interactions and adhesions. The coding sequence is located at Xp22.2 and is designated XLRS1.[12] Gene transcripts have been identified in the retina and specifically in the photoreceptor cell.[13] The protein product is comprised of two distinct regions, a putative amino terminal signal peptide and a highly conserved discoidin domain in the carboxyl terminal.[3] The majority of retinoschisin (157 amino acids) consists of a discoidin domain, which comprises exons 4 through 6 of XLRS1. Cell-cell interactions and cell-matrix interactions require the discoidin domain of the protein, a highly conserved motif, first described in Dictyostelium discoideum.[14] The discoidin motif is found in neuropilin, factor V, factor VIII, MFG-E8, and Del-1.[15,16] Additionally, discoidin domain-containing proteins are involved in neuronal development and cell-cell adhesions and may explain the loss of retinal layer integrity that is typified in congenital X-linked retinoschisis.

Congenital X-linked retinoschisis is typically inherited in an X-linked recessive pattern. In congenital X-linked retinoschisis the gene, XLRS1, is located at Xp22.2.[12] The mothers of patients are asymptomatic obligate carriers of the disease, but often have a positive family history for male members having poor vision. Spontaneous mutations do appear to occur in certain cases, but more likely represent families with previously mild disease and undiagnosed eye problems. This finding demonstrates the variability of clinical presentation that this disease represents. Familial cases of retinoschisis have been described and both autosomal dominant and autosomal recessive inheritance patterns have been reported.[19-21] The causative genes have not been elucidated in these reports, however, but may account for the small percentage of patients that are not found to have a mutation in the XLRS1 gene.

Patients with congenital X-linked retinoschisis are found to have a mutation in the XLRS1 gene >90% of the time. The XLRS1 gene consists of six exons, and the majority (>80%) of disease causing mutations occur in exons,[4-6] the discoidin domain.[5] This domain shares sequence homology with many other proteins involved in cell-cell interactions and adhesions. Upstream mutations often lead to a truncated retinoschisin product or complete lack of translation. Certain hotspots for mutations have been identified as well. The importance of this gene in establishing normal retinal structure and function is supported by the relative lack of benign polymorphisms.

A mouse model of the disease has been established. This is a retinoschisin (RS1) knock-out mouse, and demonstrates that lack of expression of the RS1 product, retinoschisin, results in significant structural abnormalities of the mouse retina. The distribution of retinoschisin has been shown to predominate in the photoreceptor outer segment, with significant concentrations in the outer plexiform layer. There is less protein concentrated in the nerve fiber layer.[22] Supporting the OCT findings in humans with congenital X-linked retinoschisis, the mouse model also demonstrates schisis in multiple layers of the retina. Additionally, this model provides support to the finding in patients of abnormal electrical conductance within the retina. Electrophysiology performed in patients with the disease demonstrates a decrease in b-wave amplitude of the ERG. The mouse model demonstrates similar abnormalities in electrical signal conductance and supports the hypothesis that loss of retinal structural integrity results in slowed cell-cell signal transduction in the visual pathway.[10]

Analysis of the distribution of both retinoschisin protein and its precursor messenger RNA (mRNA) in the developing mouse retina demonstrates expression throughout the retina.[22] The mRNA is first expressed in the retinal ganglion cells as early as postnatal day 1. The mRNA expression continues posteriorly through the developing retina in a spatial and temporal pattern. Both retinoschisin and its mRNA are expressed in all layers of the retina with the possible exception of the horizontal cells. This finding indicates that functional retinoschisin is expressed in individual retinal cells as opposed to being transported across retinal layers.[13,22]

The current mainstay of treatment for congenital X-linked retinoschisis focuses on maintaining or improving retinal structure and integrity. Laser retinopexy is used to create inflammation and scarring of the retina and underlying retinal pigment epithelium in hopes to create a mechanical adhesion and a barrier to progressing retinal schisis. This may help prevent progression of retinal detachment but is not able to close the intraretinal schisis cavities. Organized sheets of overlying vitreous also add a tractional component to the detachments and can be addressed with surgery.[23] The goal of surgical intervention is to remove the tractional components of the vitreous and close the schisis cavities. This often requires excision of the inner retina flap.[24] There is some evidence that removing the internal limiting membrane helps reduce the cystic cavities seen in foveal schisis.[8] Complete removal of the tractional forces is difficult and requires the aid of an experimental enzyme, plasmin, to cleave the non-cellular adhesions.[25] Long-term closure of the schisis cavities also requires a tamponading agent. The agent used in surgery is silicone oil. The silicone oil is left in the eye indefinitely, as removal of the oil results in reformation of the schisis detachments. Although silicone oil is an inert substance, it does cause problems, such as cataract and corneal decompensation, when left in the eye for long periods of time. The complications of silicone oil often necessitate further surgical interventions, such as cataract extraction and corneal transplant. Additionally, full-thickness detachments can and often do occur. These detachments represent particularly challenging operations, and often are not reparable by current techniques. Chronic retinal detachment may often lead to phthisis and, if the eye becomes painful, may necessitate enucleation.

OPTICAL COHERENCE TOMOGRAPHY

The development of OCT, combined with ophthalmoscopy, has changed the understanding of the retinal layers involved and how it affects retinal structure. Optical coherence tomography uses a scanning laser to evaluate the overlying hyaloid, retinal thickness, retinal layers, and underlying retinal pigment epithelium. Optical coherence tomography analysis of eyes affected by congenital X-linked retinoschisis demonstrates schisis of the retina in multiple layers and with different clinical presentations (Figs 16.1 to 16.6).

Optical coherence tomography is particularly useful in the evaluation of the patient with congenital X-linked retinoschisis. Many patients have visual loss that is greater than would be suggested by the ophthalmoscopic exam. Foveal schisis is well demonstrated in the congenital X-linked retinoschisis patient, even in mild cases (Fig. 16.1). It has been long been appreciated that significant ERG abnormalities are often seen in patients even when only foveal changes are noted by both clinical exam and fluorescein angiography. This is now understood to be due lamellar schisis that appears as attached retina by ophthalmoscopic exam, photography, and fluorescein angiography (Figs 16.2, 16.3 and 16.5). Until the development of OCT, congenital

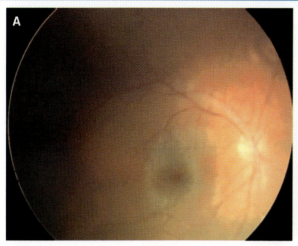
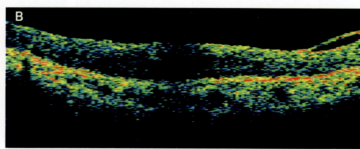

Fig. 16.1: Type I. Note foveal schisis on fundus photography and OCT.

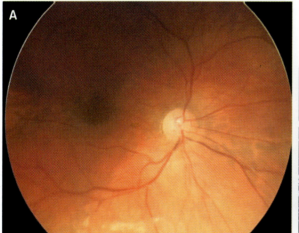
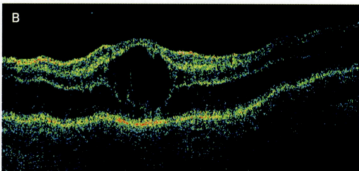

Fig. 16.2: Type II. Fundus photograph shows foveal schisis only. The OCT shows both foveal and lamellar schisis.

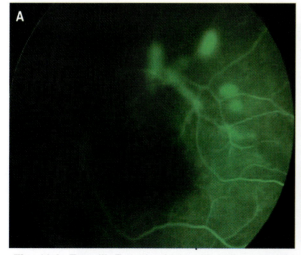
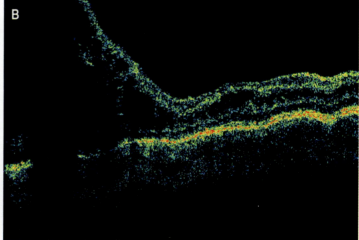

Fig. 16.3: Type III. Foveal schisis with bullous peripheral schisis adjacent to lamellar schisis is demonstrated by OCT. The lamellar schisis is only appreciated by OCT.

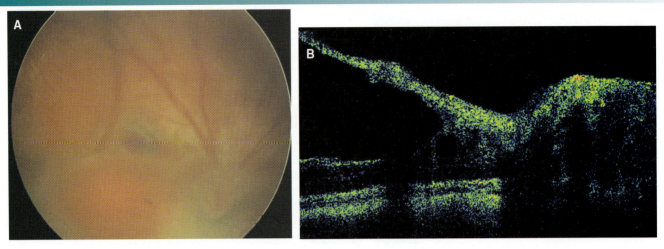

Fig. 16.4: Type IV. Foveal schisis with bullous peripheral schisis is demonstrated by both fundus photography and OCT.

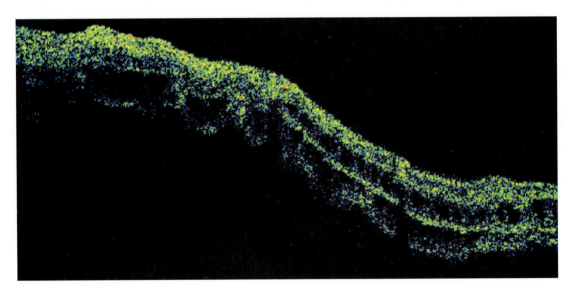

Fig. 16.5: Optical coherence tomography demonstrating lamellar schisis of the retina.

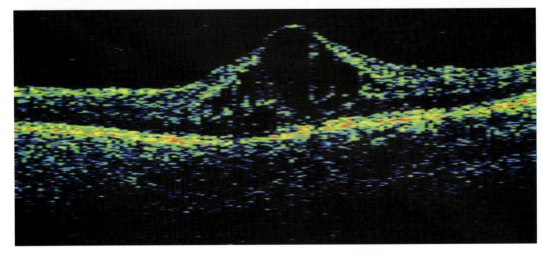

Fig. 16.6: Pronounced foveal schisis.

X-linked retinoschisis was thought to represent a splitting of the retina at the nerve fiber layer. Optical coherence tomography unequivocally shows that the schisis occurs within multiple layers of the retina, predominately at the outer plexiform layer. The potential involvement of multiple layers explains the finding of bullous and/or lamellar schisis cavities as well as foveal schisis, occurring in these patients.

The OCT findings in congenital X-linked retinoschisis have changed the understanding of the pathogenesis of the disease. The finding that retinal structure is often severely affected better explains the electrophysiology findings in patients with congenital X-linked retinoschisis. It suggests that retinoschisin plays a role in maintaining both structural integrity within the retina and plays a role in maintaining electrical conductance.

Based on these findings a new classification system has been developed (Table 16.1). Foveal is characterized by foveal schisis without other retinal findings (Figs 16.1 and 16.6). Foveal-lamellar demonstrates both foveal schisis and lamellar schisis (Fig. 16.2). Complex is the most severe form, consisting of foveal schisis, lamellar schisis and peripheral schisis (Fig. 16.3). Foveal-peripheral is characterized by foveal schisis and peripheral schisis (Fig. 16.4).

Use of the OCT-based classification system may allow for better understanding of the natural history of the disease and better correlation with genetic mutations. Earlier intervention, such as laser demarcation or vitrectomy with silicone oil tamponade, may be appropriate in patients who have traditionally been managed by observation (such as progressing lamellar schisis). Additionally, pharmacologic and genetic therapies maybe developed to replace the normal retinal adhesions and conductance.

INTERESTING CASE EXAMPLE

A 9-year-old boy presented with bilateral type III retinoschisis demonstrating significant bullous detachments OU (Fig. 16.7). Treatment consisted of vitrectomy with plasmin (an enzyme to cleave the hyaloid attachments to the retina) and surgically collapsing the schisis cavities. An inner wall retinectomy was performed and the retina flattened under air. The attached retina was barricaded with laser and the eye filled with silicone oil. Postoperative photographs and OCT analysis demonstrate significant improvement in the retinal anatomy (Figs 16.8 and 16.9)

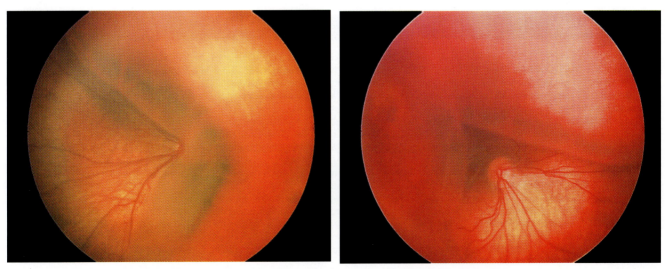

Fig. 16.7: Preoperative fundus photographs of the right (A) and left (B) eyes

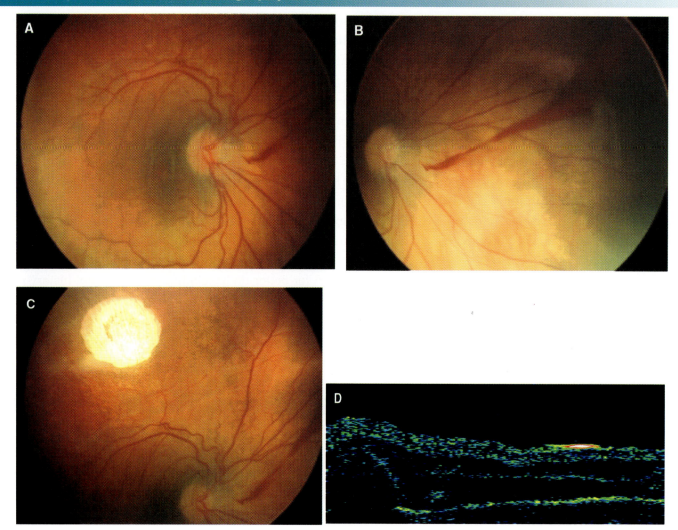

Fig. 16.8: Postoperative fundus photographs (A-C) and OCT (D) of the right eye. Note the intraretinal schisis on OCT despite an apparently flat retina

REFERENCES

1. Tanatri A, Vrabec TR, Cu-Unjieng A, et al. X-linked retinoschisis: a clinical and molecular genetic review. Surv Ophthalmol. 2004;49:214-230.
2. Sieving PA, MacDonald IM, Trese MT. Congenital X-linked retinoschisis. In Hartnett ME, Trese MT, Capone A, et al, (Eds): Pediatric Retinal Diseases: Medical and Surgical Approaches. Philadelphia: Lippincott, Williams and Wilkins, 2004.
3. Hiriyanna KT, Bingham EL, Yashar BM, et al. Novel mutations in XLRS1 causing retinoschisis, including first evidence of a putative leader sequence change. Hum Mutat 1999;14:423-427.
4. Zeng Y, Takada Y, Kjellstrom S, et al. RS-1 gene delivery to an adult RS1h knockout mouse model restores ERG b-wave with reversal of the electronegative waveform of X-linked retinoschisis. Invest Ophthalmol Vis Sci 2004;45:3279-3285.
5. The Retinoschisis Consortium. Functional implications of the spectrum of mutations found in 234 cases with X-linked juvenile retinoschisis (XLRS). Hum Mol Genet. 1998; 7:1185-1192.
6. Chan WM, Choy KW, Wang J, et al. Two cases of X-linked juvenile retinoschisis with different optical coherence tomography findings and RS1 gene mutations. Clin Experiment Ophthalmol. 2004; 32:429-432.
7. Prenner JL, Capone A, Ciaccia S, et al. Congenital X-linked retinoschisis classification system. Retina. 2005, submitted.
8. Azzolini C, Pierro L, Codenotti M, Brancato R. OCT images and surgery of juvenile macular retinoschisis. Eur J Ophthalmol. 1997;7:196-200.
9. Eriksson U, Larsson E, Holmstrom G. Optical coherence tomography in the diagnosis of juvenile X-linked retinoschisis. Acta Ophthalmol Scand 2004;82:218-223.
10. Kahn NW, Jamison JA, Kemp JA, Sieving PA. Analysis of photoreceptor function and inner retinal activity in juvenile X-linked retinoschisis. Vis Research. 2001;41:3931-3942.

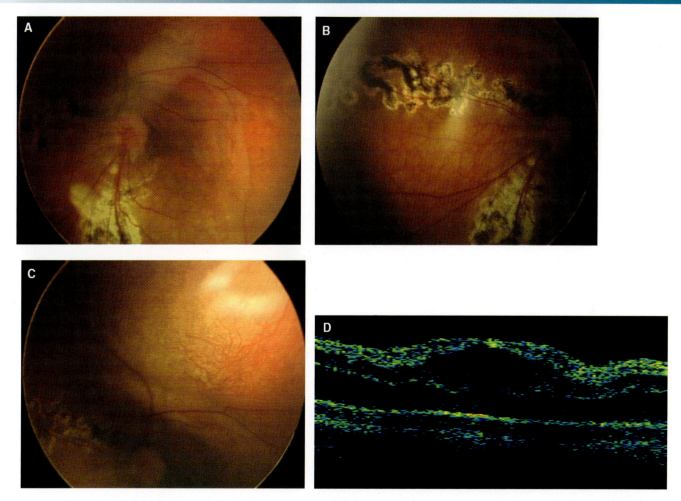

Fig. 16.9: Postoperative fundus photographs (A-C) and OCT (D) of the left eye. Intraretinal schisis is seen on OCT

11. Huang S, Wu D, Jiang F, et al. The multifocal electroretinogram in X-linked juvenile retinoschisis. Doc Ophthalmol. 2003;106:251-255.
12. Sauer CG, Gehrig A, Warneke-Wittstock R, et al. Positional cloning of the gene associated with X-linked juvenile retinoschisis. Nat Genet 1997;17:164-170.
13. Reid SNM, Akhmedov NB, Piriev NI, et al. The mouse X-linked retinoschisis cDNA: expression in photoreceptor cells. Gene. 1999; 227:257-266.
14. Reitherman RW, Rosen SD, Frasier WA, Barondes SH. Cell surface species-specific high affinity receptors for discoidin: developmental regulation in Dictyostelium discoideum. Proc Natl Acad Sci. 1975; 72:3541-3545.
15. He Z, Tessier-Lavigne M. Neuropilin is a receptor for the axonal chemorepellent semaphoring III. Cell. 1997;10:739-751.
16. Baumgartner S, Hofmann K, Chiquet-Erismann, Bucher P. The discoidin domain family revisited: new members from prokaryotes and a homology-based fold prediction. Prot Sci. 1998;7:1626-1631.
17. Hiraoka M, Trese MT, Shastry BS. Intragenic polymorphic missense mutations in the XLRS1 gene in families with juvenile X-linked retinoschisis. Hum Genet. 1999;104:526-527.
18. Sieving PA, Yashar BM, Ayyagari R. Juvenile retinoschisis: a model for molecular diagnostic testing of X-linked ophthalmic disease. Trans Am Ophthalmol Soc. 1999; 97:451-464.
19. Yassur Y, Nissenkorn I, Ben-Sira I, et al. Autosomal dominant inheritance of retinoschisis. Am J Ophthalmol. 1982;94:338-343.
20. Shimazaki J, Matsuhashi M. Familial retinoschisis in female patients. Doc Ophthalmol. 1987;65:393-400.
21. Perez Alvarez MJ, Clement Fernandez F. No X-chromosome linked juvenile foveal retinoschisis. Arch Soc Esp Oftalmol. 2002;77:443-448.
22. Takada Y, Fariss RN, Tanikawa A, et al. A retinal neuronal developmental wave of retinoschisin expression begins in ganglion cells during layer formation. Invest Ophthalmol Vis Sci. 2004; 45:3302-3312.
23. Ferrone PJ, Trese MT, Lewis H. Vitreoretinal surgery for complications of congenital retinoschisis. Am J Ophthalmol. 1997;123:742-747.
24. Trese MT, Ferrone PJ. The role of inner wall retinectomy in the management of juvenile retinoschisis. Graefe's Arch Clin Exp Ophthalmol. 1995;233:706-708.
25. Trese MT. Enzymatic Vitreous Surgery. Sem Ophthalmol. 2000;15:116-121.

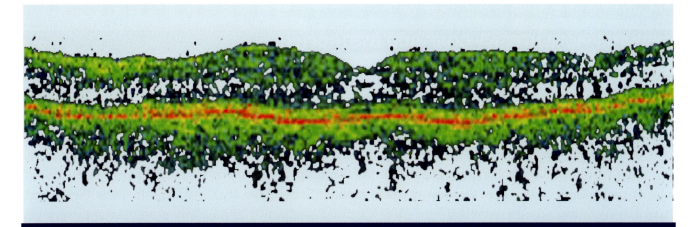

17

Retinal Degenerations and Dystrophies

Eric H Souied, Giuseppe Querques,
Gabriel Coscas, Giséle Soubrane

RETINITIS PIGMENTOSA – CONE-ROD DYSTROPHY

Retinitis pigmentosa is a heterogeneous group of inherited retinal degenerations that are characterized by progressive loss of photoreceptor.[1]

The first observation was performed by Ovelgun [2] in 1744 and subsequently by Schon. [3] In 1855, this inherited disease was called retinitis pigmentosa by Donders.[4]

Questioning of the patient represents an essential step of the examination, not only to obtain the diagnosis, but also to evaluate the functional prognosis and the handicap. Prognosis and clinical features (age of onset, rate of progression, visual loss) are related to the mode of inheritance (AD, AR, XL). Retinitis pigmentosa may also occur as an isolated sporadic disorder. Central visual acuity is generally preserved until very late stage of evolution of the disease. The presenting symptoms are commonly nyctalopia and progressive visual field loss due to rod involvement in retinitis pigmentosa, in which the disorder begins in middle periphery of the retina (rod-cone dystrophy). Initial involvement of photoreceptors leads to subsequent damage to inner retinal cells and eventual atrophy of several layers of the retina.[5] A decreased visual acuity can present early in the disease secondary mainly to cataract and cystoid macular edema or may be a result of widespread atrophy of retinal layers, late in the progression of the disease. The clinical triad of retinitis pigmentosa is arteriolar attenuation (main diagnostic feature), retinal bone-spicule pigmentation and waxy disc pallor. These signs appear on a very advanced stage of the disease and their presence is not compulsory for diagnosing retinitis pigmentosa.[6] At earlier stages, fundoscopy may, in fact, look normal but electroretinogram (ERG) is frequently altered. The opening signs observed on fundoscopy are arteriolar narrowing and decrease of the epithelial pigment charge. The aggregation of melanin in the form of osteoblasts appears secondarily, with the evolution of photoreceptor deterioration.[7,8] The alterations of the visual field, insidious and progressive, is generally symetrical. The retinal modifications starts classically at the mid-periphery. The scotoma expand to form an annular scotoma. The visual field loss leads progressively to a so-called *tubular* visual field. At an early stage, the b-wave of the electroretinogram at the scotopic phase is delayed and a and b-waves have both a reduced amplitude. At an advanced stage of the disease, there is no detectable response.[9-14] The altered rod response is the most precocious and is observed even at the earliest stages.

In a distinct phenotype of the disorder, cone-rod dystrophy, the retina degeneration begins in the macular area and progressively evolves to the periphery with early impairment of central vision.

Optical Coherence Tomography

In retinitis pigmentosa, optical coherence tomography (OCT) allows visualization of retinal atrophy in retinal thickness mode. It seems that OCT-3 scans are also able to show the loss of the outer segment layer, as it happens at first before global atrophy.

The OCT patterns appear slightly different in the two categories of retinal degeneration: retinitis pigmentosa and cone-rod dystrophies.

In retinitis pigmentosa dystrophy retinal thickness and photoreceptors' layer alterations begins at the retinal periphery and evolve concentrically to the fovea only in the late stage of the disease (Fig. 17.1). On the opposite in cone-rod dystrophy the decrease of retinal thickness begins from the center of the macula towards the retinal periphery (Fig. 17.2).

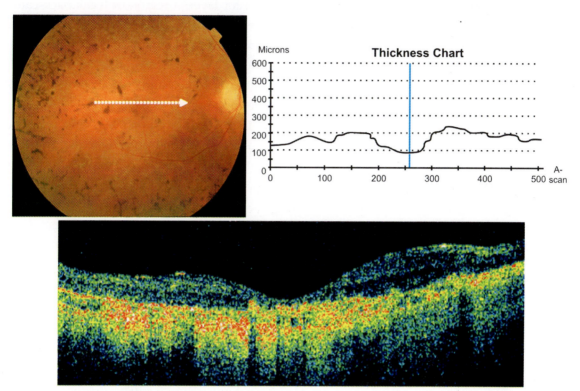

Fig. 17.1: Top left: Color fundus right eye photograph shows typical triad of retinitis pigmentosa (arteriolar attenuation, retinal bone-spicule pigmentation, waxy disc pallor) and macular atrophy. Top right: Thickness chart shows retinal thickness decrease that in retinitis pigmentosa begins at the periphery and evolve to the fovea. Bottom: OCT scan shows photoreceptors layer alterations.

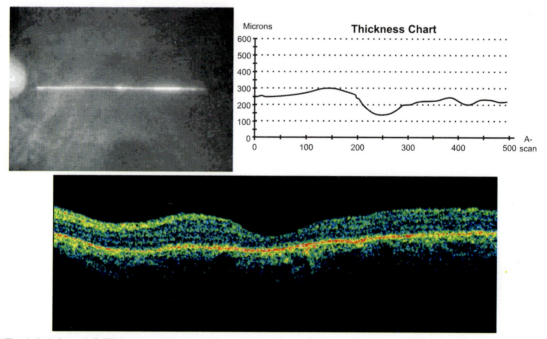

Fig. 17.2: Top left: Infrared OCT fundus left eye image shows scan direction. Top right: Thickness chart shows retinal thickness decrease that in cone-rod begins at the fovea and evolve to the periphery. Bottom: OCT scan shows photoreceptors layer alterations and accentuation of foveal depression.

On OCT scans, the presence and normality of the photoreceptor layer, a region of weak backscattering, as described by Hee and associates,[1] can be analyzed and classified as normal, reduced or not visible.

Some correlation could be made also for central retinal thickness analysis on OCT and visual acuity, as suggested for other retinal dystrophies. Anyway, the evolution of visual acuity also do not follow any particular rule.[15] This variability could be explained by the genetic, molecular and clinic heterogeneity of the disease, even when stratified by type of inheritance[16-18] or gene mutation.[19]

On the other hand, the positive correlation between retinal thickness analysis on OCT and visual acuity may confirm the hypothesis that a poor visual acuity in the absence of cataract or macular involvement (edema or atrophy) would be due to the death of photoreceptors in the macula. This hypothesis is even more reliable because of the decrease in retinal thickness is positively related to poor visibility of photoreceptor layer in OCT scans.

Moreover, it seems that OCT allows to detect retinal changes at early stage when no pigment and only mild vessel attenuation, can be seen. At this stage decreased retinal thickness is often visible on OCT scans and by retinal thickness analysis (Fig. 17.3).

Macular edema is a common complication observed in retinitis pigmentosa that severely alters visual acuity. Quantification, follow-up and response to treatment remained imprecise until OCT imaging.

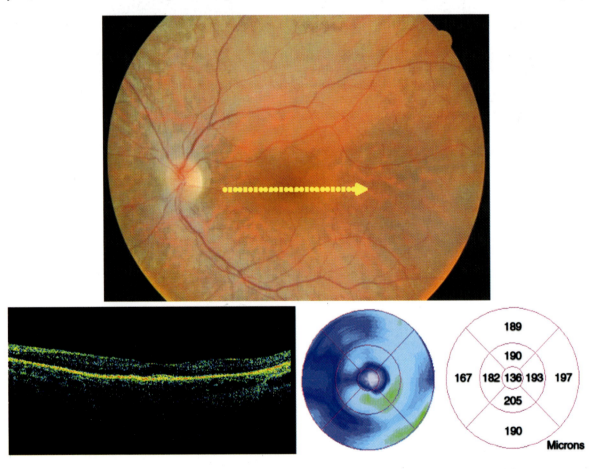

Fig. 17.3: Top: Color fundus left eye photograph shows retinal changes at early stage. Bottom left: OCT scan shows retinal atrophy. Bottom right: Retinal map analysis shows general decreased retinal thickness.

Indeed OCT is very useful to evaluate the presence and quantify macular edema in patients with retinitis pigmentosa[20] (Fig. 17.4). It also allows the follow-up of this complication and the response to treatment (Fig. 17.5). OCT seems more sensitive, in this regard, than either fluorescein angiography or fundoscopic examination and can display the evolution towards macular hole or pseudo-hole.[21] (Fig. 17.6)

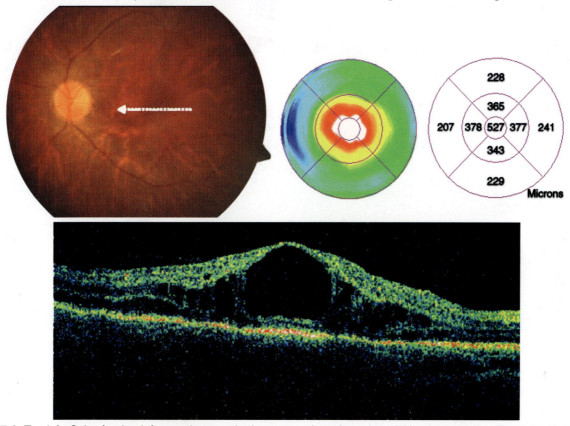

Fig. 17.4: Top left: Color fundus left eye photograph shows macular edema in retinitis pigmentosa. Top right: Retinal map shows macular thickness increase due to macular edema. Bottom: OCT scan shows cystoid macular edema.

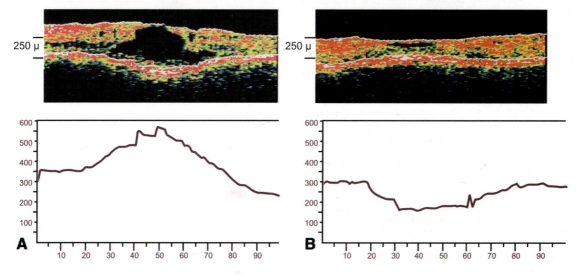

Fig. 17.5: OCT scan and thickness chart shows macular edema before (A) and during treatment (B) by acetazolamide (day 7).

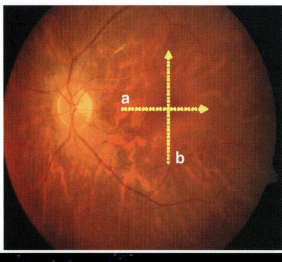

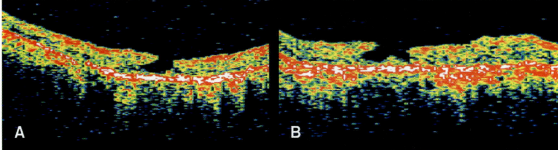

Fig. 17.6: Top: Color fundus left eye photograph shows lamellar hole in retinitis pigmentosa. Bottom: OCT horizontal (A) and vertical (B) scans show the evolution towards macular lamellar hole.

To conclude OCT has shown some interest to correlate visual function deficiency to loss of photoreceptor, but we still do not know its power as a reliable diagnostic tool for this purpose.

Provided its intersession and intra-session reproducibility and repeatability in analyzing retinal thickness,[22,24] OCT may be taken into consideration in retinitis pigmentosa evaluation and could be used as a clinical tool to assess progression, in comparison with visual field and ERG progression. Furthermore, OCT is a useful tool to quantify, to follow-up and to evaluate the efficacy of treatment of macular edema.

PROGRESSIVE CONE DYSTROPHY

Progressive cone dystrophy is a heterogeneous group of rare disorders. Patients with pure cone dystrophy initially have only cone dysfunction. Depending on the genetic defect, this inherited disorder is either limited or additional rod dysfunction may develop.[25-29]

Autosomal dominant, recessive, and X-linked inheritance patterns of inheritance have been described,[30-34] as well as sporadic cases, implying genetic and molecular heterogeneity.[35-41]

Cone dystrophies show great variability in severity and rate of progression from family to family and sometimes within the same family; several characteristic fundus pictures are seen in combination with cone dystrophy. Cone disease of the macula is shown by decreased visual acuity and very poor color discrimination.

Presentation of progressive cone dystrophy is usually in the first to third decades with gradual bilateral impairment of central and color vision associated with photophobia and fine pendular nystagmus. Visual loss precedes definite macular changes. Visual acuity usually deteriorates gradually and in advanced cases may go to hand movements.

On the basis of the fundus examination, it is sometimes difficult to differentiate sharply between progressive cone degeneration and generalized cone-rod deficiencies in which symptoms relating to the cone dysfunction predominate.

In progressive cone dystrophy, three types of macular lesions can be seen on fundus examination. First, a common type has a bull's eye appearance and consists of a sharply defined zone of atrophic pigment epithelium surrounding a central homogeneous darker area (Fig. 17.7). A second form of cone dystrophy is retinal pigment epithelium disturbance with pigment stippling and diffuse round pigment clumps in the posterior pole. Third, atrophy of the choriocapillaris and larger choroidal vessels is seen in a few patients and rarely occurs at an early age (Fig. 17.8). A temporal disc pallor and later optic atrophy is a common finding in all patients. At advanced stage, profound chorioretinal atrophy is observed in all cases. Visual field is usually normal, excepting a bilateral central scotoma.

A completely extinguished photopic and scotopic ERG is found in the most severe cases, which are often long-standing.[25] Multifocal ERG also contribute to the diagnosis, particularly in early stage and in suspicious cases.[42]

Fluorescein angiographic findings depend from the ophthalmoscopic change. In bull's eye appearance a horizontal ovoid zone of hyperfluorescence surrounding a non-fluorescent center, is observed. In case of irregular retinal pigment epithelium changes, a combination of hypo- and hyperfluorescent dots is visible, corresponding to the salt and pepper appearance. Finally, diffuse hyperfluorescence in a large part of the posterior pole or fluorescein angiographic findings like those in central choroidal atrophy can also be seen.

Optical Coherence Tomography

Optical coherence tomography images seems to correlate well with histological cross sections of the retina.[19-22, 43-45] In progressive cone dystrophy, OCT clearly reveals a large central full thickness defect that reflect a general atrophy of all retinal layers with the accentuation of physiological foveal depression.

Moreover, OCT allows evidencing the different aspects of cone dystrophy reflecting the evolution of the disease and can help differential diagnosis with other retinal dystrophies.

It seems that we can distinguish two different types with OCT-3: type 1, gradually foveal atrophy (Figs 17.7 and 17.9A); type 2, abrupt foveal atrophy (Figs 17.8 and 17.9B). In type 1 foveal thickness is more or less impaired going until the total absence of all retinal layers in foveal area, but the curve of foveal atrophy is progressive from normal thickness in periphery until total central atrophy (Fig. 17.9A). In type 2 there is an abrupt foveal atrophy and is not possible to see the progressive curve of retinal atrophy from the periphery to the center (Fig. 17.9B).

In both types progressive cone dystrophy peripheral retinal thickness is usually normal in contrast with inverse retinitis pigmentosa where a peripheral involvement can always be found in association with the macular findings (Fig. 17.10)

STARGARDT'S DISEASE AND FUNDUS FLAVIMACULATUS

Stargardt's disease is an autosomal recessive macular dystrophy of childhood, characterized by a juvenile onset, a rapidly progressive course, and a poor visual outcome.[46-48] On the other hand, fundus flavimaculatus,

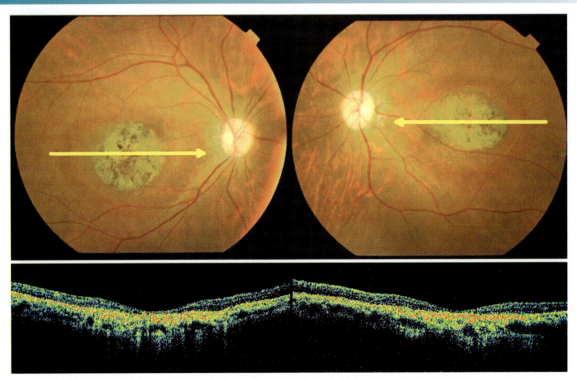

Fig. 17.7: Bull's eye appearance on color photograph (top right eye, left eye). Linear scan (5 mm) performed with OCT-3 reveals a large central full thickness defect, progressive from periphery until the center, that reflect a general atrophy of all retinal layers with the accentuation of physiological foveal depression (type 1).

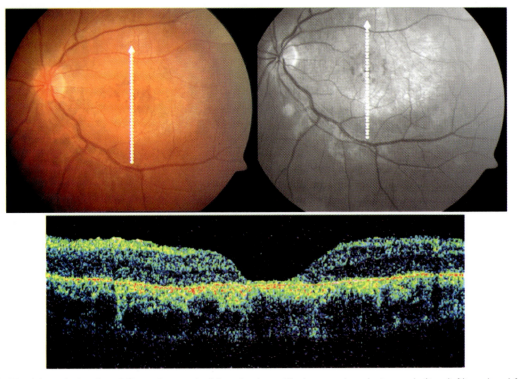

Fig. 17.8: Total foveal atrophy of the retina and of the choriocapillaris on color photograph (top left) and red-free frame (top right). OCT reveals a large abrupt central full thickness defect of the macula (type 2).

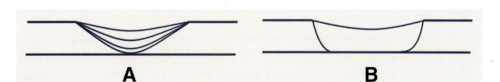

Figs 17.9A and B: Drawing of type 1 accentuation of foveal depression observed in progressive cone dystrophy. The curve of foveal atrophy is progressive from normal thickness in periphery until total central atrophy. Drawing of type 2 accentuation of foveal depression observed in progressive cone dystrophy. Abrupt foveal atrophy with the absence of the curve of retinal atrophy from the periphery to the center.

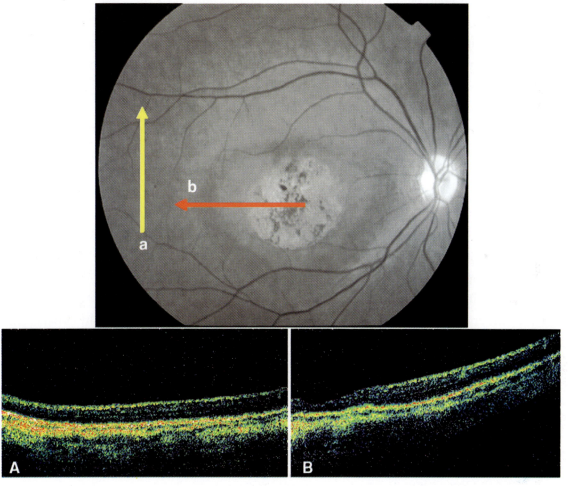

Fig. 17.10: Top: Red-free frame of cone dystrophy. Bottom left: OCT scan localized at distance from macular area (A) reveals normal retinal thickness (mean thickness 310 μm). Bottom right: OCT scan localized at the border of macular atrophy (B) shows the progressive retinal atrophy from the periphery to the center.

a Stargardt's-like phenotype, described by Franceschetti, is characterized by a late-onset and a more slowly progressive course.[49,50] Stargardt's disease and fundus flavimaculatus are variants of the same hereditary disease that affects the retinal pigment epithelium and photoreceptor layer.[46,49,50,51-57] The disease is usually termed Stargardt's disease when visual acuity loss begins in the first two decades, while the term fundus flavimaculatus is favored when the disease begins at the end of the second decade or within the third decade and has a slowly progressive course.

The general course of Stargardt's disease and fundus flavimaculatus is a progressive loss of central vision (≤ 1/10), resulting in central atrophy (Fig. 17.11) and thus loss of central visual function.[46,50,58-65]

Genetic studies demonstrated a continuum between Stargardt's disease and fundus flavimaculatus, both linked with the ABCA4 gene.[66-69] Mutations in the ABCA4 gene account for a wide range of phenotypes, e.g. retinitis pigmentosa, cone-rod dystrophy, Stargardt's disease, fundus flavimaculatus, and very late onset fundus flavimaculatus.[66,67,70,71] A second gene, ELOVL4, is also involved in Stargardt's disease and acts in elongation of very long fatty acid.[72,73]

There are few anatomo-pathologic studies except the one of Klein and Krill,[74] that found the presence of mucopolysaccharidic acid deposits (hyaluronic acid) in retinal cells. On the other hand, Eagle[75] found a massive accumulation of lipofuscin (that is composed of A2-E) in the cells of the pigmentary epithelium.

Stargardt's disease appears between the ages of 8 and 12 years with decrease of central visual acuity. In this early stage fundus is often normal. The color test shows a deutan axis (red-green), exceptional for the hereditary macular dystrophies, and this can contribute to Stargardt's diagnosis.[60-65] The first ophthalmoscopic sign, some months later, is disappearance of the foveolar reflex and a granulated aspect of the pigmentary epithelium, described as "vermillion aspect" or "snail slime."[76] Finally, a horizontal oval parafoveolar pigmentary epithelium atrophy, described as *beaten bronze atrophy*, appears.

The white yellowish perifoveal deposits called "flecks" are usual features of Stargardt's disease and fundus flavimaculatus. These flecks are polymorphous, rounded, fusiform, spearlike, pisciformes, giants, butterfly or X-shaped,[77] and can be small or large, juxta-macular or diffuse. At first, the deposits are white-yellowish and well defined. Later, in long-standing cases, the flecks become gray, fuzzy and ill-defined. At the end-stage of Stargardt's disease, there is a large retinal central atrophy extended into the deeper layers of the posterior pole. It is difficult to distinguish the flecks at this stage. The disease can appear in older patients, between the 2nd and 4th decade (fundus flavimaculatus). The evolution is usually slowly progressive. Very late onset disease, after the age of 55 years, also exists.

These forms highlight the problem to define age-related macular degeneration and Stargardt's macular dystrophy.[78] Auto-fluorescence of the flecks represents one precious effective method in the diagnosis of Stargardt's disease (Figs 17.11 to 17.14).[79-81] On the red-free photographs, adult-form vitelliform degeneration lesions are round and whitish. In the early phase, fluorescein angiography discloses early hypofluorescence, corresponding to the area of whitish material seen in the red-free photographs. In the late phase fluorescein angiography shows a central staining of variable intensity without leakage, but sometimes the hypofluorescence persists until the late phase, with no staining. Moreover fluorescein angiography reveals the characteristic phenomenon of dark-choroid and displays the entity of macular atrophy varying from discrete and bull's eye atrophy to diffuse central atrophy of the end-stage disease. On indocyanine-green angiography, the flecks are always hypofluorescent, and hypofluorescence persists until the late phase with the appearance of the characteristically hyperfluorescent "pin-points."

Visual fields show at first a relative central scotoma and later an absolute central scotoma. Time and amplitudes of the photopic and scotopic ERG are generally normal.[82]

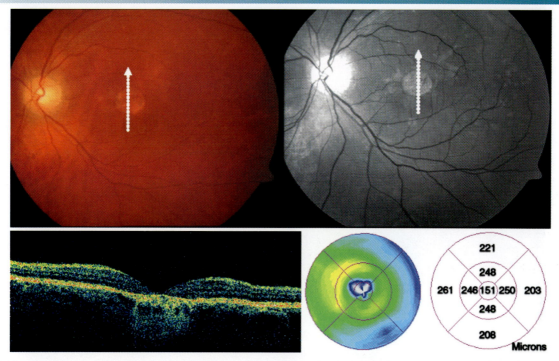

Fig. 17.11: Macular atrophy associated with Stargardt's disease. Top left: Color photograph of fundus shows both macular dystrophy and retinal flecks. Top right: Same eye, red-free frame allows a better definition and contrast of the flecks. Bottom left: OCT scan reveals a large central atrophy (macular area). Bottom right: Retinal map analysis shows a diffuse reduction foveal thickness whereas retinal thickness is globally normal around the macular area.

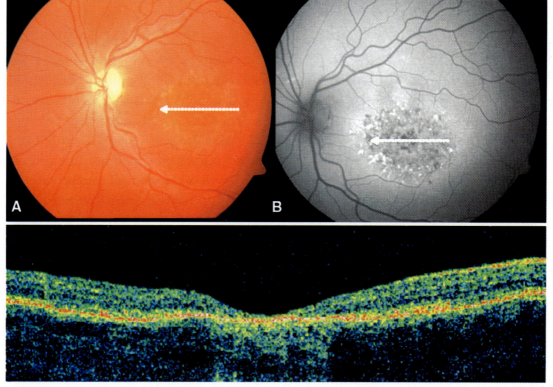

Fig. 17.12: Accentuation of foveal depression in a patient affected with Stargardt's disease. Top left: Color photograph shows macular atrophy and retinal flecks (A). Top right: Auto-fluorescent frame shows all fine retinal flecks (B). Bottom: OCT scan shows global irregularities and defects within the photoreceptor layer.

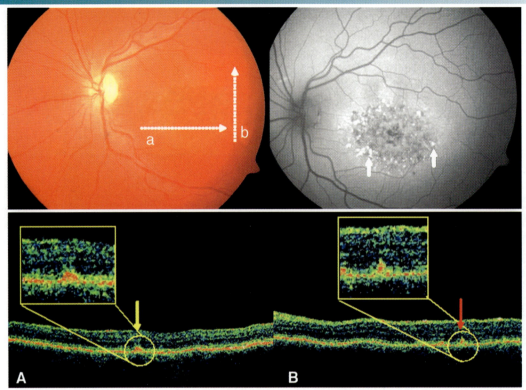

Fig. 17.13: Visualisation of elevated dots at the level or above the retinal pigment epithelium layer. Top left: Color photograph shows macular atrophy and retina flecks (a, b). Top right: Auto-fluorescent frame shows all fine retinal flecks. Bottom: OCT scans show little hyper-reflective dots at the level of retinal pigment epithelium layer (red and yellow arrows). These little dots seem to correspond to the accumulation of auto-fluorescent material and could be interpreted as retinal flecks.

Optical Coherence Tomography

Optical coherence tomography images seem to correlate well with histological cross sections of the retina in animal experiment.[83-87] In Stargardt's disease/ fundus flavimaculatus, OCT-3 usually reveals irregularities or defect at the level of photoreceptors layers in macular area (Fig. 17.12). At advanced stages of the disease a profound atrophy of all retinal layers can be observed at the posterior pole (Figs 17.11 to 17.14).

Thus *in vivo* visualization and quantification of transverse, central photoreceptor loss and correlation with visual function seems possible.[88] In fact it seems that lower visual acuity well corresponds to a greater transverse photoreceptor loss, which also correlates with the extent of changes seen in fluorescein angiography and in fundus autofluorescence. Furthermore reduced retinal thickness does not correlate with the transverse extent of photoreceptor loss; although a progressive atrophy of intraretinal layers an intact photoreceptor layer, leads to better visual acuity.[88]

Moreover, OCT-3 sometimes allows visualization of hyper-reflective dots that could be interpreted as the presence of material. When comparing OCT scans and color photograph of the fundus, the localization of the hyper-reflective dots seems to correlate with the localization of the retinal flecks. We tried to classify the deposits according to their localization within the retina with 2 pattern types:

1. Little dots at the level or just above the retinal pigment epithelium (Figs 17.13 and 17.14).
2. Little dots at the level of to the outer nuclear layer (Figs 17.15 and 17.16).

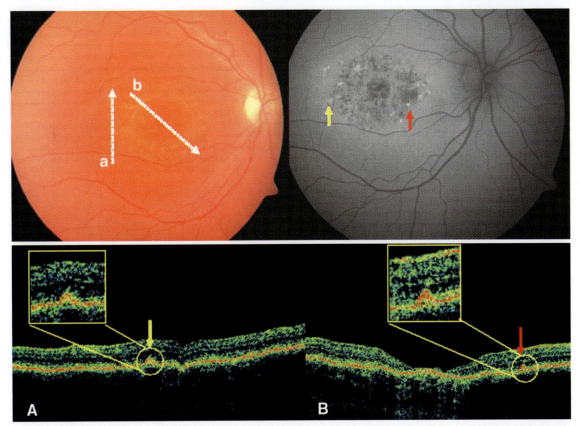

Fig. 17.14: Visualisation of elevated dots at the level or above the retinal pigment epithelium layer. Top left: Color photograph shows macular atrophy and retina flecks (a, b). Top right: Auto-fluorescent frame shows all fine retinal flecks. Bottom: OCT scans show little hyper-reflective dots at the level of retinal pigment epithelium layer (red and yellow arrows). These little dots seem to correspond to the accumulation of auto-fluorescent material and could be interpreted as retinal flecks. Note that retinal thickness appears normal besides the macular area (bottom left) whereas a profound atrophy observed in macular area (bottom right).

In most cases, the retinal pigment epithelium layer appears more reflective than the material. However, in some cases, the reflectivity of the retinal pigment epithelium and the material was very close and thus cannot be distinguishable by OCT. Optical coherence tomography examination could be performed using lower intensity energy (300~400µW), thus reducing reflectivity of the two structures and allowing their differentiation. The retinal pigment epithelium band usually appears linear and continuous without retinal pigment epithelium detachment and no edema, retinal cysts, retinal thickening or serous detachment is found on OCT examination.

In conclusion, OCT seems to allow quantitative *in vivo* assessment of the photoreceptor layer in patients with Stargardt's disease and to correlate it with visual acuity,[88] providing interesting information about morphology of retina and localization of flecks.

BEST'S VITELLIFORM DYSTROPHY

Best's vitelliform dystrophy has been initially described by Adams in 1883. In 1905, Best published a family of 59 members and described then the principal stages of the disease.[89] Zanen and Rausen in 1950 described the typical "Egg Yolk" aspect and introduced the term "vitelliform".[90]

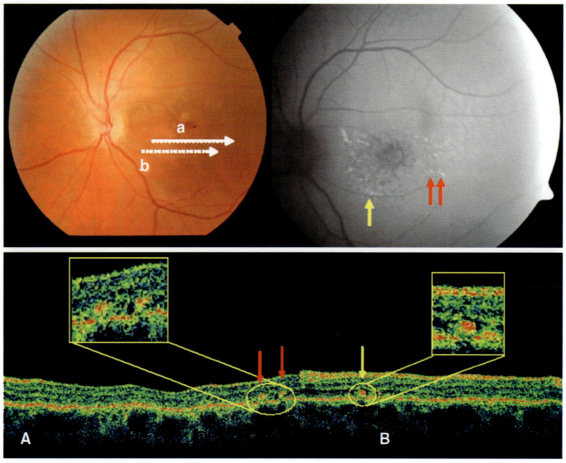

Fig. 17.15: Visualisation of elevated dots at the level of outer nuclear layer. Top left: Color photograph shows macular atrophy and retina flecks (a, b). Top right: Auto-fluorescent frame shows all fine retinal flecks. Bottom left and right: Hyper-reflective dots are observed at the level of outer nuclear layer by OCT-3 and seems to correspond to retinal flecks (A, B). Retinal thickness is normal.

Best's macular dystrophy is a hereditary disease, autosomal dominant with strong penetrance but variable expressivity. The onset takes place mainly in childhood but late onset cases have been described. The gene VMD2 (Vitelliform Macular Dystrophy – 2) [91] located on the chromosome 11q13 has been associated with the disease. It codes for the protein "bestrophin", [92] which plays a role in the ionic transmembrane canals.[93,94]

In literature some histological lesions have been reported such as diffuse alterations of the pigment epithelium,[95-97] excessive lipofuscin deposit, geographic atrophy of the retinal pigment epithelium, abnormal fibrillary material deposition similar to drusen and ruptures of the Bruch's membrane and development of choroidal neovascular membrane.[98,99] Gass referred two cases from the literature where histopathology was available that gave the hint that Best's disease is a generalized "abnormality" of the retinal pigment epithelium associated with accumulation of granules of lipofuscin at the level of the pigment epithelium and in the macrophages of the subretinal and choroidal space.

Presentation of Best's disease is usually in the first to second decades (7-12 years) with uni- or bilateral gradual impairment of central vision and metamorphopsia.[100,101] Juvenile Best's disease evolves gradually through five-six stages, described on the basis of fundus examination:

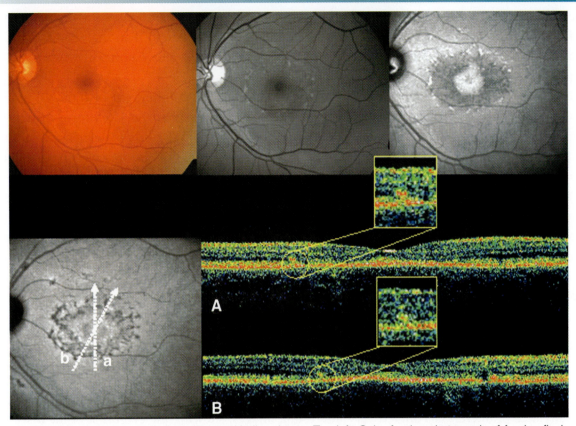

Fig. 17.16: Little dots above the retinal pigment epithelium layer. Top left: Color fundus photograph of fundus flavimaculatus. Retinal flecks appear yellow and poorly contrasted. Top middle: On red-free frame, the perimacular flecks appear more contrasted. No profound macular atrophy is visible. Top right: Perifoveal flecks appear auto-fluorescent on Heidelberg retinal angiogram frame as well as macular area. Bottom left: Late stage of ICG sequence (30 min) the flecks are hypo-fluorescent, more numerous and well defined. Some hyper-fluorescent pin-points are visible on their borders. Bottom right A and B: Some hyper-reflective dots are observed at the level of outer nuclear layer. These dots are clearly separated from retinal pigment epithelium layer. Again they could correspond to the retinal flecks.

- *Previtelliform stage* is characterized by normal fundus or sometimes a bullous aspect. The electro-oculogram (EOG) is usually abnormal with an Arden ratio of <140%.[102,103]

- *Vitelliform stage* or egg yolk stage is characterized by a yellowish or orange macular elevation creating an "egg-yolk "aspect.[104] The lesion is centered on the fovea and is 0.5 to 2 disc diameters in size. The visual acuity is typically preserved.

- *Vitelliruptive stage*, also called pseudohypopyon stage, is characterized by a horizontal sedimentation of the vitelliform material.[105] A horizontal level is obvious with the material on the lower part and pigment epithelial changes on the upper part. During this stage, visual acuity begins to decline.

- *Scrambled eggs' stage* is characterized by inhomogeneous dispersion of the vitelliform material. The visual acuity continues to decrease during this stage.

- *Atrophy stage* is the final stage of the disease, characterized by a homogenous plaque of atrophy centered on the macula. The atrophy involves mainly the retinal pigment epithelium with a salt and pepper aspect, as well as the chorioretinal layer. Without history of Best's disease, positive diagnosis is difficult at this stage.

- *Stage of fibrosis*, also called retractile stage, is in fact an alternative evolution of the disease that often coexists with atrophy. The lesion is white-yellow, and appears more rigid than the vitelliform material. Visual acuity depends on the location of the fibrosis in rapport to the foveola. Choroidal neovascularisation, when complicating Best's disease, most frequently occurs at this stage.

Angiographic features correlate well with fundus aspects.[106] First, autofluorescent frames are of major diagnostic importance because of the characteristic autofluorescence that the vitelliform material.[107] At vitelliform stage, fluorescein angiography reveals a hypofluorescent disc, with complete blocked fluorescence of the choroidal background. At pseudohypopyon stage, a normo or hyperfluorescence is visible on the upper part of the lesion, where the material is absent, contrasting with the hypofluorescence in the lower part of the lesion, where the sediment material lies. At scrambled eggs' stage, scattered areas of hypo and hyperfluorescence are observed according with the dispersion of the material. At atrophic stage, the typical window defect aspect of the retinal pigment epithelium atrophy is observed. At fibrotic stage, intense early hyperfluorescence of the fibrosis is shown by fluorescein angiography, which helps in the differential diagnosis with the material in vitelliform stage. Hyperfluorescence is due to staining of the fibroglial material and a window defect due to retinal pigment epithelium changes. Indocyanine green angiography is useful in case of suspicion of associated CNV.

Optical Coherence Tomography

Optical coherence tomography has been particularly helpful for the understanding of retinal abnormalities in Best's vitelliform macular dystrophy.[108] The capacity for visualization of the structures of the affected retina at any area of interest has offered very interesting images, showing the evolution of the disease from one stage to the other.

- At previtelliform stage, OCT is most often normal. Rarely, an aspect of discrete elevation of retinal pigment epithelium-Bruch's membrane complex can be observed.
- At vitelliform stage an elevated, dome shaped aspect of the whole retina is observed. The neurosensory retina preserves its thickness and structure (Fig. 17.17).
- At pseudohypopyon stage, OCT clearly distinguishes two different zones (Figs 17.18 and 17.19). In the upper part of the lesion, the OCT scan shows a zone optically empty (hypo-reflectivity) giving an aspect of duplication of the retinal pigment epithelium-Bruch's complex. In fact several interpretations could be given to these images. It is also possible that the outer hyper-reflective layer of this complex could be the "envelope" or the "cover" of the vitelliform lesion. Anyway, the retinal pigment epithelium seems to have lost its regularity. In the lower part of the lesion, where the material is still visible, OCT scan exhibits a hyper-reflectivity pattern; witch seems located between the retinal pigment epithelium and Bruch's membrane. Again, another explanation of these images could be that the materiel is enclosed between the cover of the lesion (outer part) and the retinal pigment epithelium (inner part).

There is scarce bibliography on the location of the vitelliform material in respect to the retinal pigment epithelium. According to Coscas and associates,[109] the vitelliform material could be localized under the retinal pigment epithelium layer, which seems mildly thickened and protruding forwards giving rise to accentuation of the hyper-reflectivity of the retinal pigment epithelium band. The photoreceptor layer is spared, which explains preservation of visual acuity at this stage.

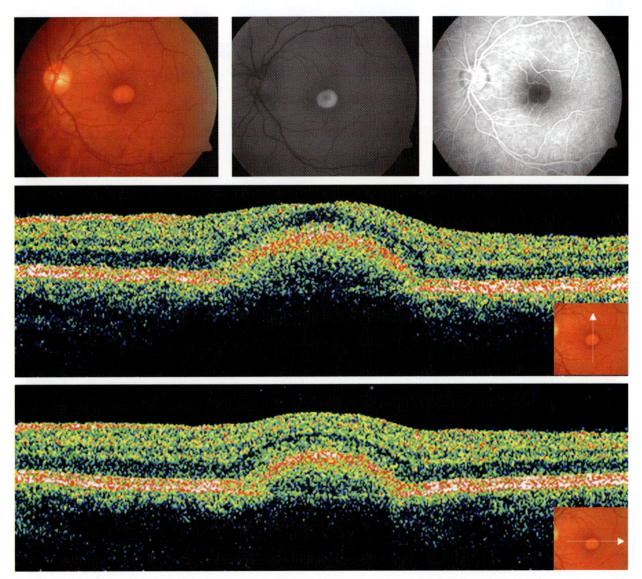

Fig. 17.17: Vitelliform stage: Color photograph of the fundus (top left) shows the well-delineated, round, orange-yellow vitelliform lesion. The lesion harbors homogeneous auto fluorescence (top middle). On fluorescein angiography (top right), the lesion is hypofluorescent, with complete blocked fluorescence of the choroid background. Linear vertical OCT scan (5 mm) reveals an elevation of the neurosensory retina that keeps its normal thickness and structure (middle). Horizontal 5 mm scan crossing the upper part of the lesion shows a hyper-reflective dome-shaped elevation in the macular region with total integrity of the retina (lower).

- At scrambled eggs stage, an optically empty lesion is visible on OCT, comparable with the upper part of the pseudohypopyon. Furthermore, on some parts, where the residual material is still present, OCT scan reveals a hype-reflective mottling stuck on the retinal pigment epithelium layer (Figs 17.20 and 17.21).
- At atrophic stage, OCT reveals thinning of all the retinal layers with enhancement of reflectivity of the retinal pigment epithelium, which seems to spread far behind it (Fig. 17.22).
- Finally, at fibrosis stage, the fibroglial lesion shows a characteristic configuration of a prominent very hyper-reflective thickening at the level of the retinal pigment epithelium accompanied by thinning of the

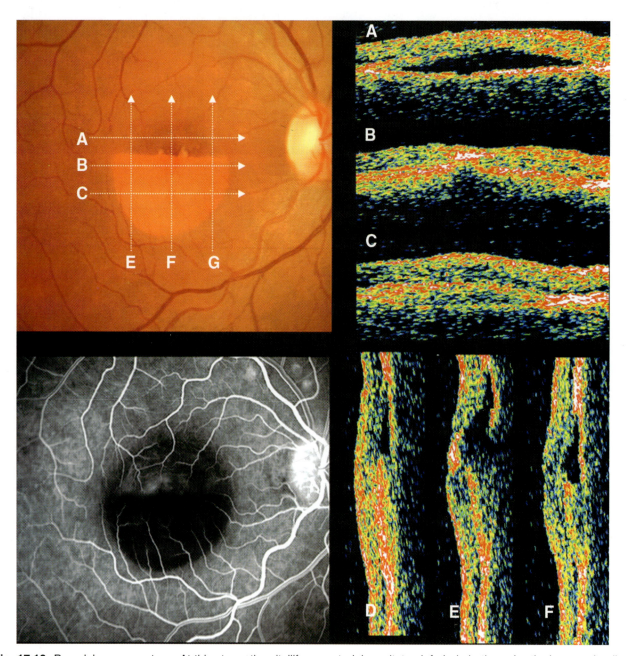

Fig. 17.18: Pseudohypopyon stage. At this stage, the vitelliform material gravitates inferiorly in the subretinal space, leading to a horizontal level dividing the macular lesion on fundus examination (top left). On fluorescein angiography, the inferior part is hypofluorescent, due to the blocked fluorescence effect of the sediment vitelliform material, whereas the superior part is slightly hyperfluorescent due to a window defect caused by retinal pigment epithelium changes (bottom left). A, B and C lines illustrates 3 horizontal cross sections of the macular area, from the top to the bottom. On the superior part, OCT scans demonstrate an optically empty zone, comprised between 2 hyper-reflective layers. On the inferior part of the lesion, the sediment material appears as a dense hyper reflective structure. D, E and F lines illustrates 3 vertical cross sections, from the temporal to the nasal part of the macula. The transition between the empty area and the material is abrupt.

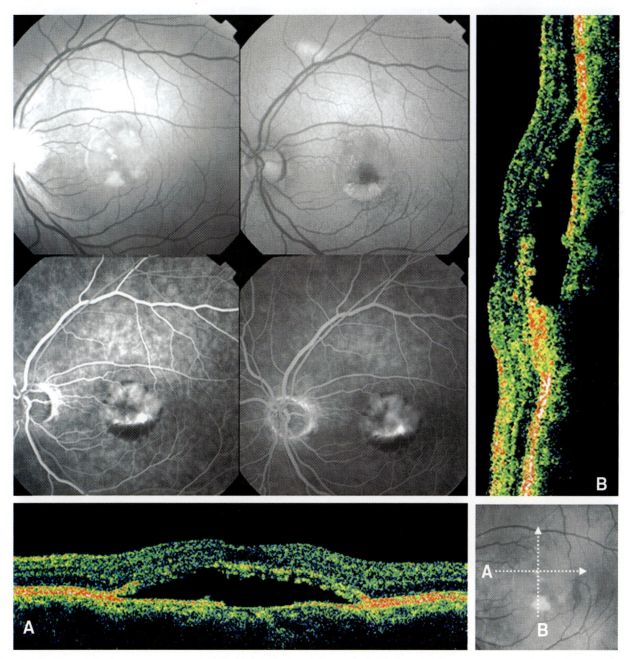

Fig. 17.19: Pseudohypopyon: advanced stage. Here, the material is partially degraded, with few residual material accumulated in the lower part of the macular area. Red free and autofluorescent frames (top left and top middle) allow localizing the remaining material. On fluorescein angiography, the material appears hypofluorescent because of a blocking effect (early phase and late phase, middle). A and B respectively represents horizontal and vertical 5 mm OCT scans. The superior part of the lesion appears hypo reflective, included between two hyper-reflective layers (A, bottom). Few remaining material appears hyper reflective, on the lower part of the lesion (B, right).

sensory retina above it (Fig. 17.23). In these fibroglial forms, OCT reveals a hyper-reflective mass, continuous with the retinal pigment epithelium but inducing thickening and marked anterior bulging. The inner layers of the retina are markedly thinned at this stage. This protruding lesion is easily

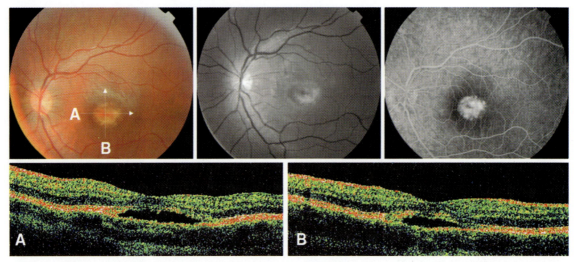

Fig. 17.20: Scrambled egg stage: On fundus examination, the lesion appears irregular and heterogeneous (color picture and red free frames, top left and top middle panels respectively). On fluorescein angiography, an irregular appearance of hyperfluorescence is seen, with early staining but without any leakage. Horizontal and vertical OCT scan show a hyporeflective aspect included between two hyper-reflective layers.

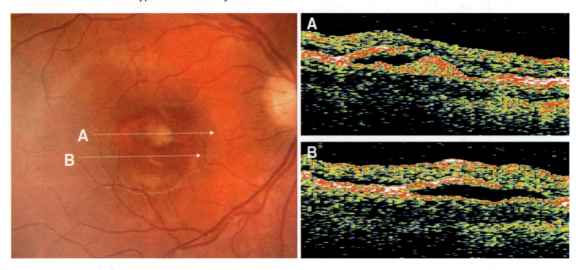

Fig. 17.21: Scrambled egg stage with residual material. Here, the apparent residual material in the centre of the lesion appears as a hyper-reflective deposit stuck on the outer hyper reflective layer on OCT-1 (A). The rest of the lesion is hyporeflective (B).

distinguished from that seen at the vitelliform stage. Therefore, OCT contributes to the differential diagnosis in cases with doubtful findings on fundus examination.

ADULT-ONSET FOVEOMACULAR VITELLIFORM DYSTROPHY

Adult-onset foveomacular vitelliform dystrophy (AFVD) was first described by Gass in 1974 and subsequently analyzed and clinically defined by many authors.[110-114] AFVD differs from vitelliform dystrophy (Best's disease) by many characteristics: late onset (40-70 years of age), moderate symptoms, normal or subnormal electro-oculogram, and an indeterminate genetic inheritance. While some authors suggest an autosomal dominant

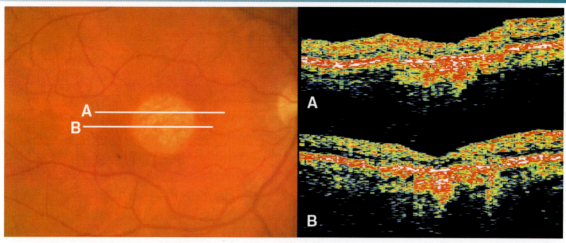

Fig. 17.22: Atrophic stage: Fundus examination reveals a regular, disciform, atrophic area centered on the fovea (left). This profound atrophy involves the deeper layers such as the choriocapillaris, exposing large choroidal vessels. On OCT-1 scans (A and B, right), we observe thinning of the inner and outer retinal layers, with extended hyper-reflectivity of the retinal pigment epithelium-Bruch's membrane-choriocapillaris complex towards the underlying choroid.

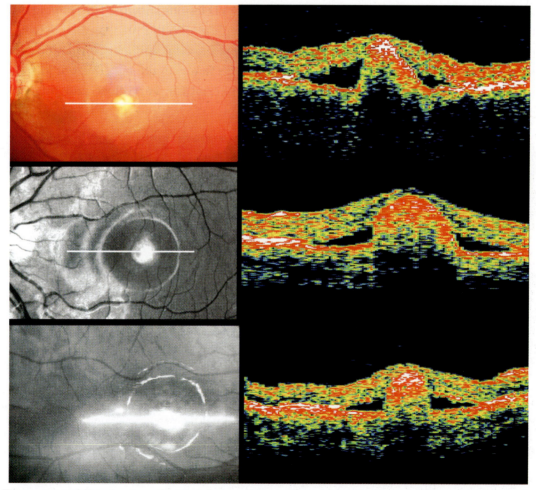

Fig. 17.23: Three cases of fibrosis stage. On the left side, 3 color picture or red free frames of 3 unrelated patients with fibrotic lesions show yellowish, retractile, and rigid fibrous lesions. On the right side of the figure, the 3 corresponding OCT-1 scans show hyper-reflective masses, continuous with the retinal pigment epithelium. The inner layers of the retina are markedly thinned at this stage.

inheritance, others emphasize that many cases are sporadic, with no evidence of a familial inheritance pattern. [115-117] The age of onset is comprised between 35 and 55 years, and visual acuity usually ranges from 20/50 to 20/25 at presentation. The main symptoms of the disease are a relative scotoma, metamorphopsia or it can be simply discovered during a standard control.

On fundus examination, AFVD is characterized by a subretinal deposit of yellowish material that is oval or round, elevated, localized in the macular area, and often centered by a pigmented spot. [111-117] The size of the vitelliform lesion is between ¼ and 1 disc diameter. Small hard drusen are often associated. Natural course involves progressive fragmentation of the material and slow evolution towards atrophy, or development of choroidal neovascular membrane, in 5 to 15% of cases. The lesion is typically autofluorescent. On fluorescein angiography examination, the material is hypofluorescent on early phases, surrounded by a hyperfluorescent ring. A progressive staining is observed and the material becomes hyperfluorescent on late stage of fluorescein angiography, without leakage. On indocyanine green angiography, the material is always hypofluorescent.

Optical Coherence Tomography

Two types of lesions can be distinguished by OCT. [118-121] In AFVD lesions showing late staining on fluorescein angiography, the yellowish material appears on OCT as a highly reflective area, located between the hypo-reflective photoreceptor layer and the hyper-reflective retinal pigment epithelial layer (type 1; Fig. 17.24). In most cases, the retinal pigment epithelial layer is more reflective than the material, but in some cases, the reflectivity of the retinal pigment epithelium and the material are very close and thus could not be distinguishable by OCT.

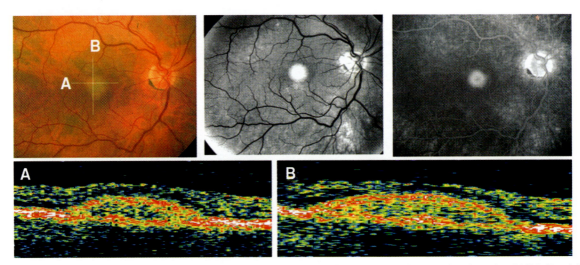

Fig. 17.24: Optical Coherence Tomography in AFVD, type I: Right eye of a 68-year-old man, visual acuity: 20/63. Top left: Color photograph, showing the round yellowish foveal lesion of AVFD Top middle: Red-free photograph showing the whitish foveal lesion. Top right: Fluorescein angiogram, late phase, showing staining of the pseudovitelliform lesion. Bottom left: 3 mm horizontal scan: the pseudo-vitelliform lesion is shown as a hyper-reflective structure, close to the retinal pigment epithelium reflectivity, lying on the retinal pigment epithelium. Bottom right: 3 mm vertical scan: the deposit of material raises the hyporeflective photoreceptor layer, thus leading to the disappearance of the foveal depression. The retinal pigment epithelium layer located under the material looks less reflective than usual, probably due to attenuation of the signal by the material.

Lesions presenting with persistence of central hypofluorescence without late staining on fluorescein angiography, appear as a focal thickening of the retinal pigment epithelium on OCT, associated with a shadow effect (type 2; Fig. 17.25). The major differences between the morphology of these two groups observed by OCT may be explained by the different stages of AFVD. In advanced stages, a foveal thinning observed by OCT is possibly related with the progressive visual loss.

MALATTIA LEVENTINESE

Familial drusen is thought to represent an early manifestation of age-related macular degeneration. Malattia Leventinese (ML) or Doyne honeycomb retinal dystrophy (DHRD) is an inherited autosomal dominant macular degeneration that results in progressive vision loss. In 1925, Vogt described a form of familial drusen observed in patients living in the Leventine valley in the Ticino Canton of southern Switzerland.[122] These drusen progressed to form a mosaic pattern, named "honeycomb choroiditis" by Doyne.[123]

The gene responsible for ML has been localized on 2p21-p16. [124,125] Recently, Stone and associates [126,127] identified a single nonconservative mutation (arg345trp) in the EFEMP1 (EGF-containing fibrillin-like extracellular matrix protein) gene in 5 families affected with ML/DHRD. The EFEMP1 gene encodes fibulin-3, a member of the fibulin family. Malattia Leventinese is an infrequent disorder but of major interest because of the presence of drusen, a feature shared with age-related macular degeneration (AMD), the most common cause of irreversible vision loss in the developed world.

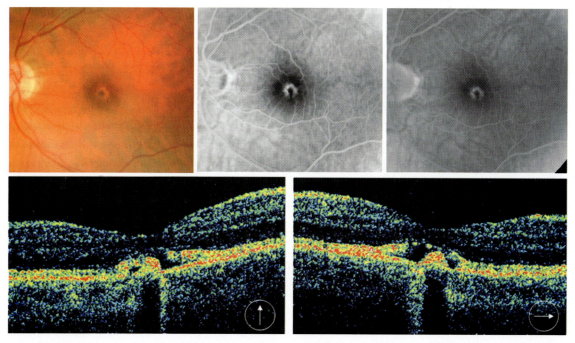

Fig. 17.25: Optical Coherence Tomography in AFVD, type II. Left eye of a 65-year-old woman, BCVA: 20/100. Top left: Color photograph showing the small brown foveal lesion, surrounded by a halo of retinal pigment epithelium atrophy Top middle: Early frame of the fluorescein angiogram showing the foveal hypofluorescence associated with a ring of hyperfluorescence due to retinal pigment epithelium atrophy. Top right: Persistence of the foveal hypofluorescence on late frame. Bottom left: Vertical OCT scan showing a hyper-reflective aspect, inside outer layer of the foveal pseudoviteliform lesion. This hypereflective deposit leads to the masking of the OCT signal in the deep choroidal layers. Bottom right: Similar aspect on horizontal OCT scan.

Diagnosis of ML is usually based on fundus examination, showing small discrete drusen which radiate into the peripheral retina.[128-130] Later, these drusen usually become confluent, leading to the honeycomb appearance.[131] The progression of this macular dystrophy is usually slow except when choroidal neovascularisation (CNV) occurs. Several histopathological report have been published, showing deposits, external to the basement membrane of the retinal pigment epithelium, that occupy the entire thickness of Bruch's membrane.[132,133]

The lesions typically appear in the third decade, and are bilateral and asymmetric. Best corrected visual acuity (BCVA) ranges from 20/25 to 20/200. Metamorphopsia is usually present. Fundus examination shows yellow-white drusen of different size, localized in the macular area and in the peripapillary area (Figs 17.26 and 17.27). There is partial sparing of the central part of the macular area in a heterogeneous pattern. The largest drusen are round, confluent, and localized beside the macular area (also called Forni's verrucosities).[134] Most of the drusen are not well-defined, because of fuzzy limits between each other. The smallest drusen are mainly visible in the peripheral part of the lesion, and are arranged in a radial distribution. Some pigmentary changes, with focal atrophy and pigment mottling, are observed in the macular area.

Optical Coherence Tomography

Multiple vertical and horizontal scans give optimal evaluation of the shape and reflectivity of the material and its location, as well as the reflectivity and appearance of the retinal pigment epithelium, retinal changes and retinal thickness. A hyper-reflective thickening of the retinal pigment epithelium–Bruch's membrane complex can be observed on the scans of the large juxta-central drusen (see Figs 17.1 and 17.2). The largest drusen can be distinguished by a localized dome-shaped elevation, the retinal pigment epithelium–Bruch's membrane complex, which is mainly located parapapillary.[134,137] Retinal thickness and morphology of the inner layers of the retina appear well-preserved above drusen, although some waves of the surface of the retina are observed. Foveal thickness is usually preserved. This preservation probably explains the relative conservation of BCVA despite the importance of the lesions observed in the fundus. In some cases, an appearance of separation between retinal pigment epithelium and Bruch's membrane in the macular area can be observed with a hypo reflective space (see Fig. 17.1A). One hypothesis could be that these drusen, or a lipidic component amalgamated with Bruch's membrane and create a hydrophobic barrier between retinal pigment epithelium and Bruch's membrane,[130] leading to an accumulation of fluid between both the layers. Despite this dissociation, Bruch's membrane is still reflective, containing hyper-reflective elevations on its internal side. In these cases drusen seem to be localized at the inner side of Bruch's membrane. A localized elevation of drusen is sometimes visible and is consistent with the hypothesis of a confluence of the drusen in these patients (see Figs 17.1A, 17.2 and 17.5). The small peripheral radial drusen cannot be clearly identified on OCT. Imaging of these drusen remains rarely described, except in few reports, when associated with CNV.

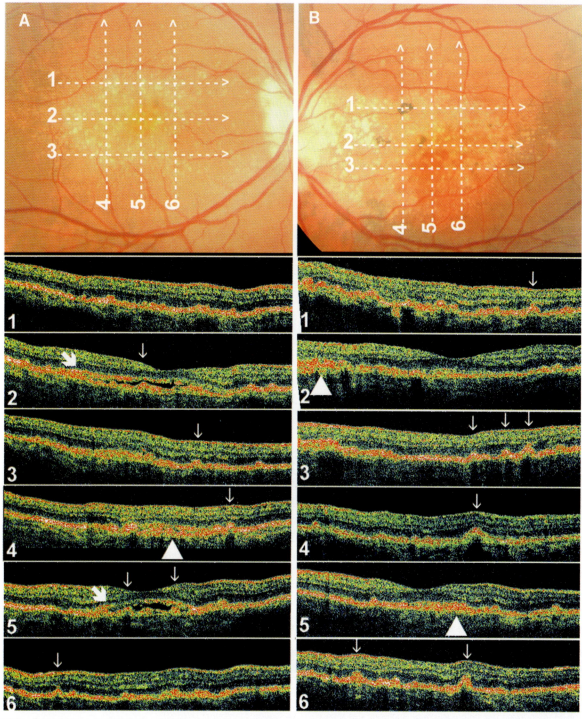

Fig. 17.26: Doted lines indicate the localisation of the OCT scans. Numbers indicate the OCT lines. On the right eye (A), we observe an aspect of separation between the retinal pigment epithelium layer and the Bruch's membrane layer on the center of the macula (scans #2 and #5, oblique white arrows). In both eyes (A and B) vertical thin arrows indicate the presence of limited little zones of elevation of the Bruch's membrane that correspond to the localisation of the large drusen. On the area of the duplication of retinal pigment epithelium-Bruch's membrane, the drusen are clearly localized on the inner part of the Bruch's membrane (A, scan #5). White triangles indicate the presence of a thickening of the retinal pigment epithelium -Bruch's membrane complex. It is notable that the neurosensory layers of the retina and the foveal depression (scans #2 and #5) seem to be well preserved, in both eyes.

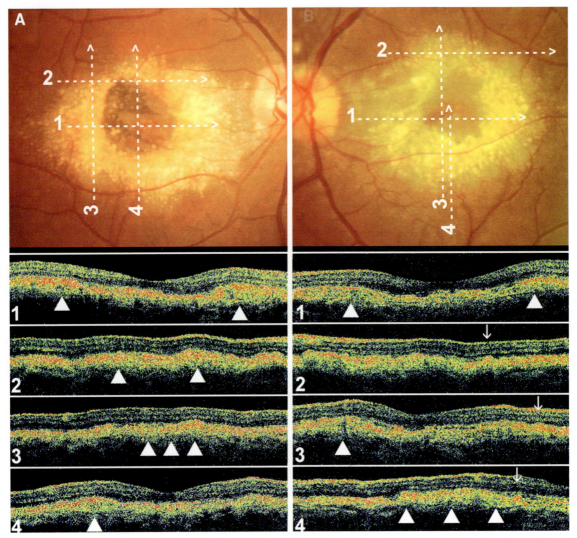

Fig. 17.27: On the right eye (A), the retinal pigment epithelium-Bruch's membrane complex (large white triangles) around the macular area is globally thickened. It is notable that the layers of the neurosensory retina are still preserved in both macular and juxta-macular areas. No limited zone of elevation of the Bruch's membrane is observed in any of the scan for this eye, possibly explained by a confluence of the drusen. On the left eye (B), a similar aspect of thickening of the retinal pigment epithelium-Bruch's membrane complex (large white triangles) is observed with a relative preservation of the layers of the neurosensory retina and some little elevations of Bruch's membrane (vertical thin arrows).

REFERENCES

1. McKusick VA. Mendelian inheritance in man. 9th ed. Baltimore, Johns Hopkins University Press. 1990:974-975.
2. Ovelgün. Nyctalopia haerediotria. Acta Physico Med (Nuremburg). 1744;7:76-77.
3. Schon M. Handbuch der pathologischen. Anatomie des menschlichen Auges. Hamburg. 1828;202.
4. Donders FC. Torpeur de la retine congénitale héréditaire. Ann Ocul (Paris). 1855;34:270-273.
5. Weleber RG, Gregory-Evans K. Retinitis Pigmentosa and allied Disorders. In Ryan SJ (ed.). Retina, Vol. 1, 3rd ed., St. Louis, CV Mosby, 2001; p362.
6. Berson EL. Retinitis pigmentosa without pigment. Arch Ophthalmol. 1969;81:453.
7. Pearlman JT, Axelrod RN, Tom A. Frequency of central visual impairment in retinitis pigmentosa. Arch Ophthalmol 1977;95:894.
8. Friberg TR. Natural course of retinitis pigmentosa over a three-year interval. Am J Ophthalmol 1985;100:621-622.
9. Andreasson S. Electroretinographic studies of families with dominant retinitis pigmentosa. Acta Ophthalmol 1991;69:162-168.
10. Massof RW, Wu L, Finkelstein D, et al. Properties of electroretinographic intensity-response functions in retinitis pigmentosa. Doc Ophthalmol. 1984;57:279-296.

11. Andreasson SO, Sandberg MA, Berson EL. Narrow-band filtering for monitoring low-amplitude cone electroretinograms in retinitis pigmentosa. Am J Ophthalmol 1988;105:500-503.
12. Fahle M, Steuhl KP, Aulhorn E. Correlations between electroretinography, morphology and function in retinitis pigmentosa. Graefe's Arch Clin Exp Ophthalmol 1991;229:37-49.
13. Miller S, Sandberg MA. Cone electroretinographic change during light adaptation in retinitis pigmentosa. Invest Ophthalmol Vis Sci. 1991;32:2536-2541.
14. Foerster MH, Kellner U, Wessing A. Cone dystrophy and supernormal dark-adapted b-waves in the electroretinogram. Graefe's Arch Clin Exp Ophthalmol 1990;228:116-119.
15. Hee MR, Izatt JA, Swanson EA, et al. Optical coherence tomography of the Human Retina. Arch Ophthalmol 1995;113:325-332.
16. Massof RW, Benzschawel T, Emmel T, et al. The spread of retinal degeneration in retinitis pigmentosa. Invest Ophthalmol Vis Sci 1984; 25 (suppl):196.
17. Berson EL, Sandberg MA, Rosner B, et al. Natural Course of Retinitis Pigmentosa over a three-Year Interval. Am J Ophthalmol. 1985;99:240-251.
18. Berson EL, Rosner B, Simonoff E. Risk factors for Genetic Typing and Detection in Retinitis Pigmentosa. Am J Ophthalmolol 1980;86:763-775.
19. Sullivan LJ, Makris GS, Dickinson P, et al. A new codon 15 rodopsin gene mutation in autosomal dominant retinitis pigmentosa is associated with sectorial disease. Arch Ophthalmol 1993,111:1512-1517.
20. Rumen F, Souied E, Oubraham H, et al. Optical coherence tomography in the follow up of macular edema treatment in retinitis pigmentosa. J Fr Ophtalmol. 2001;24:854-859.
21. Apushkin MA, Fishman GA, Janowicz MJ. Monitoring cystoid macular edema by optical coherence tomography in patients with retinitis pigmentosa. Ophthalmology 2004;111:1899-1904.
22. Massin P, Vicaut E, Haouchine B, et al. Reproducibility of retinal mapping using optical coherence tomography. Arch Ophthalmol 2001;119:1135-1142.
23. Koozekanani D, Roberts C, Katz SE, Herderick EE. Intersession repeatability of macular thickness measurements with the Humphrey 2000 OCT. Invest Ophthalmol Vis Sci 2000;40:1486-1491.
24. Muscat S, Parks S, Kemp E, Keating D. Repeatability and reproducibility of macular thickness with the Humphrey OCT system. Invest Ophthalmol Vis Sci 2002;43:490-495.
25. Krill AE, Deutman AF. Dominant macular degenerations: the cone dystrophies. Am J Ophthalmol. 1972;73:352.
26. Francois J, De Rouck A, De Laey JJ. Progressive cone dystrophies. Ophthalmologica. 1976;173:81-101.
27. Gouras P, Eggers HM, MacKay CJ. Cone dystrophy, nyctalopia, and supernormal rod responses. A new retinal degeneration. Arch Ophthalmol. 1983;101:718-724.
28. Ripps H, Noble KG, Greenstein VC, et al. Progressive cone dystrophy. Ophthalmology. 1987;94:1401-1409.
29. Additional evidence for a gene locus for progressive cone dystrophy with late rod involvement in Xp21.1-p11.3. Genomics. 1993;18:463-464.
30. Bergen AA, Meire F, ten Brink J, et al. X-linked progressive cone dystrophy. Clinical characteristics of affected males and female carriers. Ophthalmology. 1989;96:885-895.
31. Hong HK, Ferrell RE, Gorin MB. Clinical diversity and chromosomal localization of X-linked cone dystrophy (COD1). Am J Hum Genet. 1994;55:1173-1181.
32. Bergen AA, Pinckers AJ. Localization of a novel X-linked progressive cone dystrophy gene to Xq27: evidence for genetic heterogeneity. Am J Hum Genet. 1997;60:1468-1473.
33. Sohocki MM, Sullivan LS, Mintz-Hittner HA, et al. A range of clinical phenotypes associated with mutations in CRX, a photoreceptor transcription-factor gene. Am J Hum Genet. 1998;63:1307-1315.
34. Downes SM, Holder GE, Fitzke FW, et al. Autosomal dominant cone and cone-rod dystrophy with mutations in the guanylate cyclase activator 1A gene-encoding guanylate cyclase activating protein-1. Arch Ophthalmol. 2001;119:96-105.
35. Krill AE, Deutman AF, Fishman, M. The cone degenerations. Doc Ophthalmol 1973;35:1.
36. Sadowski B, Zrenner E. Cone and rod function in cone degenerations. Vision Res. 1997;37:2303-2314.
37. Simunovic MP, Moore AT. The cone dystrophies. Eye. 1998;12:553-565.
38. Holopigian K, Seiple W, Greenstein VC, et al. Local cone and rod system function in progressive cone dystrophy. Invest Ophthalmol Vis Sci. 2002;43:2364-2373.
39. Michaelides M, Aligianis IA, Holder GE, et al. Cone dystrophy phenotype associated with a frameshift mutation (M280fsX291) in the alpha-subunit of cone specific transducin (GNAT2). Br J Ophthalmol 2003;87:1317-1320.
40. Ladewig M, Kraus H, Foerster MH, Kellner U. Cone dysfunction in patients with late-onset cone dystrophy and age-related macular degeneration. Arch Ophthalmol 2003;121:1557-1561.
41. Ebenezer ND, Michaelides M, Jenkins SA, et al. Identification of Novel RPGR ORF15 Mutations in X-linked Progressive Cone-Rod Dystrophy (XLCORD) Families. Invest Ophthalmol Vis Sci 2005;46:1891-1898.
42. Hubsch S, Graf M. Foveal cone dystrophy: diagnostic ranking of the multifocal electroretinogram. Klin Monatsbl Augenheilkd 2002;219:370-372.
43. Drexler W, Sattmann H, Hermann B, et al. Enhanced visualization of macular pathology using ultrahigh resolution optical coherence tomography. Arch Ophthalmol 2003;121:695-706.
44. Gloesmann AM, Hermann B, Schubert C, et al. Histological correlation of pig retinal stratification with ultrahigh resolution optical coherence tomography. Invest Ophthalmol Vis Sci 2003;44:1696 -1703.
45. Drexler W, Morgner U, Ghanta RK, et al. Ultrahigh resolution ophthalmologic optical coherence tomography. Nat Med. 2001;7:502-507.
46. Anger EM. Unterhuber A, Hermann B, et al. Ultrahigh resolution optical coherence tomography of the monkey fovea: identification of retinal sublayers by correlation with semi-thin histology sections. Exp Eye Res. 2004;78:1117-1125.
47. Stargardt K. Ueber familiare progressive degeneration in der makulagegend des Auges. Albrecht V. Graefes. Arch Ophthalmol 1909;71:534-550.
48. Cibis GW, Morey M, Karris DJ. Dominantly inherited macular dystrophy with flecks (Stargardt), Arch Ophthalmol. 1980;98:1785.
49. Merlin S, Landau J. Abnormal findings in relatives of patients with juvenile hereditary macular degeneration (Stargardt's disease). Ophthalmologica 1970;161:1.

50. Francheschetti A: Ueber tapcto-retinale Degenerationen im Kindesaltcr. In: Entwicklung und Fortschritt in derAugenheilkunde Stuttgart, Enke, 1953.
51. Franceschetti A, Francois J. Fundus flavimaculatus. Arch Ophtalmol (Paris). 1965;25:505.
52. Krill AE, Deutman AF. The various categories of juvenile macular degeneration. Trans Am Ophthalmol Soc. 1972;70:220.
53. Stargardt K. Zur Kasuistik der "familiaren, progressiven Degeneration in der Makulagegcnd des Auges," Z Augenheilkd. 1916;35:249.
54. Stargardt K. Ueber familiare Degeneration in der Maculagegend des Auges, mit und ohne psychische Storungen. Arch Psychiatr Nervenk 1917;58:852.
55. Stargardt K. Em Fall von familiarer progressiver Makuladegeneration. Klin Monatsbl Augenheilkd. 1925;75:246.
56. Mylius K. Ueber Fundusveranderungen ausserhalb des Foveagebietes bei der Heredodegeneration der „Makula" (Behr). Klin Monatsbl Augenheilkd. 1955;126:539.
57. Klien BA, Krill AE. Fundus flavimaculatus: clinical, functional and histopathologic observations. Am J Ophthalmol. 1967;64:3.
58. Kniazeva M, Chiang MF, Morgan B, et al. A new locus for autosomal dominant Stargardt-like disease maps to chromosome 4. Am J Hum Genet. 1999;64:1394.
59. Aaberg TM. Stargardt's disease and fundus flavimaculatus: evaluation of morphologic progression and intrafamilial co-existence. Trans Am Ophthalmol Soc. 1980;84:453-487.
60. Isashiki Y, Ohba N. Fundus flavimaculatus: Polymorphic retinal change in siblings. Br J Ophthalmol. 1985;69:522-524.
61. Noble KG, Carr RE. Stargardt's disease and fundus flavimaculatus. Arch Ophthalmol. 1979;97:1281-1285.
62. Rotenstreich Y, Fishman GA, Anderson RJ. Visual acuity loss and clinical observations in a large series of patients with Stargardt's disease. Ophthalmology. 2003;110:1151-1178.
63. Armstrong TD, Meyer D, Xu S, et al. Long-term follow-up of Stargardt's disease and fundus flavimaculatus. Ophthalmology. 1998;105:448- 458.
64. Fishman GA, Farber M, Patel BS, et al, Visual acuity loss in patients with Stargardt's macular dystrophy. Ophthalmology. 1987;94:809-814.
65. Irvine AR, Wergeland FL. Stargardt's hereditary progressive macular degeneration. Br J Ophthalmol. 1972;56:817-826.
66. Hadden O, Gass JDM. Fundus flavimaculatus and Stargardt's disease. Am J Ophthalmol. 1976;82:527-539.
67. Allikmets R, Singh N, Sun H, et al. A photoreceptor cell-specific ATP-binding transporter gene (ABCR) is mutated in recessive Stargardt's macular dystrophy, Nature Genet. 1997;15:236-246.
68. George ND, Yates, JR, Moore, AT. Clinical features in affected males with X-linked retinoschisis, Arch Ophthalmol 1996;114:274-280.
69. Gerber S, Rozet JM, Bonneau E, et al. A gene for late-onset Fundus Flavimaculatus with macular dystrophy maps to chromosome 1p13. Am J Hum Genet. 1995;56:396-399.
70. Kaplan J, Gerber S, Larget-Piet D, et al. A gene for Stargardt's disease (fundus flavimaculatus) maps to the short arm of chromosome 1. Nature Genet. 1993;5:308-311.
71. Cremers FP, van de Pol DJ, van Driel M, et al. Autosomal recessive retinitis pigmentosa and cone-rod dystrophy caused by splice site mutations in the Stargardt's disease gene ABCR. Hum Mol Genet. 1998;7:355-362.
72. Rozet JM, Gerber S, Souied E, et al. Spectrum of ABCR gene mutations in autosomal recessive macular dystrophies. Eur J Hum Genet. 1998;6:291-295.
73. Bernstein PS, Tammur J, Singh N, et al. Diverse macular dystrophy phenotype caused by a novel complex mutation in the ELOVL4 gene. Invest Ophthalmol Vis Sci. 2001;42:3331-3336.
74. Zhang K, Kniazeva M, Han M, et al. A 5-bp deletion in ELOVL4 is associated with two related forms of autosomal dominant macular dystrophy. Nat Genet. 2001;27:89-93.
75. Klein BA, Krill AE. Fundus flavimaculatus. Clinical, functional and histopathological observations. Am J Ophthalmol. 1967;64:3-23.
76. Eagle RC, Lucier AC, Bernadrdino VB, Yanoff M. Retinal pigment epithelial abnormalities in fundus flavimaculatus. Ophthalmology. 1980;87:1189-1200.
77. Doyne RW. Peculiar condition of choroiditis occurring in several members of the same family. Trans Ophthalmol Soc UK. 1899;19:71.
78. Lois N, Holder GE, Bunce C, et al. Phenotypic subtypes of Stargardt's macular dystrophy-fundus flavimaculatus. Arch Ophthalmol. 2001;119:359-369.
79. Allikmets, R, Shroyer, NF, Singh, N, et al. Mutation of the Stargardt's disease gene (ABCR) in age-related macular degeneration, Science 1997;277:1805-1807.
80. Holz FG. Auto fluorescence imaging of the macula. Ophthalmologe. 2001;98:10-18
81. Von Ruckmann A, Fitzke FW, Bird AC. In vivo autofluorescence in macular dystrophies. Arch Ophthalmol. 1997;115:609-615.
82. Bellmann C, Hvlz FG, Schapp O, et al. Topography of fundus auto fluorescence with a new confocal scanning laser ophthalmoscope. Ophthalmologe. 1997;94:385-391.
83. Stavrou P, Good PA, Misson GP, et al. Electrophysiological findings in Stargardt's-fundus flavimaculatus disease. Eye. 1998;12:953-958.
84. Drexler W, Sattmann H, Hermann B, et al. Enhanced visualization of macular pathology using ultrahigh resolution optical coherence tomography. Arch Ophthalmol. 2003;121:695-706.
85. Gloesmann A, Hermann B, Schubert C, et al. Histological correlation of pig retinal stratification with ultrahigh resolution optical coherence tomography. Invest Ophthalmol Vis Sci. 2003;44:1696 -1703.
86. Drexler W, Morgner U, Ghanta RK, et al, ultrahigh resolution ophthalmologic optical coherence tomography. Nat Med. 2001;7:502-507.
87. Anger EM. Unterhuber A, Hermann B, et al. Ultrahigh resolution optical coherence tomography of the monkey fovea: identification of retinal sub layers by correlation with semi-thin histology sections. Exp Eye Res. 2004;78:1117-1125.
88. Ergun E, Hermann B, M Wirtitsch M, et al. Assessment of Central Visual Function in Stargardt's Disease/Fundus Flavimaculatus with Ultrahigh-Resolution Optical Coherence Tomography. Invest Ophthalmol Vis Sci. 2005; 46: 310-316.
89. Sayag D, Souied E, Pawlak D, et al. Contribution of OCT for analysing the white-yellowish fleks in Stargardt's disease. Journal Francaise d'Ophtalmologie. 2003; 26:series number1:1S215.
90. Best F. Uber eine hereditare maculaafektion; Beitrage zur verergslehre. Zschr. Augenheilk. 1905;13:199-212.
91. Zanen J, Rausin G. Kyste vitelliforme congénital de la macula. Bull Soc Belge Ophthalmol. 1950;96:544-549.
92. Stone EM, Nichols BE, Streb LM, et al. Genetic linkage of vitelliform macular degeneration Best's disease to chromosome 11q13. Nat. Genet. 1992;1:246-250.

93. Petrukhin K, Koisti MJ, Bakall B, et al. Identification of the gene responsible for Best's macular dystrophy. Nat Genet. 1998;19:241-247.
94. Sun H, Tsunenari T, Yau KW, Nathans J. The vitelliform macular dystrophy protein defines a new family of chloride channels. Proc Natl Acad Sci USA. 2002;99:4008-4013.
95. Marmorstein AD, Marmorstein LY, Rayborn M, et al. Bestrophin, the product of the Best vitelliform macular dystrophy gene (VMD2), localizes to the basolateral plasma membrane of the retinal pigment epithelium. Proc Natl Acad Sci USA. 2000;97:127: 58-63.
96. Weingeist TA, Kobrin JL, Watzke RC. Histopathology of Best's macular dystrophy. Arch Ophthalmol. 1982;100:1108-1114.
97. Patrinely JR, Lewis RA, Font RL. Foveomacular vitelliform dystrophy, adult type. A clinicopathologic study including electron microscopic observations. Ophthalmology. 1985;92:1712-1718.
98. Dubovy SR, Hairston RJ, Schatz H, et al. Adult-onset foveomacular pigment epithelial dystrophy: clinicopathologic correlation of three cases. Retina. 2000;20:638-649.
99. Turut P, Malthieu D, Lenski C. [Vitelliform degeneration of the macula and neovascular choroidal membrane] Bull Soc Ophtalmol Fr. 1982;82: 587-590.
100. Miller SA, Bresnick GH, Chandra SR. Choroidal neovascular membrane in Best's vitelliform macular dystrophy. Am J Ophthalmol. 1976; 82:252-255.
101. Turut P, Chaine G, Puech B, et al. Francois P. Les dystrophies hereditaires de la macula. Bull Soc Ophtalmol. 1991: (Suppl) 97 -110.
102. Turut P, Hache JC, Francois P. [Early change of macular function in vitelliform degeneration of the macula]. Bull Soc Ophtalmol Fr. 1972; 72:1121-1124.
103. Krill AE, Morse PA, Potts AM, Klien BA. Hereditary vitelliruptive macular degeneration. Am J Ophthalmol. 1966;61:1405.
104. François J, De Rouck A, Fernandez-Sasso D. Electro-oculography in vitelliform degeneration of the macula. Arch Ophthalmol. 1967;77:726-733.
105. Francois P, Turut P. [Vitelliform degeneration of the macula] Arch Ophtalmol Rev Gen Ophtalmol. 1975;35:609-626.
106. Godel V, Chaine G, Regenbogen L, Coscas G. Best's vitelliform macular dystrophy. Acta Ophthalmol Suppl. 1986;175:1-31.
107. Gass JMD. Stereoscopic atlas of macular diseases diagnosis and treatment. St. Louis, 1987, CV Mosby Co, 3 ed.
108. Barr DB, Beirouty ZA. Auto fluorescence in a patient with adult vitelliform degeneration. Eur J Ophthalmol. 1995;5:155-159.
109. Pianta MJ, Aleman TS, Cideciyan AV, et al. In vivo micropathology of Best's macular dystrophy. Invest Ophthalmol Vis Sci. 2002 ;43(suppl):1165.
110. Coscas G. Atlas d'angiograpie en indocyanine confrontations FLUO-ICG-OCT. Bullettin des Societes d'Ophtalmologie de France, rapport annuel – Novembre 2004.
111. Brecher R, Bird AC. Adult vitelliform macular dystrophy. Eye. 1990;4:210-215.
112. Gass JDM. A clinicopathologic study of peculiar foveomacular dystrophy. Trans Am Ophthalmol Soc 1974;72:139-156.
113. Marmor MF, Byers B. Pattern dystrophy of the pigment epithelium. Am J Ophthalmol 1977; 83:32-44.
114. Vine AK, Schatz H. Adult onset foveomacular pigment epithelial dystrophy. Am J Ophthalmol 1980;89:680-691.
115. Lim JI, Enger C, Fine SL. Foveomacular dystrophy. Am J Ophthalmol 1994;117:1-6.
116. Fishman GA, Trimble S, Rabb MF, Fishman M. Pseudovitelliform macular degeneration. Arch Ophthalmol 1977;95:73-76.
117. Cohen SY, Chretien P, Cochard C, Coscas GJ. Monozygotic twin sisters with adult vitelliform macular dystrophy. Am J Ophthalmol 1993;116:246-247.
118. Sabates R, Pruett RC, Hirose T. Pseudovitelliform macular degeneration. Retina 1982;2:197-205.
119. Benhamou N, Souied E, Zolf R, et al. Adult-onset foveomacular vitelliform dystrophy- a study by optical coherence tomography. Am J Ophthalmol. 2003; 135:362-367.
120. Pierro L, Tremolada G, Introini U, et al. OCT findings in adult onset foveomacular vitelliform dystrophy. Am J Ophthalmol 2002;134:675-680.
121. Benhamou N, Souied E, Zolf R, et al. Adult-onset Foveomacular Vitelliform Dystrophy : A study by optical coherence tomography. Am J Ophthalmol. 2003 ;135:362-367.
122. Benhamou N, Messas-Kaplan A, Cohen Y, et al. Adult-onset foveomacular vitelliform dystrophy with OCT 3. Am J Ophthalmol. 2004;138:294-6.
123. Vogt A. Die Ophthalmoskopie im rotfreien Licht.In: Graefe A,Saemisch T (eds.). Handbuch der gesammten Augenheilkunde.Untersuchungsmethoden. Berlin: Leipez, Verlag von Wilhelm Engelman (3rd ed.) 1925:1-118.
124. Doyne RW. Peculiar condition of choroiditis occurring in several members of the same family. Trans Ophthalmol Soc UK 1899;19:71.
125. Heon E, Piguet B, Munier F, et al. Linkage of autosomal dominant radial drusen (malattia leventinese) to chromosome 2p16-21. Arch Ophthalmol 1996;114:193-198.
126. Gregory CY, Evans K, Wijesuriya SD, et al. The gene responsible for autosomal dominant Doyne's honeycomb retinal dystrophy (DHRD) maps to chromosome 2p16.Hum Mol Genet. 1996;5:1055-1059.
127. Stone EM, Lotery AJ, Munier FL, et al. A single EFEMP1 mutation associated with both Malattia Leventinese and Doyne honeycomb retinal dystrophy. Nat Genet 1999;22:199-202.
128. Matsumoto M, Traboulsi EI. Dominant radial drusen and Arg345Trp EFEMP1 mutation. Am J Ophthalmol 2001;131:810-812.
129. Piguet B, Haimovici R, Bird AC. Dominantly inherited drusen represent more than one disorder: a historical review. Eye 1995;9:34-41.
130. Deutman AF, Jansen LM. Dominantly inherited drusen of Bruch's membrane. Br J Ophthalmol 1970;54:373-382.
131. Pauleikhoff D, Zuels S, Sheraidah GS, et al. Correlation between biochemical composition and fluorescein binding of deposits in Bruch's membrane. Ophthalmology 1992;99:1548-1553.
132. Zech JC, Zaouche S, Mourier F, et al. Macular dystrophy of malattia leventinese. A 25-year follow up. Br J Ophthalmol. 1999;83:1195-1196.
133. Holz FG, Owens SL, Marks J, et al. Ultrastructural findings in autosomal dominant drusen. Arch Ophthalmol 1997;115:788-792.
134. Marmorstein LY, Munier FL, Arsenijevic Y, et al. Aberrant accumulation of EFEMP1 underlies drusen formation in Malattia Leventinese and age-related macular degeneration. Proc Natl Acad Sci USA. 2002; 99:13067-13072.
135. Gaillard MC, Wolfensberger TJ, Uffer S, et al. Optical coherence tomography in Malattia Leventinese. Klin Monatsbl Augenheilkd 2005; 222:180-185.
136. Leveziel N, Souied E, Coscas G, Soubrane G. Imaging of Malattia Leventinese. Invest Ophthalmol Vis Sci 2005 46: E-Abstract 3296.
137. Souied EH, Leveziel N, Letien V, et al. Optical coherance tomography features of Malattia Leventinese. Am J Opthalmol (In press).

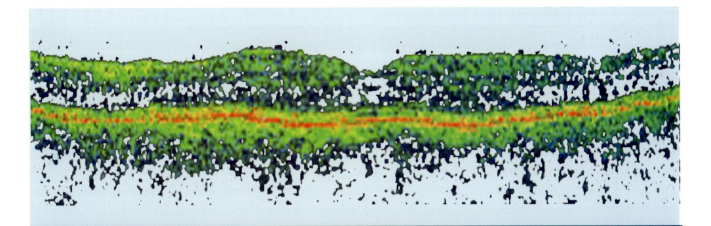

CHAPTER
18

Ocular Oncology

**Carol L Shields, Miguel A Materin,
Jerry A Shields**

INTRODUCTION

There are several tumors that can occur in the posterior segment of the eye.[1,2] They are generally classified based on the main tissue involved such as the choroid, retinal pigment epithelium, or retina. The spectrum of tumors in each tissue varies. For example, tumors in the choroid include the melanocytic nevus, melanoma, metastasis, cavernous hemangioma, and other less common tumors such as lymphoma, neurilemoma, leiomyoma, and osteoma. [1,2] Lesions of the retinal pigment epithelium include congenital hypertrophy, congenital simple hamartoma, combined hamartoma, reactive hyperplasia, adenoma, and adenocarcinoma. Those affecting the retina include capillary hemangioma, cavernous hemangioma, racemose hemangioma, vasoproliferative tumor, astrocytic hamartoma, and retinoblastoma. The differentiation of these tumors by experienced clinicians is made primarily by indirect ophthalmoscopy. Ancillary testing with intravenous fluorescein angiography, indocyanine green angiography, ultrasonography, optical coherence tomography (OCT), color Doppler testing, magnetic resonance imaging, computed tomography, and fine needle aspiration biopsy can assist in confirming the diagnosis.[1,2] In this chapter, the OCT findings of selected intraocular tumors will be presented.

Optical coherence tomography provides cross sectional imaging of the retina and retinal pigment epithelium primarily, and deeper tissues, including the choroid and sclera, show poorer resolution. With this in mind, OCT of retinal and retinal pigment epithelium tumors show good resolution whereas OCT of choroidal tumors show only superficial information of the choroidal tumor, but more extensive information of the overlying retina and retinal pigment epithelium.

CHOROIDAL TUMORS

Choroidal Nevus

Choroidal melanocytic nevus is a benign tumor that is seen with increasing frequency in the latter decades of life. It is estimated that between 4% to 6% of caucasians manifest a uveal nevus.[3] It can occur in the iris, ciliary body, or choroid, and is most frequent in the posterior choroid. Choroidal nevus varies in size from a fraction of a millimeter to several millimeters in base. The degree of pigmentation can extend from dark brown to slate gray to completely yellow, or amelanotic. The shape of a choroidal nevus is generally round to oval, and it usually manifests smooth regular margins, but slightly irregular margins can be found. Overlying degenerative changes of the retina and retinal pigment epithelium can occur with the most common being drusen, retinal pigment epithelial atrophy and hyperplasia, and clumped orange pigment. Less commonly, subretinal neovascularization and serous and hemorrhagic detachments of the retina and retinal pigment epithelium can occur.

Most choroidal nevi are less than 2 mm in thickness. It is often difficult to differentiate those nevi that are near 2 mm in thickness from small choroidal melanoma. Risk factors predictive of small melanoma have been identified and include tumor thickness greater than 2 mm, overlying orange pigment, associated subretinal fluid, symptoms of flashes, floaters, or blurred vision, and location of the mass at the optic disc.[4-6] The presence of three or more of these five risk factors imparts greater than 50% risk that the tumor will grow, a sign of malignant melanoma.

In general, a choroidal nevus is poorly imaged on OCT due to its location deep in the choroid; however, the overlying retina can show several alterations. In an assessment of 120 eyes with choroidal nevus using

OCT, Shields and associates[7] found related retinal findings that included overlying retina edema (15%), subretinal fluid (26%), retinal thinning (22%), drusen (41%), and retinal pigment epithelial detachment (12%) (Figs 18.1 to 18.3). Furthermore, OCT permitted classification of the overlying retinal edema as focal cystoid (3%), diffuse cystoid (8%), coalescent cystoid (3%), and noncystoid edema (1%). By OCT, the overlying retina was normal thickness (32%), thinned (22%), or thickened (45%) and photoreceptor loss or attenuation was noted in 51% of cases. Specific OCT findings of the choroidal nevus were limited to its anterior surface with minimal information deeper within the mass. These findings included increased thickness of the retinal pigment epithelium/choriocapillaris layer (68%) and optical qualities within the anterior portion of the nevus of hyporeflectivity (62%), isoreflectivity (29%), and hyper reflectivity (9%). Hypo-reflectivity was observed in 68% of pigmented nevi and 18% of non pigmented nevi. (Table 18.1) When comparing OCT to clinical examination, these authors concluded that OCT was more sensitive in the detection of related retinal edema, subretinal fluid, retinal thinning, photoreceptor attenuation, and retinal pigment epithelium detachment. [7]

Table 18.1: Optical coherence tomography in 120 eyes of 120 patients with choroidal nevus: Correlation between nevus pigmentation and OCT findings.[7]		
Findings	*Pigmented choroidal nevus n=109*	*Non-pigmented choroidal nevus n=11*
Retinal findings		
Retinal edema	16 (15%)	2 (18%)
Retinal thinning	22 (22%)	4 (40%)
Photoreceptor layer loss or thinning	55 (50%)	5 (45%)
RPE/choriocapillaris findings		
RPE/choriocapillaris thickening	76 (70%)	6 (55%)
RPE/choriocapillaris hyper-reflectivity	58 (53%)	4 (36%)
RPE/choriocapillaris fragmentation	16 (15%)	7 (64%)
RPE/choriocapillaris surface irregularity	48 (44%)	7 (64%)
Choroidal findings		
Anterior choroid reflectivity*		
Hyporeflective	61 (68%)	2 (18%)
Isoreflective	23 (26%)	6 (55%)
Hyper-reflective	6 (7%)	3 (27%)

* Information on anterior choroid reflectivity was available only for 101 nevi. There were 19 pigmented and 0 non-pigmented nevi where the data was unavailable.

RPE: Retinal pigment epithelium

The findings on OCT of retinal edema, retinal pigment epithelium alterations, photoreceptor loss, and retinal pigment epithelium detachment are related to chronic retinal degeneration and suggest a stable, chronic choroidal nevus.[7] On the other hand, the presence of subretinal fluid and photoreceptor preservation suggests a more acute situation and potentially a more active lesion with risk for growth into melanoma.[8]

Choroidal Melanoma

Malignant melanoma of the choroid is uncommon, found in 6 persons per million population.[1,2,9,10] Melanoma usually grows as a localized elevated mass protruding toward the vitreous cavity on its inner aspect and limited by the sclera on its outer aspect. Occasionally, it will grow into a mushroom configuration or grow horizontally as a diffuse, flat lesion.[11] As the tumor grows it may become associated with widespread

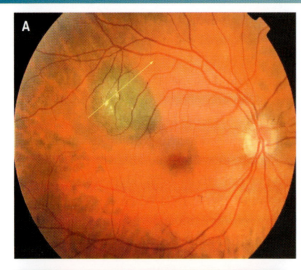

Fig. 18.1: Choroidal nevus; A. Pigmented choroidal nevus displays overlying drusen. Optical coherence tomography shows thickening and hyper-reflectivity of the retinal pigment epithelium/ choriocapillaris layer and hyporeflectivity (optical shadowing) of the choroid at the site of the nevus. Note the subtle multifocal elevations at the level of the retinal pigment epithelium/ choriocapillaris suggestive of drusen.

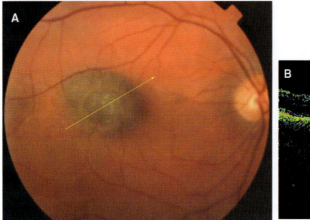

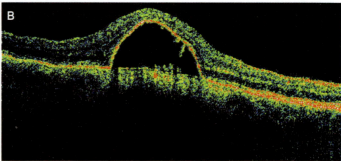

Fig. 18.2: Choroidal nevus: A. Pigmented choroidal nevus shows overlying retinal pigment epithelium detachment outlined with subtle orange pigment. B. Optical coherence tomography shows obvious overlying retinal pigment epithelium detachment with debris in the subpigment epithelial space.

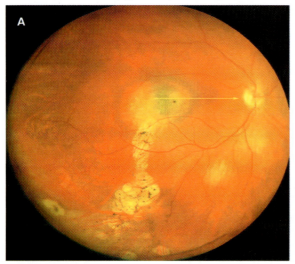

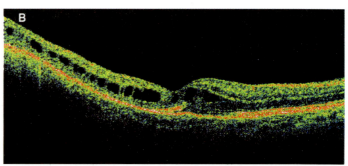

Fig. 18.3: Choroidal nevus: A. Lightly pigmented choroidal nevus displays chronic retinal pigment epithelium alterations inferiorly suggestive of resolved subretinal fluid. B. Optical coherence tomography reveals diffuse cystoid retinal edema over the elevated portion of the nevus and extending into the fovea.

changes in the overlying retinal pigment epithelium including atrophy and degeneration, clumped orange pigment, serous retinal pigment epithelium detachment, sensory retinal detachment, sensory retinal infiltration or erosion, cystoid retinal edema, and occasionally hemorrhage.

Choroidal melanoma, in general, is poorly imaged on OCT. However, detection of overlying subretinal fluid by OCT could be important in confirming the suspicion of melanoma in eyes with borderline small or intermediate size tumors.[8] This confirms the previous clinical observations that presence of subretinal fluid is a risk factor for eventual growth of the tumor.[4-6] Espinoza and associates[8] showed that OCT findings of subretinal fluid might have a predictive value in identifying choroidal melanocytic tumors that are likely to grow. In an assessment using OCT on 30 eyes with suspicious choroidal melanocytic lesions, tumor growth was found in only 8% of those with no subretinal fluid, 50% of those with active subretinal fluid, and 11% of those with retinal atrophy or edema.

Optical coherence tomography is particularly useful for determining the presence and degree of radiation-related maculopathy or papillopathy following radiotherapy of choroidal melanoma. Radiation retinopathy is the most common cause of irreversible visual loss in patients treated with plaque or charged particle radiotherapy for choroidal melanoma. The clinical manifestations of radiation retinopathy appear as slow onset occlusive retinal vasculopathy leading to intraretinal edema, exudation, hemorrhage and eventual retinal atrophy. Optical coherence tomography can detect intraretinal edema before it is visually symptomatic or clinically appreciable. Optical coherence tomography is also useful in monitoring resolution of radiation-induced macular edema following therapy with laser photocoagulation or intravitreal triamcinolone acetonide (Fig. 18.4). In an assessment of 31 patients with plaque-irradiated choroidal melanoma and radiation maculopathy, foveal thickness by OCT at the time of clinical detection of maculopathy was a mean of 417 mm and following intravitreal triamcinolone acetonide, the thickness decreased to 207 mm at 1 month, 305 mm at 6 months, and 273 mm at 12 months.[12] The long-term effects of intravitreal triamcinolone for radiation maculopathy are not known, but monitoring of the macular edema with OCT is informative and provides an objective guideline for documentation of treatment results.

Choroidal Metastasis

Cancer metastatic to the choroid is probably more common than generally realized.[1,2,13] It typically originates from breast carcinoma or lung carcinoma. Choroidal metastases can be unilateral and unifocal or bilateral and multifocal. The bilateral lesions are related to breast carcinoma in nearly 70% of cases.[13] Lung carcinoma metastasis is usually unifocal. Most choroidal metastases occur posterior to the equator of the fundus in the macular or paramacular regions. It generally appears as a flat or slightly elevated amelanotic lesion with poorly discernible margins. Scattered clumps of brown pigment can be seen over the lesion, which correlates histopathologically with lipofuscin pigment within macrophages at the level of the retinal pigment epithelium. Overlying retinal pigment epithelium changes and sensory retinal detachment can accompany these lesions.

Like other choroidal tumors, choroidal metastasis is not well imaged by OCT, but the overlying retinal and retinal pigment epithelial changes can be illustrated. Optical coherence tomography can depict overlying subretinal fluid, retinal pigment epithelial hyperplasia, retinal pigment epithelial detachment, and clumps of orange pigment. Resolution of subretinal fluid on OCT can be documented following therapy of the metastasis (Fig. 18.5).[14]

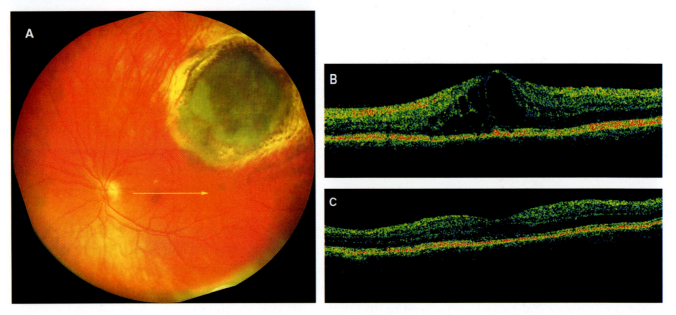

Fig. 18.4: Choroidal melanoma: A . Twelve months following plaque radiotherapy for a choroidal melanoma, tumor regression was achieved but radiation maculopathy was noted. B. At that time, OCT revealed cystoid macular edema of 446 microns and intravitreal triamcinolone acetonide was injected. C. Four months after injection, the foveal anatomy was restored with foveal thickness of 207 microns.

Choroidal Hemangioma

Choroidal hemangioma is considered a hamartomatous vascular tumor and is usually not clinically detectable until the second or third decade of life.[1,2,15-17] This lesion appears typically as a round or oval, slightly elevated, orange-colored tumor. It can vary in size from 2 mm to several 8 or 10 mm in diameter, with a mean of 6 mm diameter and 3 mm in thickness at the time of discovery.[15] Classically, choroidal hemangioma occurs in the posterior pole.[15] It usually exhibits slow enlargement in early life and by young adulthood it can develop overlying atrophic changes in the retinal pigment epithelium, cystoid degeneration of the sensory retina, and sensory retinal detachment. The diffuse choroidal hemangioma which permeates throughout the entire choroid is frequently associated with facial hemangioma (Sturge-Weber disease).

On OCT, choroidal hemangioma is imaged with poor resolution of the mass itself. The mass appears to be optically reflective at its anterior surface with little detail deeper into the choroidal mass. On the other hand, OCT is quite beneficial for imaging the overlying retina and ascertaining the reason for visual loss. Visual loss occurs due to subretinal fluid, intraretinal edema, chronic photoreceptor loss, induced hyperopia, tilt of the fovea on the elevated mass as well as long-standing related amblyopia. Newly active choroidal hemangioma shows subretinal fluid and preserved photoreceptor layer with minimal intraretinal edema.[18] Chronically leaking choroidal hemangioma displays additional photoreceptor attenuation and overlying intraretinal edema and even bullous retinoschisis.[19] When a tumor is discovered with newly active or chronic features causing visual loss, treatment is advised. Options for treatment include laser photocoagulation, transpupillary thermotherapy, application of a radiation plaque, and most recently, photodynamic therapy. Optical coherence tomography is an important tool in depicting resolution of subretinal fluid and foveal edema following therapy. This is especially helpful for those eyes that receive photodynamic

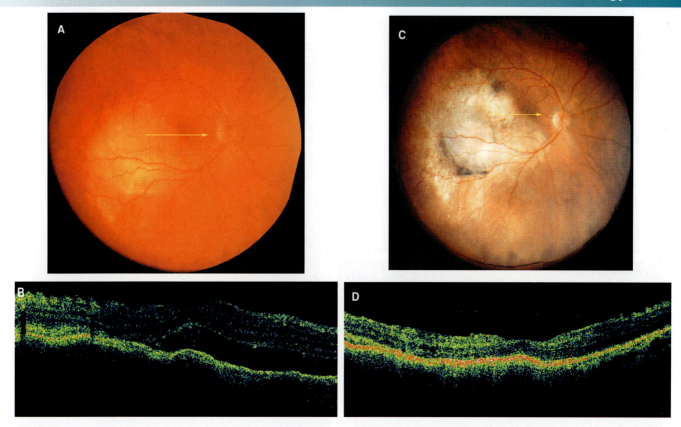

Fig. 18.5: Choroidal metastasis: A. Amelanotic choroidal metastasis in the foveal region produced subretinal fluid. B. Optical coherence tomography before therapy demonstrates subfoveal fluid. C. Following 9 months of hormonal therapy, the choroidal metastasis regressed. D. Following 9 months of hormonal therapy, the subretinal fluid regressed.

therapy for management of choroidal hemangioma as the subretinal or intraretinal fluid generally resolves rapidly and parallels return of visual acuity (Figs 18.6 and 18.7). [18,19]

Choroidal Osteoma

Choroidal osteoma is a benign intraocular tumor comprised of mature bone that typically replaces the full thickness choroid. This tumor classically manifests as an orange-yellow plaque deep to the retina in the juxtapapillary or macular region. [20-23] It most often occurs as a unilateral condition in teen-aged or young adult females. Unfortunately, the etiology and pathogenesis of this tumor is poorly understood. Despite its benign histopathology, it can compromise visual acuity. Aylward and associates[22] analyzed 36 affected patients and found the 10 year probability for tumor growth was 41%, related choroidal neovascularization was 47%, and poor visual acuity was 58%. Shields and associates[23] later reported in a group of 74 affected eyes the 10-year probability for tumor growth was 51%, tumor decalcification was 46%, related choroidal neovascularization was 31%, visual acuity loss was 45%, and poor visual acuity was 56%. Since this condition typically occurs in otherwise healthy young patients, most can anticipate experiencing one or many of these outcomes. [23]

The OCT features of choroidal osteoma include preservation of the inner retinal layers with atrophy of the outer layers, especially the photoreceptor layer of the retina. Often subretinal fluid or separation of the

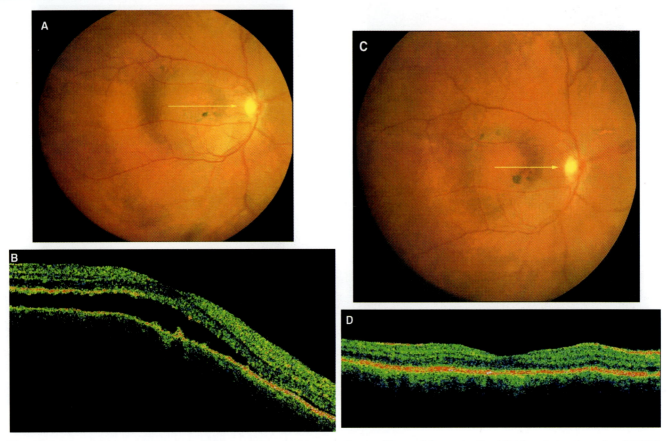

Fig. 18.6: Choroidal hemangioma: A. Subfoveal choroidal hemangioma with overlying subretinal fluid and visual acuity of 20/50 is noted. B. Subretinal fluid and focal retinal pigment epithelial hyperplasia is documented on OCT. C. Following photodynamic therapy, the tumor regressed and visual acuity returned to 20/20. D. Following photodynamic therapy, the subretinal fluid resolved on OCT.

neurosensory retina from the excavation underlying choroidal tumor is noted. The retinal pigment epithelium layer is indistinct as both the calcified tumor and retinal pigment epithelium layer appear as one layer of bright signal.[24,25] Abrupt elevation of the choroidal tumor at its margin, dense optical reflectivity, and complete shadowing are characteristic of the choroidal osteoma. Areas of elevation and excavation can be found (Fig. 18.8). In the areas of osteoma decalcification, where the lesion clinically appears atrophic and white, there is mild transmission of light through the tumor, whereas in areas where the osteoma is calcified and appears orange, light transmission is blocked and more complete shadowing is noted.[25]

LESIONS OF THE RETINAL PIGMENT EPITHELIUM

The lesions affecting the retinal pigment epithelium which will be discussed in this section are congenital hypertrophy of the retinal pigment epithelium, congenital simple hamartoma of the retinal pigment epithelium, and combined hamartoma of the retinal pigment epithelium and retina. Other lesions of the retinal pigment epithelium are well documented in the literature.[26]

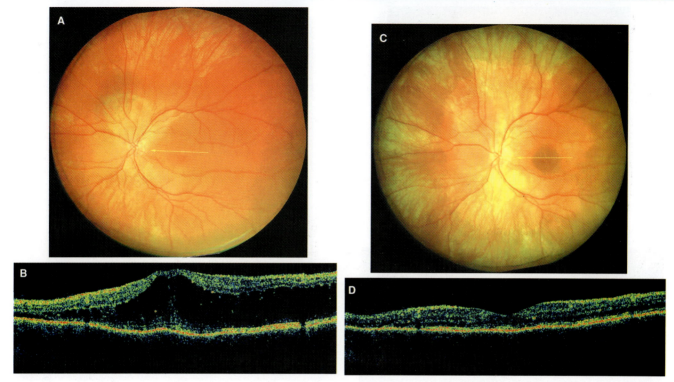

Fig. 18.7: Choroidal hemangioma: A. Juxtapapillary choroidal hemangioma with cystoid macular edema accounted for visual acuity of 20/200. B. Optical coherence tomography shows extensive cystoid macular edema. C. Following photodynamic therapy, the tumor appears atrophic and visual acuity improved to 20/25. D. Following photodynamic therapy, the cystoid edema resolved on OCT.

Congenital Hypertrophy of the Retinal Pigment Epithelium

Congenital hypertrophy of the retinal pigment epithelium (CHRPE) is a flat, heavily pigmented benign lesion that varies in diameter from 1 to several mm and may be found anywhere in the fundus (Fig. 18.9). [27] This lesion displays sharp margins that may be associated with a surrounding clear halo, which, in turn, is surrounded by a halo of pigmentation. Patchy round areas of hypopigmentation within the central portion of the lesion are termed lacunae. Occasionally, more than one retinal pigment epithelium can be seen in the eye and these congenital lesions can rarely occur bilaterally. Slight growth of CHRPE over many years has been documented. [1,2,27] Histopathologically, these lesions represent hypertrophy of the RPE with the enlarged retinal pigment epithelial cells containing large round melanosomes. Rarely, adenoma or adenocarcinoma can develop within CHRPE. [28]

By OCT, CHRPE shows slight increased thickness of the retinal pigment epithelium layer with slight shadowing deep to the lesion. The overlying retina is thinned and there is loss of the photoreceptor layer (Fig. 18.9). This tumor is typically difficult to image by OCT as it is usually located in the peripheral fundus.

Congenital Simple Hamartoma of the Retinal Pigment Epithelium

Simple hamartoma of the retinal pigment epithelium is an uncommon, presumed congenital lesion that has been recently recognized to have characteristic ophthalmoscopic, angiographic, and OCT features. [29,30] On

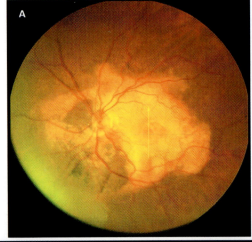

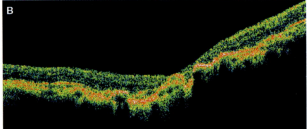

Fig. 18.8: Choroidal osteoma: A. Panoret™ image shows calcified circumpapillary choroidal osteoma. B. Optical coherence tomography demonstrates preservation of the inner retinal layers but loss of photoreceptor layer of the retina overlying the irregular choroidal mass. The slightly nodular appearance to the retinal pigment epithelium layer could represent retinal pigment epithelial hyperplasia or irregular surface of the choroidal osteoma.

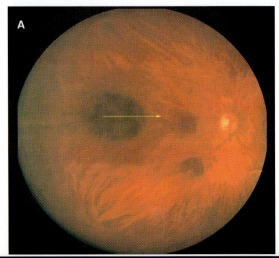

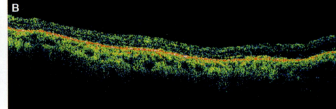

Fig. 18.9: Congenital hypertrophy of the retinal pigment epithelium (CHRPE): A. Panoret™ image shows CHRPE temporal to the fovea. B. Optical coherence tomography shows slight thickening and increased reflectivity of the retinal pigment epithelium layer with thinned overlying retina and loss of photoreceptors in the region of the flat CHRPE. Note the normal adjacent retina with lucent photoreceptor layer.

clinical examination, this circumscribed benign tumor appears as a small black mass in the macular region measuring a mean of 0.8 mm in basal dimension and 1.6 mm thickness, involving full thickness retina and protruding into the vitreous. Minimally dilated retinal vessels feeding the mass and mild retinal traction can be noted. The lesion blocks fluorescence on angiography and often manifests a ring of staining around the small tumor. There is only one report in the literature on the OCT of this tumor and the features included an abruptly elevated, dome-shaped, optically dense mass protruding from the retina into the vitreous cavity, with complete shadowing of the deeper levels (Fig. 18.10). [30]

Combined Hamartoma of the Retina and Retinal Pigment Epithelium

The combined hamartoma of the retina and retinal pigment epithelium represents a disorganized proliferation of glial and vascular elements of the retina along with retinal pigment epithelial cells.[31] It is generally associated with vitreoretinal interface disturbance and retinal folds or striae. While most commonly found adjacent to the disc, it can also occur in the macula or mid periphery.

The combined hamartoma of the retinal pigment epithelium and retina shows many interesting findings on OCT. In 2002, Ting and associates[32] reported the first OCT observations of in two adult patients with this

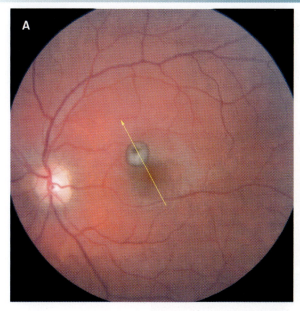

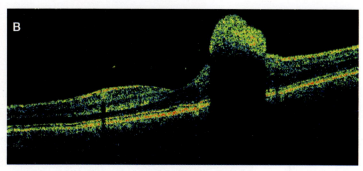

Fig. 18.10: Congenital simple hamartoma of the retinal pigment epithelium: A. The hamartoma appears as a small black mass in the foveal retina. B. On OCT, the mass shows a domed, reflective appearance protruding into the vitreous cavity with abrupt shadowing of deeper tissues and barely sparing the foveola.

tumor. They noted important findings such as a thickened retinal mass with a hyper reflective (high backscatter) surface and deep shadowing and they commented that the adjacent retina appeared normal and separate from the mass. Cystoid edema was found in one case. Shields and associates reported a series of 11 patients, eight of whom were teenagers or children.[33,34] They found a distinct epiretinal membrane with secondary retinal folds and striae in nearly all 11 cases.[34] The membrane showed horizontal traction in all cases and in 2 cases the membrane was configured in multiple peaks, suggesting vertical traction into the vitreous cavity (Fig. 18.11). The membrane, suspected to be glial tissue, was preretinal with no evidence of intertwining into the tumor. It was associated with soft, undulating retinal folds on OCT consistent with the clinical features of retinal traction. Additional findings on OCT included full thickness retinal disorganization in all cases. Interestingly, the adjacent retina was normal in architecture and seemed to gradually thicken into the disorganized tissue. One might speculate that the tractional component from the epiretinal membrane was the sole source for the distorted retinal findings.[34] On the other hand; others have speculated that the epiretinal component could be secondary to the retinal tumor.[35]

TUMORS OF THE RETINA AND OPTIC DISC

There are six different entities mentioned in this discussion of tumors of the sensory retina and disc: (i) capillary hemangioma, (ii) cavernous hemangioma, (iii) racemose hemangioma, (iv) astrocytic hamartoma, (v) retinoblastoma, and (vi) melanocytoma.

Capillary Hemangioma

Retinal capillary hemangioma is a vascular hamartoma that may involve the optic disc and/or retina.[1,2,36-38] It can be sporadic or can have a dominant hereditary pattern. When associated with similar lesions of the

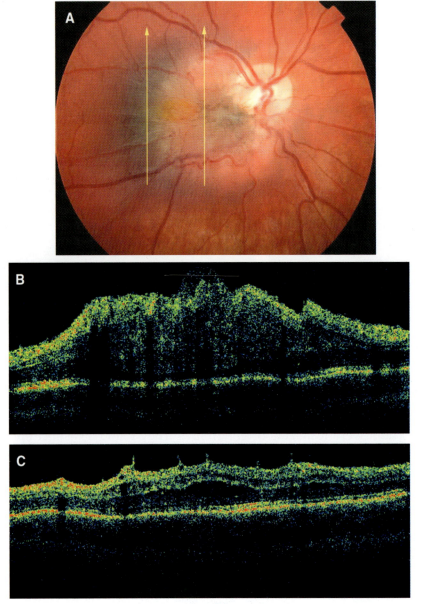

Fig. 18.11: Combined hamartoma of the retina and retinal pigment epithelium: A. The hamartoma is located in the papillomacular bundle with visual acuity of 20/100. B. Vertical OCT through the center of the mass shows retinal disorganization and thickening of 990 microns. Peaks of retinal traction towards the vitreous are noted. C. Vertical OCT through the temporal margin of the mass shows fine retinal traction peaks and relative preservation of the retinal microarchitecture with outer retinal tenting.

central nervous system, it is called von Hippel-Lindau syndrome. [1,2,36-38] Retinal capillary hemangioma located away from the disc is usually associated with one or more feeding arteries and draining veins. Lipid exudation in the macula and retinal detachment are common accompanying manifestations. At the disc the tumor may occur as an inner retinal (endophytic) or deep retinal (exophytic) juxtapapillary lesion. It appears as reddish-orange tumor of variable size, ranging from less than 1 mm to several mm in diameter. Intraretinal and subretinal lipid exudation may extend into the macula, even if the tumor rests in the far periphery. Histopathologically, it is characterized by dilated and hyperplastic capillaries and typical clear cells called foam cells.

With OCT, retinal capillary hemangioma displays thickening and disorganization of the retinal layers. The lesion is optically dense due to multiple interfaces of the diffuse capillary channels within the vascular mass. Slight shadowing of deeper tissues is often seen. Optical coherence tomography is most beneficial in detecting subretinal fluid, intraretinal edema, and preretinal fibrosis in the macular region that can accompany retinal capillary hemangioma (Fig. 18.12). Chronic cases with intraretinal edema can manifest with a cystoid appearance and even the appearance of retinoschisis. Chronic subretinal fluid shows thinning of the photoreceptor layer. Optical coherence tomography is used to monitor the response to therapy with resolution of the macular subretinal fluid and edema.

Cavernous Hemangiomas

Cavernous hemangioma of the retina or optic nerve is an uncommon tumor that appears as dark grape-like lesion in the sensory the retina.[1,2,36,37] It can vary in size from a few vascular clusters to a larger lesions 10-15 mm in diameter. Intraretinal and subretinal exudation are not generally associated with this lesion although occasionally vitreous hemorrhage can occur. There is occasionally a familial tendency, with a autosomal dominant pattern of inheritance in in which cases intracranial and cutaneous hemangiomas can be present. The tumor is relatively stable and rarely shows true growth. Histopathologically, it is characterized by a cluster of thin-walled dilated veins that replace the normal architecture of the retina or optic nerve head.

Optical coherence tomography of retinal cavernous hemangioma shows an optically dense mass with a lobulated surface. Preretinal fibrosis from chronic vitreous hemorrhage can be seen. If the aneurysms are large, a cystic appearance might be suggested on OCT; however, the anterior reflectivity might cause shadowing and blunt the visibility of deeper levels.

Racemose Hemangioma

The retinal racemose hemangioma is actually a congenital — arteriovenous malformation that can be a simple communication or a complex array of intertwining vessels.[1,2,36,37,39] The involved vessels are dilated, tortuous, and often more numerous than in the normal eye. Visual function can be normal, and spontaneous hemorrhage rarely occurs. Branch retinal vascular obstruction is a concern at the site of crossing of the large angiomatous vessels.[40] When this arteriovenous malformation is associated with similar midbrain, mandibular, maxillary or pterygoid fossa lesions, it is called the Wyburn-Mason syndrome. With OCT, the racemose hemangioma appears as a relatively large intraretinal cystic mass due to the dilated vessels.[39] Rarely, surrounding retinal changes of retinal atrophy, edema, and hemorrhage can be found (Fig. 18.13).

Astrocytic Hamartoma of the Retina

Astrocytic hamartoma is a retinal lesion typically seen in patients who have tuberous sclerosis.[1,2,36,37] It occurs in the superficial retina or optic disc as a white, round or oval, elevated mass with occasional intralesional calcification imposing a mulberry-like appearance. Mild associated retinal traction can be found. The astrocytic hamartoma is frequently multiple and, despite its white color, is usually highly vascularized. It carries minimal growth potential. Histopathologically, it is usually composed of fibrillary astrocytes, although a giant cells variant is occasionally seen.

With OCT, retinal astrocytic hamartoma shows gently sloping irregular surface overlying an optically dense, disorganized mass replacing the retinal architecture. If there is calcification within the astrocytic hamartoma, then the reflectivity of the mass is high and deep shadowing is noted (Fig. 18.14).

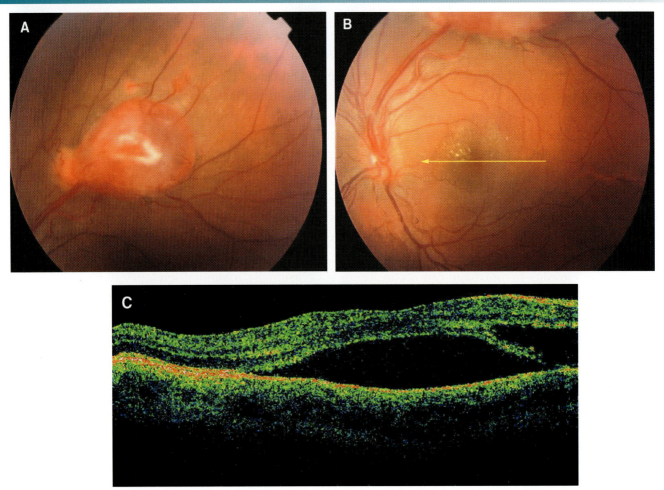

Fig. 18.12: Retinal capillary hemangioma: A. Multiple hemangiomas are noted along the superotemporal vascular arcade. B. Macular exudation and edema from the hemangiomas are shown. C. Optical coherence tomography shows subretinal fluid in the foveal region and intraretinal edema in the perifoveal area.

Retinoblastoma

Retinoblastoma is the most common intraocular malignancy of childhood.[1,2,41,42] This tumor grows in either an endophytic or exophytic pattern. The endophytic retinal mass usually has a vascular, cauliflower appearance with scattered tumor nodules along the inner retinal surface and in the vitreous cavity. In the exophytic form there is marked prominence of the vasculature of the tumor and the overlying retina. Histopathologically, retinoblastoma is composed of well differentiated to undifferentiated neuroblastic cells, with scanty cytoplasm, and sometimes characteristic rosettes.

During the very early phases of the fluorescein angiogram, vascular hyperfluorescence is evident from the large vessels which course throughout this cellular tumor. As the study continues, there is leakage from the tumor vasculature causing an increasing hyperfluorescence diffusely within the mass. On OCT, retinoblastoma shows an optically dense appearance with shadowing of the deep tissues. Intralesional calcification can cause higher internal reflectivity (backscattering) and denser shadowing posterior to the tumor. There is abrupt transition of the normal retinal architecture to the retinal mass. If the mass is

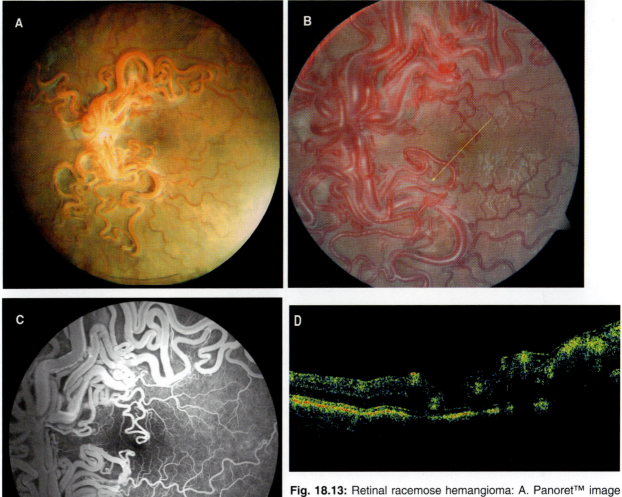

Fig. 18.13: Retinal racemose hemangioma: A. Panoret™ image showing snake-like configuration of the arteriovenous malformation. B. The mass obscures a view of the optic disc. C. Fluorescein angiography demonstrates the nonleaking, widely dilated vessels. D. OCT shows irregularity to the retinal surface from the large caliber vessels and shadowing of the deeper structures. There is a faint epiretinal membrane.

intraretinal, full thickness retina is involved (Fig. 18.15). An endophytic retinoblastoma may be difficult to image due to overlying vitreous seeds. An exophytic tumor shows retinal detachment overlying the neoplasm. In rare cases, intraretinal empty cavities can be visualized and these are usually found in well differentiated portions of the tumor (Fig. 18.15). [43] OCT is a useful test in monitoring reasons for visual loss following treatment of retinoblastoma. Causes for visual loss include retinal atrophy, retinal edema, persistent retinal detachment, optic disc edema or atrophy, macular tumor scar, cataract, corneal dryness and scarring, and amblyopia. In some instances, eyes with total retinal detachment from retinoblastoma have recovered complete function of the retina both clinically and anatomically, confirmed on OCT (Fig. 18.16). [44]

Melanocytoma of the Optic Nerve

Melanocytoma is a heavily pigmented benign tumor that is usually located on the optic disc. [1,2,45] It can vary in size from less than 1 disc diameter to a much larger lesion extending into the overlying vitreous and adjacent

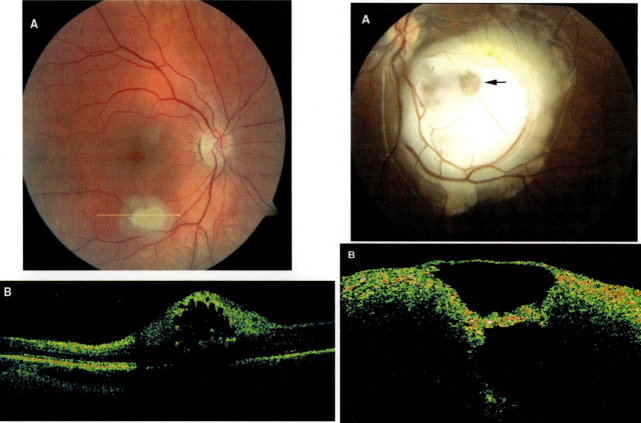

Fig. 18.14: Retinal astrocytic hamartoma: A. A calcified retinal astrocytic hamartoma is noted inferior to the macula. B. Optical coherence tomography shows an intraretinal mass with anterior homogeneous appearance but with deeper "moth eaten" appearance and abrupt reflectivity and shadowing consistent with nodules of calcification.

Fig. 18.15: Retinoblastoma: A. Retinoblastoma with cavities (arrow) was found in a 4-year-old girl. B. Optical coherence tomography shows a dense homogeneous retinal mass with cavities anteriorly.

retina and choroid. Histopathologically, it is composed of large pigmented melanocytes found near the region of the lamina cribrosa.

Because of the heavily pigmented cells, this lesion shows hypofluorescence throughout fluorescein angiogram. On OCT, melanocytoma is found to occupy the anterior portion of the optic nerve in a sessile or dome-shaped fashion (Fig. 18.17). There is disorganization of the normal optic nerve features. Shadowing of deeper tissues is present. The mass often spills over into and under the adjacent retina. By OCT, the retinal involvement appears as optically dense material in the nerve fiber layer and the choroidal involvement appears as slight elevation of the choroid, sometimes with subretinal fluid.

Optical coherence tomography is a useful technique for imaging the primary and secondary effects of intraocular tumors. It is most suited for information regarding tumors of the retina and retinal pigment epithelium. Information regarding details of choroidal tumors is currently limited due to lack of penetration of the light into the choroid. Optical coherence tomography is especially helpful in imaging the retina following treatment of intraocular tumors and provides important information on the reasons for visual acuity change.

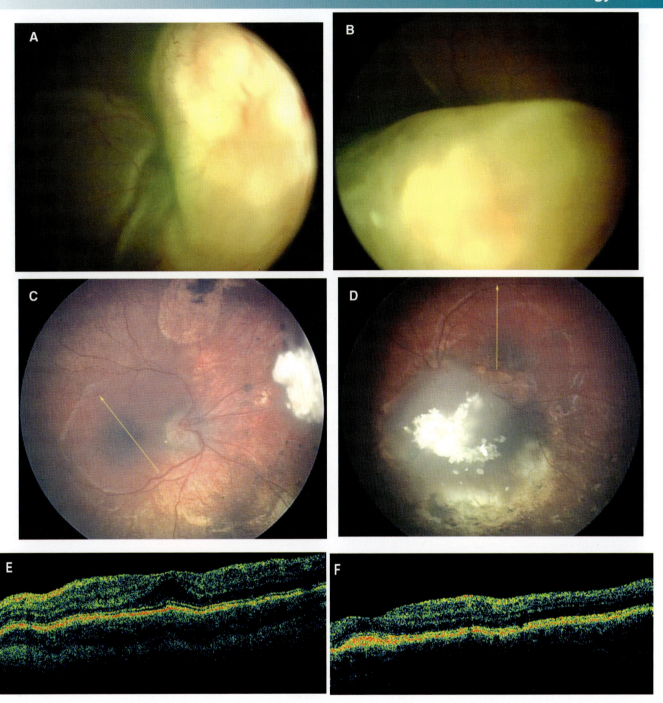

Fig. 18.16: Retinoblastoma: A. Advanced retinoblastoma with total retinal detachment in the right eye. B. Advanced retinoblastoma with total retinal detachment in the left eye. C. Following chemoreduction and thermotherapy, the tumors regressed and the retina flattened in the right eye. D. Following chemoreduction and thermotherapy, the tumors regressed and the retina flattened in the left eye. E. Six years following stable regression, OCT of the right eye shows normal macular architecture without edema or subretinal fluid but with blunted foveal depression. F. Six years following stable regression, OCT of the left eye shows normal superotemporal macular architecture without edema or subretinal fluid and with normal foveal depression, but with retinal pigment epithelial thickening.

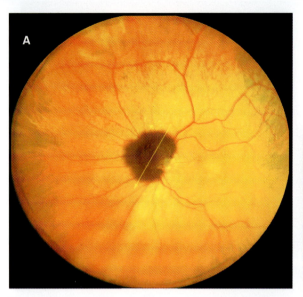

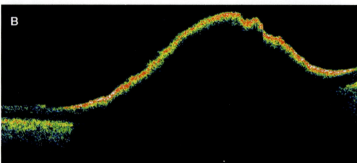

Fig. 18.17: Optic disc melanocytoma:A. Panoret™ image shows the darkly pigmented optic nerve mass with adjacent retinal infiltration. B. Optical coherence tomography shows a thin, delicate, echogenic line delineating the anterior aspect of the melanocytoma with abrupt and complete shadowing behind, obscuring all details of the optic nerve and adjacent retina.

REFERENCES

1. Shields JA, Shields CL. Intraocular Tumors: A Text and Atlas. Philadelphia: WB Saunders, 1992.
2. Shields JA, Shields CL. Atlas of Intraocular Tumors. Philadelphia, Lippincott Williams and Wilkins, 1999.
3. Sumich P, Mitchell P, Wang JJ. Choroidal nevi in a white population: the Blue Mountains Study. Arch Ophthalmol. 1998;116: 645-650.
4. Shields C, Shields JA, Kiratli H, et al. Risk factors for growth and metastasis of small choroidal melanocytic lesions. Ophthalmology. 1995;102:1351-1361.
5. Shields CL, Cater JC, Shields JA, et al. Combination of clinical factors predictive of growth of small choroidal melanocytic tumors. Arch Ophthalmol. 2000;118:360-364.
6. Shields CL, Demirci H, Materin MA, et al. Clinical factors in the identification of small choroidal melanoma. Can J Ophthalmol. 2004;39:351-357.
7. Shields CL, Mashayekhi A, Materin MA, et al. Optical coherence tomography of choroidal nevus in 120 consecutive patients. Submitted.
8. Espinoza G, Rosenblatt B, Harbour JW. Optical coherence tomography in the evaluation of retinal changes associated with suspicious choroidal melanocytic tumors. Am J Ophthalmol. 2004;137: 90-95.
9. Shields JA, Shields CL, Donoso LA. Management of posterior uveal melanomas. Surv Ophthalmol 1991;36:161-195.
10. Shields CL, Shields JA. Recent developments in the management of choroidal melanoma. Curr Opin Ophthalmol 2004; 15: 244-251.
11. Shields CL, Shields JA, DePotter P, et al. Diffuse choroidal melanoma: Clinical features predictive of metastasis. Arch Ophthalmol 1996;114:956-963.
12. Shields CL, Demirci H, Dai V, et al. Intravitreal triamcinolone acetonide for radiation maculopathy following plaque radiotherapy for choroidal melanoma. (submitted for publication).
13. Shields CL, Shields JA, Gross N, et al. Survey of 520 uveal metastases. Ophthalmology, 1997;104:1265-1276.
14. Manquez ME, Shields CL, Karatza EC, Shields JA. Regression of choroidal metastases from breast carcinoma using aromatase inhibitors. Arch Ophthalmol. (in press).
15. Shields CL, Honavar SG, Shields JA, et al. Circumscribed choroidal hemangioma. Clinical manifestations and factors predictive of visual outcome in 200 consecutive cases. Ophthalmology 2001;108:2237-48
16. Mashayekhi A, Shields CL. Circumscribed choroidal hemangioma. Curr Opin Ophthalmol 2003; 14: 142-149.
17. Shields JA, Shields CL, Materin MA, et al. Changing concepts in management of circumscribed choroidal hemangioma. The 2003 J Howard Stokes Lecture, part 1. Ophthalmic Surg Lasers 2004;35:383-393.
18. Materin MA, Shields CL, Marr BP, Shields JA. Restoration of anatomic fovea following photodynamic therapy (PDT) for circumscribed choroidal hemangima. (Submitted for publication).
19. Shields CL, Materin MA, Marr BP, et al. Resolution of advanced cystoid macular edema following photodynamic therapy of choroidal hemangioma. Ophthalmic Surg Laser Imaging. (in press).
20. Gass JD, Guerry RK, Jack RL, Harris G. Choroidal Osteoma. Arch Ophthalmol 1978;96:428-435.
21. Shields CL, Shields JA, Augsburger JJ. Choroidal osteoma. Surv Ophthalmol 1988;33:17-27.
22. Aylward GW, Chang TS, Pautler SE, Gass JD. A long-term follow-up of choroidal osteoma. Arch Ophthalmol 1998;116:1337-1341.

23. Shields CL, Sun H, Demirci H, Shields JA. Choroidal osteoma: factors predictive of tumor growth, tumor decalcification, choroidal neovascularization, and visual outcome in 74 eyes. (Submitted for publication).
24. Ide T, Ohguro N, Hayashi A, et al. Optical coherence tomography patterns of choroidal osteoma. Am J Ophthalmol. 2000; 130: 131-134.
25. Fukasawa A, Iijima H. Optical coherence tomography of choroidal osteoma. Am J Ophthalmol. 2002;133:419-421.
26. Shields JA, Shields CL, Gunduz K, Eagle RC Jr. Neoplasms of the retinal pigment epithelium. The 1998 Albert Ruedemann Sr. Memorial Lecture. Part 2. Arch Ophthalmol. 1999;117:601-608.
27. Shields CL, Mashayekhi A, Ho T, et al. Solitary congenital hypertrophy of the retinal pigment epithelium: Clinical features and frequency of enlargement in 330 patients. Ophthalmology. 2003;110:1968-1976.
28. Shields JA, Shields CL, Singh AD. Acquired tumors arising from congenital hypertrophy of the retinal pigment epithelium. Arch Ophthalmol. 2000;118:637-641.
29. Shields CL, Shields JA, Marr BP, et al. Congenital simple hamartoma of the retinal pigment epithelium. A study of five cases. Ophthalmology 2003;110:1005-1011.
30. Shields CL, Materin MA, Karatza E, Shields JA. Optical coherence tomography (OCT) of congenital simple hamartoma of the retinal pigment epithelium. Retina. 2004;24:327-328.
31. Schachat AP, Shields JA, Fine SL, et al, the Macula Society Research Committee. Combined hamartomas of the retina and retinal pigment epithelium. Ophthalmology. 1984;91:1609-1614.
32. Ting TD, McCuen BW 2nd, Fekrat S. Combined hamartoma of the retina and retinal pigment epithelium: optical coherence tomography. Retina. 2002;22:98-101.
33. Shields CL, Mashayekhi A, Dai VD, et al. Optical coherence tomography findings of combined hamartoma of the retinal pigment epithelium in 11 patients. (Submitted for publication).
34. Shields CL, Mashayekhi A, Luo CK, et al. Optical coherence tomography in children. Analysis of 44 eyes with intraocular tumors and simulating conditions. (Submitted for publication).
35. Stallman JB. Visual improvement after pars plana vitrectomy and membrane peeling for vitreoretinal traction associated with combined hamartoma of the retina and retinal pigment epithelium. Retina. 2002;22:101-104.
36. Shields JA, Shields CL. Tumors of the retina and optic disc. In Regillo CD, Brown GC, Flynn HW Jr, eds. Vitreoretinal Disease. The Essentials. New York: Thieme Medical Publisheres, Inc, 1999:439-454
37. Shields CL, Shields JA. Phakomatoses. In Regillo CD, Brown GC, Flynn HW Jr, eds. Vitreoretinal Disease. The Essentials. New York: Thieme Medical Publisheres, Inc, 1999:377-390.
38. Singh AD, Shields CL, Shields JA. Major review: Von Hippel-Lindau disease. Surv Ophthalmol. 2001;46:117-142.
39. Materin MA, Shields CL, Marr BP, et al. Retinal racemose hemangioma. (Submitted for publication).
40. Shah GK, Shields JA, Lanning R. Branch retinal vein obstruction secondary to retinal arteriovenous communication. Am J Ophthalmol. 1998;126:446-448.
41. Shields CL, Shields JA. Recent developments in the management of retinoblastoma. J Ped Ophthalmol Strabismus. 1999;36:8-18.
42. Shields CL, Meadows AT, Leahey AM, Shields JA. Continuing challenges in the management of retinoblastoma with chemotherapy. Editorial. Retina. (in press).
43. Mashayekhi A, Shields CL, Eagle RC Jr, Shields JA. Cavitary changes in retinoblastoma. Relationship to chemoresistence. (Submitted for publication).
44. Shields CL, Materin MA, Shields JA. Restoration of foveal anatomy and function following chemoreduction for bilateral retinoblastoma with total retinal detachment. Arch Ophthalmol (in press).
45. Shields JA, Demirci H, Mashayekhi A, Shields CL. Melanocytoma of the optic disc in 115 cases. The 2004 Samuel Johnson Memorial Lecture. Ophthalmology. 2004;111:1739-1746.

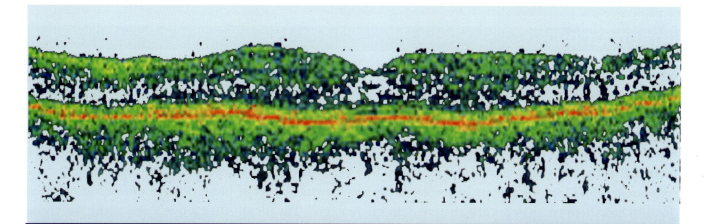

CHAPTER
19

Posterior Segment Trauma

Carsten H Meyer, Peter Kroll

INTRODUCTION

Non-penetrating or closed-globe injuries may occur by several mechanisms thus damaging a variety of different retinal structures. The *Ocular Trauma Classification Group* defined a standardized classification for frequently used terms based on standard terminology and features of ocular injuries, which have demonstrated prognostic significance. In a closed-globe injury the eye wall does not have a full-thickness wound and the mechanism of injury may be grouped into two main categories: the direct (anterior) type occurring at the site of the impact and an indirect (posterior) type at the contre-coup injury, which is more commonly found. Several groups investigated the mechanical impact of blunt ocular trauma and reported theories how defined anatomical structures can be damaged (Fig. 19.1). After a traumatic event the vision can be unaffected or completely lost, depending on the location of the damaged anatomical structure e.g.: choroidal vessels, choriocapillaris, Bruch's membrane, retinal pigment epithelium and neuroretinal.[1-7]

This chapter demonstrates a variety of closed-globe injuries on optical coherent tomography (OCT), fluorescein angiography and fundus photography.

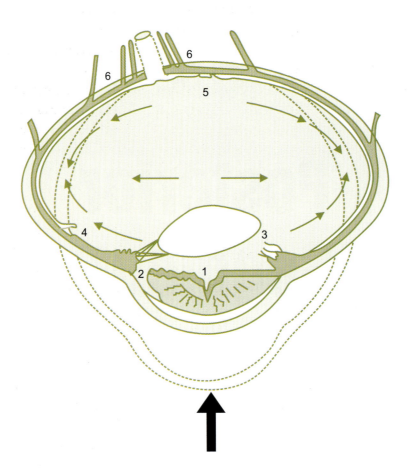

Fig. 19.1: Non-penetrating or closed-globe injuries may occur by several mechanisms thus damaging a variety of different retinal structures including the iris (1), trabecular mash work (2), lens fibers (3), retina (4), posterior pole (5) or optic nerve with the posterior ciliary vessels (6).

CHOROIDAL FOLDS

Choroidal folds are visible striae at the posterior pole that radiate across the macula arranged in a parallel and horizontal fashion as dark and light lines. They were first described by Nettleship in 1884, and were initially considered as foldings of the entire retina.[8] However, later Norton investigated the typical fluorescein angiographic appearance and defined a clear distinction between choroidal and retinal folds.[9] The anatomical structure of choroidal folds can be explained by the typical fluorescein pattern traversing the folded choroidal vessels. Hyperfluorescent streaks occur in the early arteriovenous phase and persist throughout the late venous phase with no leakage. A stretching and atrophy of the retinal pigment epithelium induces an increased filling of the choriocapillaris overlying this peak of the choroidal fold. Hypofluorescent streaks are on the bases of inclinated retinal pigment epithelium in the valley of the fold, resulting from a compression of the pigment-containing base of the retinal pigment epithelial cells and blockage of the underlying choroidal fluorescence. Histologic studies confirmed a folding at the level of the retinal pigment epithelium, Bruch's membrane and choroid giving the retina above a "brain-like" configuration. Cross-sectional imaging by computer tomography (CT) or B-scan ultrasonography reveal an abnormal flattening of the posterior pole, a thickening of the sclera and consecutive axial shortening of the globe.[10-11] This characteristic picture is associated with a variety of orbital and ocular conditions including trauma, hypotony, orbital tumors, thyroid disease, papillitis, or uveal effusion syndrome.

Fluorescein traversing the folded choroid vessels demonstrated hyperfluorescent streaks in the early and late phase with no signs leakage while adjacent hypofluorescent streaks remained dark throughout the entire angiography (Fig. 19.2A). *In-vivo* measurements by OCT determined a significant folding of the hyper reflective retinal pigment epithelium-choriocapillaris-complex of approximately 45mm height (Fig. 19.2B) in the papillomacular area.[12] The thickness, reflectivity and surface contour of the retina appeared within normal limits.

On the other side patients with ocular hypotony may face severe impaired vision with metamorphopsia. On fundus examination there is a significant tortuous beading of the retinal and venous vessels (Fig. 19.2C). Fluorescein angiography demonstrates a fussy fluorescence in the early and late phase (Fig. 19.2D). Optical coherence tomography delineates a mountain-like folding of the entire retina (X) with moderate hyporeflective areas in the subretinal space corresponding with subretinal fluid (Fig. 19.2E). Between the retinal pigment epithelium and the sclera there are flat large areas corresponding with choroidal fluid (*).

COMMOTIO RETINAE

Commotio retinae, first described by Berlin in 1873, is defined as a transient gray-white opacification at the level of the deep sensory retina occurring after blunt ocular trauma.[13] The whitening and elevation of the retina appears immediately after a trauma and can be limited to the central retina although it may even involve extensive areas of the peripheral retina progressing to retinal necrosis and chorioretinitis sclopetaria.[14]

Commotio retinae are grouped in two variations: a milder type (retinal concussion) with less dramatic gray-white changes and no visible pigment alterations, which later may progress to scarring. The more severe type (retinal contusion or chorioretinitis sclopetaria) can occur anterior at the point of impact (coup) or posterior at the remote impact site (contre-coup). A coup damage is therefore caused by local trauma

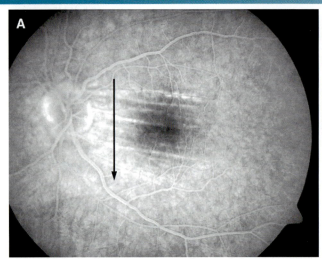

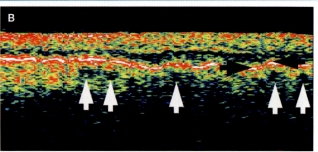

Fig. 19.2A: In the late venous phase of the fluorescein angiography there are multiple parallel and horizontal lines of different fluorescence in the macular area. The hyperfluorescent streaks persist with no leakage and are caused by an increased filling of the choriocapillaris overlying the peak of the choroidal fold. The hypofluorescent streaks are in the valley of the fold, where the compressed retinal pigment epithelium blocks the underlying choroidal fluorescence. The black arrow indicates the location and direction of the corresponding linear OCT scan.

Fig. 19.2B: The vertical OCT scan of the choroidal folds in the papillomacular area. The inner surface of the retina is flattened by image analysis using Abobe Photoshop, so that the choroidal folds become more prominent. The neuroretina in the papillomacular bundle has a moderate reflectivity and normal thickness of approximately 225 mm. There is no intraretinal or subretinal fluid. The folded hyper reflective band, in red to white colors, corresponds to the retinal pigment epithelium-choriocapillaris complex and is firmly attached to the underlying sclera, with no signs of pigment epithelium detachment (PED). Each fold has a height of approximately 45 mm (black arrows). The dark and hyporeflective spots in the deep scleral layer under each fold (white arrows) may either correspond to compressed tissue or shadowing of the folded retinal pigment epithelium-choriocapillaris complex.

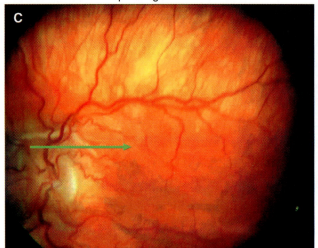

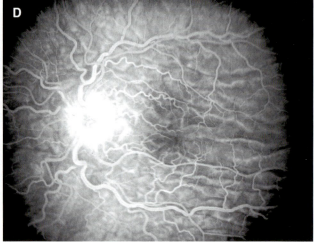

Fig. 19.2C: Fundus image of the right eye in a patients with severe hypotony after blunt ocular trauma. Funduscopy demonstrates a chorioretinal folding of the entire retina.

Fig. 19.2D: Fluorescein angiography demonstrates a moderate elevation of the retina with mild leakage.

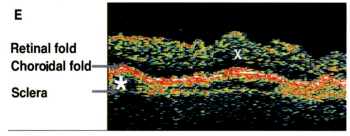

Fig. 19.2E: On OCT there is a significant folding of the entire neuroretina (X) with some hyporeflective areas in under the retina corresponding with subretinal fluid. Under the hyper-reflective retinal pigment epithelium-choriocapillaris-complex there is a broad hyper reflective area (*) presenting a second fluid compartment in the choroid adjacent to the sclera.

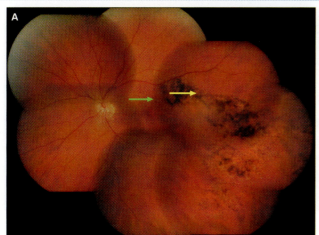

Fig. 19.3A: Fundus image of the left posterior pole. Chorioretinitis sclopetaria results from a localized destruction of both the retina and choroid adjacent to the impact site. These damaged structures are subsequently replaced by a connective tissue response.

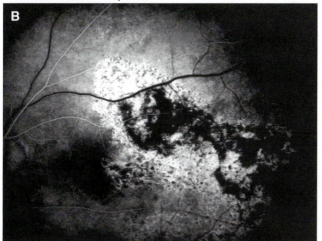

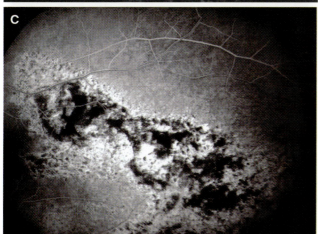

Figs 19.3B and C: On fluorescein angiography the filling of the choriocapillaris is irregular and partially obstructed by connective tissue plaques.

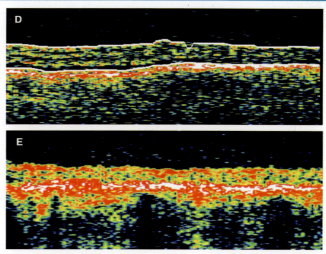

Figs 19.3D and E: On OCT there is a marked thinning of the entire neuroretina. The retinal thickness in the sclopetaria area is 75–95 mm whereas 280–320 mm in the adjacent unaffected area.

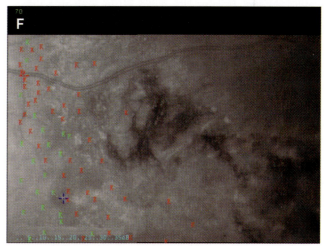

Fig. 19.3F: Multifocal ERG demonstrates residual field defects corresponding to the area of retinal capillary non-perfusion and chorioretinitis sclopetaria.

directly at the site of impact, while a contusive counter-coup injury occurs at the opposite site of the blunt trauma creating damage at tissue interfaces. The consecutive whitening is more severe and a creamy discoloration of the retinal pigment epithelium appears within 48 hours after the injury. Fluorescein angiography typically demonstrates an alternated retinal vascular permeability, a bright leakage due to a partially breakdown of the outer blood-retina-barrier at the level of the retinal pigment epithelium. Visual acuity may be transiently

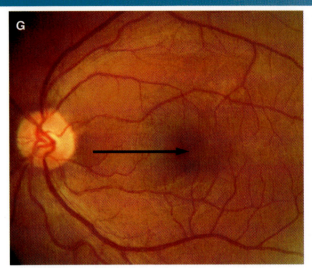

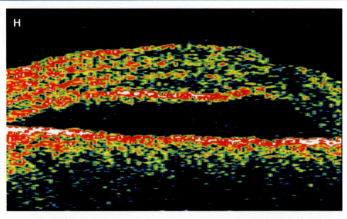

Fig. 19.3G: Fundus image of the left posterior pole. The optic disc has a sharp margin and the foveal reflex is vanished. There is a mild retinal elevation in the papillomacular region. The black arrow indicates the location and direction of the corresponding linear OCT-scan (From Meyer CH, Rodrigues EB, Mennel S. Acute commotio retinae determined by cross-sectional optical coherence tomography. Eur J Ophthalmol. 2003;13:816-818, reprinted with permission.)

Fig. 19.3H: Horizontal OCT scan in the papillomacular area demonstrates a detachment of the entire neuroretina with hyporeflective space underneath, corresponding with subretinal fluid. The structure of the neuroretina appears hyporeflective and less dense compact with a mean retinal thickness of 285 mm (190 mm-345 mm). The foveola has a thickness of 70 mm (white arrow). The outer retina appears as a hyper reflective band in reddish to orange colors, corresponding to the layer of the photoreceptors. (From Meyer CH, Rodrigues EB, Mennel S. Acute commotio retinae determined by cross-sectional optical coherence tomography. Eur J Ophthalmol. 2003;13:816-818, reprinted with permission.)

or permanently reduced. The visual prognosis is good if the damaged location is outside the fovea. However, if the fovea is involved, vision loss may be permanent (Fig. 19.3F).[15, 16]

The clinicopathologic features of retinal contusion or chorioretinitis sclopetaria include direct traumatic chorioretinal damage followed by marked fibrovascular proliferation with variable replacement of vascular and neuroretinal tissue (Fig. 19.3A). A visible retinal opacity at the site of the contre-coup injury is considered to be a severe injury. It may later progress to a "salt-and-pepper" appearance accompanied by a hypofluorescence on fluorescein angiography. The chorioretinal circulation disturbance corresponds with a delayed filling and narrowing of the choroidal veins and changes in choroidal vasculature causing obstruction and occlusion of the choriocapillaris (Figs 19.3B and C). The breakdown of the outer blood-retinal barrier in the retinal pigment epithelium may increase the permeability of the choriocapillaris.

Histopathologic studies demonstrated a partial loss of the nerve fiber and ganglion cell layers and loss of the photoreceptors with hypertrophy and hyperplasia of the retinal pigment epithelium. Although the sclera and a long posterior ciliary nerve remained intact, a marked ingrowth of fibrovascular tissue may extended from the choroid into the subretinal space where it was covered by retinal pigment epithelium. On OCT there is a marked thinning of the neuroretina in the affected area compared to the unaffected adjacent areas (Figs 19.3D and E).[17-20]

There have been conflicting reports on histopathologic features of Berlin's edema or commotio retinae. Although Berlin originally hypothesized, that the loss of the outer retinal transparency may relate to an extracellular edema, the origin and underlying pathogenesis remains controversial. Several postmortem studies on human and animal eyes confirmed a disruption of photoreceptor outer segments followed by phagocytosis of fragmented outer segments by the retinal pigment epithelium. While some authors reported a direct damage to the neurosensory retina as seen by swelling of Müller food processes and mitochondria in the nerve fiber layer. The gross anatomy revealed swollen inner segments with mitochondrial deposits of resembling calcium, indicating an increased permeability of the plasma membranes. The blunt ocular trauma may generate mechanical contre-coup distortion of the retina via vitreo-retinal attachments. Mansour and associates[21] hypothesized, that hydraulic forces stretch the neuroretina at the level of the outer segments, while intact Müller cells hold the rest of the retina together.

In-vivo measurements by OCT revealed a traumatic lesion at the level of the photoreceptor-retinal pigment epithelium-complex, disclosing a detached sensory retina with fluid in the subretinal space.[22,23] The reflectivity of the neuroretinal tissue was reduced and the architecture less compact. The neuroretina, held together by the Müller food processes, appears to be intact up to the photoreceptors. The uncommon hyper reflective inner retinal band possibly represents the photoreceptor inner segments, with less reflective outer segments underneath and in the subretinal space. Although the neuroretinal thickness was increased, the foveolar indentation remained still visible (Fig. 19.3G). Fundus biomicroscopy revealed a mild retinal elevation at the level of neurosensory retina and the retinal pigment epithelium in the fovea with white concentric lines (Fig. 19.3H). The retinal pigment epithelium phagocytosis damages the outer segments and restores central vision within weeks. We determined a full anatomical and functional recovery of the macular lesion within 3 months. The patient's vision returned to 20/20 OU 5 months later.

CHOROIDAL RUPTURE

Choroidal rupture, first described by von Graefe in 1854, is a tear of Bruch´s membrane, the choroid and the retinal pigment epithelium secondary to a blunt ocular trauma.[24] They can be divided into two main categories:

A direct (anterior) type occurring at the site of the impact and are oriented parallel to the ora serrata. Indirect ruptures, which are more common, occur predominantly at the posterior pole away from the site of impact. The rupture is here usually crescent-shaped and concentrically aligned to the optic disc, with the convexity away from the optic disc. The majority (82%) of ruptures run temporal to the optic disc may involve the macula.

Mechanical or vascular mechanisms are the two must frequently cited hypothesizes explaining the damages in choroidal ruptures. While the elasticity of the retina normally resists its tearing, the strength of the sclera prevents rupturing and protects the globe from mechanical compression or sudden hyper expansion. However, the inelastic Bruch´s membrane along with the apposed retinal pigment epithelium and choriocapillaris lacks of both: strength and elasticity and thus is most likely to rupture first after a severe compressive and contusional injury of the eye, inducing a marked deformation of the globe. In blunt injury the energy is transmitted across the globe either through the vitreous gel or via the wall of the globe, consequently inducing a rupture of Bruch's membrane. Between 5 and 10% of all blunt ocular trauma lead to indirect choroidal ruptures. [25]

Patients with choroidal ruptures are predisposed to develop choroidal neovascularization (CNV) as a common feature during the later healing process, as it may be observed in angoid streaks. The severity of the visual impairment depends on the location of the choroidal rupture and size of CNV as well as damage of additional structures. Morphometric analysis of traumatized eyes by Secètan and associates [26] demonstrated that ruptures greater than 4000 mm in length and located within 1500mm of the center of the fovea is more frequently associated with CNV.

Fluorescein angiography demonstrates a crescent-shaped delay filling that peaked at the site of the choroidal rupture. Early on there is a hypoperfusion of the choroidal artery. Evidence of the choroidal rupture hyperfluorescent streak occurred in the late phase of the fluorescein angiography at the site of the choroidal rupture. Indocyanine green angiography may also disclose a hypofluorescent rim along the choroidal veins as signs of an increased permeability of the choriocapillaris. Flower and associates [27] speculated that new proliferations originate from choroidal vessels of the Sattler layer. These feeder vessels seem to have a greater caliber, a higher tendency to proliferate and are therefore more resistant to photodynamic therapy and selective feeder vessel treatment as recently demonstrated by us in another patient. [28]

The primary tear consists of a rupture of Bruch's membrane and the adjacent superficial or deep layers. The lesion may be obscured in the beginning by subretinal hemorrhages from the choroid. However, when the blood resorbs the rupture appears as a yellow strip surrounded by red hemorrhages. Often the rupture transforms into a sharply defined white streak with pigmented edges encircled by atrophic retinal pigment epithelium, while adjacent hemorrhages may organize a large fibrovascular scar (Figs 19.4 A to C). The covering retina may remain intact, although choroidal vessels may pass from the base of the rupture. Superficial retinal vessels usually remain undisturbed from the rupture. Late complications may include ingrowth of fibrovascular tissue, migration of retinal pigment epithelial cells, epiretinal membrane-formation, and loss of photoreceptors, optic atrophy and retinal detachment.

Histopathologic studies by Aguilar and Green demonstrated, that choroidal ruptures are followed by fibrovascular tissue proliferation and retinal pigment epithelium-hyperplasia. [29] The overlying retina is variably affected, from a loss of the outer layers to a full-thickness fibrovascular scar formation. A discontinuity of the overlying retinal layers may occur with atrophic retina pulled down into the flat choroidal defect. Abrupt ending of the retinal pigment epithelium at the edges of the rupture in Bruch's membrane, without signs of proliferation or migration of retinal pigment epithelium across the defect are common histopathologic features.

An OCT highlight the cross sectional features of choroidal ruptures. The first case demonstrated a mounted subretinal lesion corresponding with fibrovascular scar tissue. The superficial neuroretina appeared normal in contour, thickness and reflectivity pattern (Figs 19.4A to C).

In the second case there was a hyper reflective band radiating from the subretinal space through the entire neuroretina to the retinal surface, indicating a transretinal migration of fibrovascular cells. The irregular hyper reflective contour of the retinal surface corresponded to a mild epiretinal membrane as seen on the fundus image (Figs 19.4D to G).

VALSALVA RETINOPATHY

The term 'Valsalva retinopathy' was first used in 1972 by Duane to describe preretinal hemorrhages in association after vomiting, coughing, heavy lifting, or straining stool, although in some instances no initiating event can be ruled out. [30] A well-circumscribed, round or dumbbell-shaped mound of preretinal blood is seen in or near the central macular area.

The presumed mechanism of preretinal hemorrhages is a rupture of superficial retinal capillaries due to increased sudden intrathoracic pressure associated with a decreased venous return, by forced exhalation against a closed glottis. The most common site for this hemorrhage is the posterior pole, where the premacular bursa provides a preexisting anatomic space. [31] In addition the internal limiting membrane has no firm

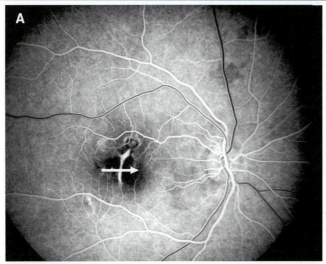

Fig. 19.4A: Fluorescein angiography in the early phase demonstrates a dark hypofluorescence and delayed filling in the foveal area of the choroidal rupture.

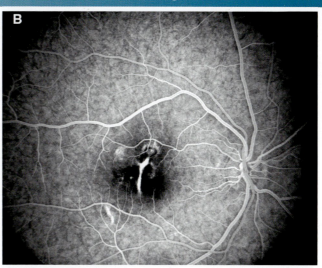

Fig. 19.4B: Fluorescein angiography late phase. During the late phase there is a sharp crescent-like hyperfluorescence in the area of the choroidal rupture.

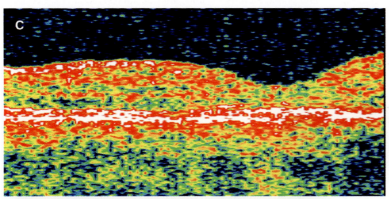

Fig. 19.4C: Horizontal OCT image at the choroidal rupture delineates a broadened hyper reflective retinal pigment epithelium-choriocapillaris complex, corresponding with a subretinal dome shaped fibrovascular scar formation. The superficial retina has a normal contour reflectivity and no signs of an epiretinal membrane formation.

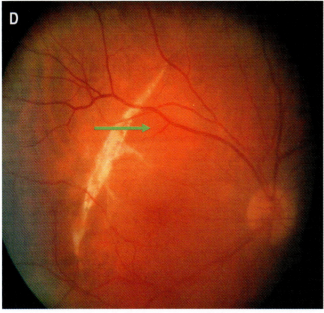

Fig. 19.4D: Fundus image demonstrates a white crescent-like rupture of the choroid in the superotemporal quadrant. The superficial retina appears to be damaged. The lesion has a length of approximately 3000mm and a maximal width of 250 mm. The arrow indicates the location and direction of the corresponding OCT-scan.

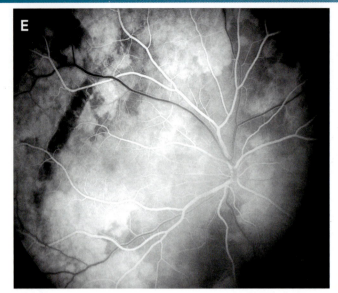

Fig. 19.4E: Fluorescein angiography early phase. During the arteriovenous phase there is an incomplete filling of the choroidal vasculature. A lobular hypofluorescence indicates a partial delay of the choroidal vasculature. The retinal vessels demonstrate a normal filing. In the area of the choroidal rupture there is a dark hypofluorescence visible consistent with the rupture and loss of choroidal vessels.

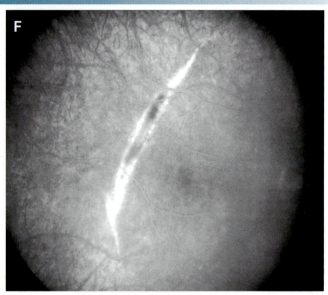

Fig. 19.4F: Fluorescein angiography late phase. During the late phase there is a homogeneous fluorescence of the choroid except the area of the choroidal rupture, where a sharp crescent-like hyperfluorescence becomes visible. The fluorescence present leakage of choroidal vessels and a window defect at the choroidal rupture.

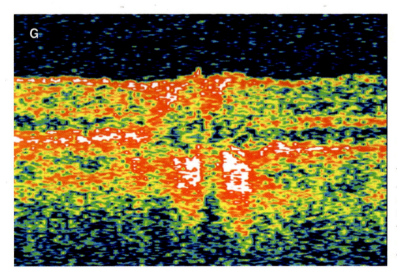

Fig. 19.4G: Horizontal OCT image at the choroidal rupture demonstrated two hyper reflective areas at the deep choroid corresponding to the scar formation at the edge of the choroidal rupture. The retina has a normal thickness, however there is a hyper reflective band extending from the outer retinal to throughout the entire retina to the retinal surface. A hyper reflective band on the retinal surface corresponds to a fine epiretinal membrane on the retinal surface.

attachments to the retina at the posterior pole, thus predisposing hemorrhagic detachments between both layers (Figs 19.5A and B).

It is generally agreed that the sharply demarcated hemorrhage is located at the vitreo-retinal interface either directly under the posterior hyaloid of the vitreous or under the internal limiting membrane itself. The exact location of cannot be determined biomicroscopically, although subhyaloid blood tents to shift by changing the head from an up-right to flat position, and sublaminar retinal hemorrhage remains still (Figs 19.5C and D). [32]

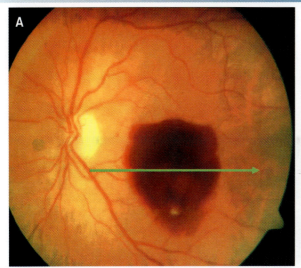

Fig. 19.5A: Fundus image of the left posterior pole. A well-circumscribed, round or dumbbell-shaped mound of preretinal blood is seen in or near the central macular area.

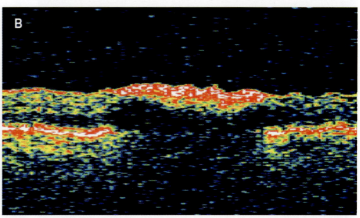

Fig. 19.5B: The entrapped blood under the internal limiting membrane presents on OCT a hyper reflective band in the retina surface obscuring the underlying retinal structures.

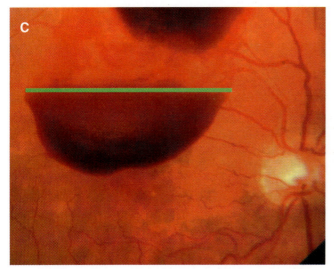

Fig. 19.5C: Fundus image of the right taken in an up-right position. The preretinal hemorrhage has a horizontal direction.

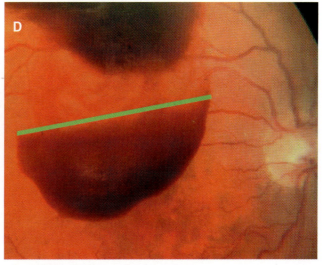

Fig. 19.5D: Fundus image of the right taken after the head was tilted to the right side. The preretinal blood has shifted to the right side in an oblique direction

Patients commonly describe a sudden spontaneous loss of their vision. Part of the blood may decent in the preretinal bursa and turn yellow after several days. Resorption of the entrapped blood tends to be slow and may result in long standing visual impairment. With a spontaneous rupture of the membrane vision recovers rapidly. However, if the spontaneous resorption of preretinal blood is slow, laser puncturing or photodisruption of the posterior hyaloid face or the limiting membrane has been described by means of argon laser coagulation [33] or Nd:YAG laser [34] as an alternative to vitrectomy. The laser puncturing enables a drainage through the focal opening of entrapped premacular blood into the vitreous cavity, where it is resorbed more quickly (Figs 19.5E and F).

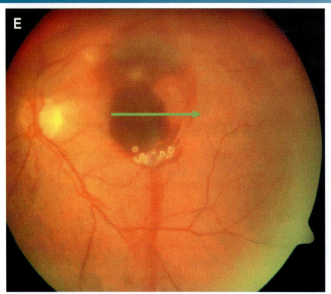

Fig. 19.5E: Fundus image of the left posterior pole. The laser puncturing enables drainage through the focal opening of entrapped premacular blood into the vitreous cavity

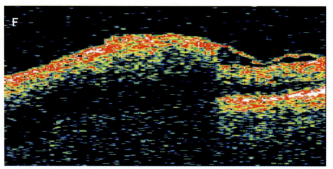

Fig. 19.5F: OCT demonstrates a remaining blood on the retinal surface as a brought hyper reflective band. Temporal to the fovea there is a small thin hyper reflective band probably corresponding to detached internal limiting membrane.

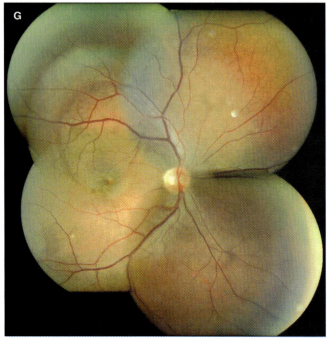

Fig. 19.5G: Fundus picture of the left eye 3 month after Argon laser treatment. There is a moderate epiretinal membrane in the fovea with pigment alterations. Fine retinal striae radiate perpendicular along the retinal surface to the periphery. A giant translucent cavity extends form the superior arcade to the inferior macula. The white arrow indicates the length and direction of the corresponding OCT scan.

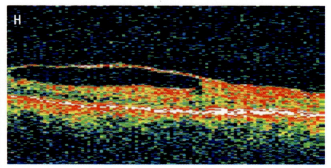

Fig. 19.5H: The horizontal OCT scan demonstrates a persisting preretinal bursa in the area of the previously entrapped preretinal blood.

We previously presented a case, where a premacular hemorrhage was drained into the vitreous cavity.[35] A 52-years old patient complained about decreased visual acuity (VA) after a Valsava maneuver. His VA was counting fingers OD and 20/20 OS. On fundus examination OD there was a premacular hemorrhage extending from the superior arcade to the macula. A focal membranotomy created by Argon laser coagulation at the inferior margin immediately released the hemorrhage into the inferior vitreous so that VA improved to 20/30.

The patient returned 6 months later complaining about decreased VA with metamorphopsia. On fundus examination there was a moderate epiretinal membrane on the retinal surface with a superficial prominent sheen-like membrane (Fig. 19.5G). Optical coherence tomography determined an epiretinal membrane on the retinal surface and a hyper reflective convex shaped prominent cavity in the area of macula (Fig. 19.5H). During pars plana vitrectomy the cortical vitreous was remarkably adherent to the retinal surface. This prominent membrane had no contact to the retinal surface and was also removed by aspiration. When indocyanine green dye (ICG) was injected intravitreally prior to internal limiting membrane-peeling,[36] it was not possible to stain the retinal surface in the area of the removed sheen-like membrane.[37] There is evidence that the preretinal hemorrhage was between the retinal nerve fiber layer and the internal limiting membrane:

- First, the dome-shaped preretinal membrane was difficult to penetrate by laser, indicating a substantial structure, such as the internal limiting membrane.
- Second, after the entrapped hemorrhage was released the preretinal cavity remained intact for months and no posterior vitreous detachment developed.
- Third, on OCT the convex shaped membrane was hyper reflective, possibly corresponding to the internal limiting membrane.
- Fourth, it is known, that intraoperatively injected ICG selectively stains the internal limiting membrane but not the bare retinal surface.

The submembranous blood was therefore released by a laser membranotomy. Proliferating cells on the internal limiting membrane and retinal surface may have sealed the membranotomy, so that the convex cavity persisted. Our two layered membrane theory in premacular hemorrhages was recently confirmed by Garcia-Arumi and associates [38] They performing a vitrectomy and histology in preretinal hemorrhages and determined multiple layers of cells on the inside of the dome-shaped membrane.

TRAUMATIC OPTIC PIT MACULOPATHY

Congenital pits of the optic nerve head result from an imperfect closure of the embryonic fissure. An unequal growth on both sides causes a delayed closure of the fissure at approximately 5 weeks of gestation. Optic pits appear as crater-like indentations on the surface of the optic nerve head usually with a steep temporal wall. [39] Anatomical the most anterior component of the optic nerve head contains the retinal nerve fiber layer (RNFL), composed of approximately 1.2 million unmyelinized retinal ganglion cell axons extending from all regions of the retina. Congenital optic pits have an incomplete axonal outgrowth of ganglion cells so that the primitive epithelial papilla contains with aberrant nerve fibers.[40] Histological sections defined rudimentary retinal tissue and aberrant nerve fibers in the pit.

A first patient with an optic pit presented a significant darker papillomacular bundle (Fig. 19.6A), extending from the edge of the optic nerve head to the macula, which appeared clinically like a severe RNFL-loss. [41] Optical coherence tomography was performed to determine the RNFL-thickness at the side of the pit and the corresponding papillomacular bundle. Circular OCT disclosed a predominant reduced RNFL-thickness in the temporal quadrant (Fig. 19.6B). There were no signs of a schisis-like retinal detachment on OCT. The imperfect closure and lack of papillomacular nerve-fiber bundles represent a 'loco minoris resistenciae' in optic pits, predisposing the development of a spontaneous schisis-like detachment during aging.

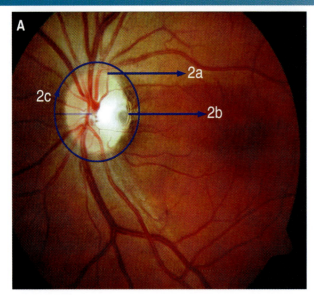

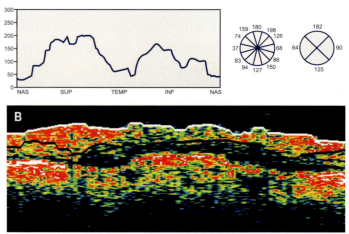

Fig. 19.6A: Fundus picture of the left eye presents an optic disc with a grey oval pit at the temporal side and a darker area in the papillomacular bundle appeared. The green line indicates the location of the corresponding circular OCT scan.

Fig. 19.6B: The cylindrical OCT scan started nasally and measured clockwise around the optic nerve with a diameter of 2.0. The unfolded section displayed as flat cross-sectional, two-dimensional false-color image. The mean thickness of the RNFL 64mm in the nasal quadrant. There is a markedly reduced RNFL of 48mm at the 4 o'clock position consistent with the location of the optic pit.

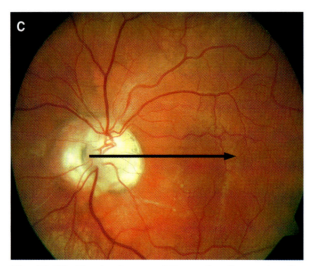

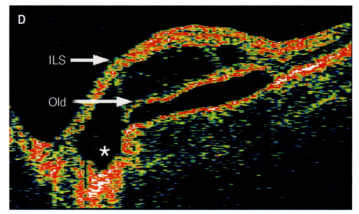

Fig. 19.6C: Fundus image of the optic pit maculopathy demonstrates an inferotemporal pit with a shallow retinal detachment extending to the macula. The arrow indicates the location and direction of the corresponding OCT scan. (From Meyer CH, Rodrigues EB. Optic disc pit maculopathy after blunt ocular trauma. Eur J Ophthalmol. 2004 ;14:71-73, reprinted with permission.)

Fig. 19.6D: Horizontal OCT image of the optic disc and the papillomacular region demonstrates an inner layer separation (ISL) as a thick hyper reflective orange to reddish color, consistent with nerve fiber detachment. It extends from the mid of the optic nerve across the papillomacular region to the margin of the fovea. The temporal edge of the optic nerve has a deeper hyper reflective reddish lesion, corresponding to the optic pit (white star). The outer layer detachment (OLD) of the neuroretina from the retinal pigment epithelium can be seen in a second hyper reflective band. The non-reflective space between the ILS and the OLD responds to a large schisis-like cavity. The retinal pigment epithelium–choriocapillaris-complex represents as a third hyper reflective band. The fluid under the OLD can leak through a hole in the outer layer into the subretinal space. (From Meyer CH, Rodrigues EB. Optic disc pit maculopathy after blunt ocular trauma. Eur J Ophthalmol. 2004;14:71-73, reprinted with permission.)

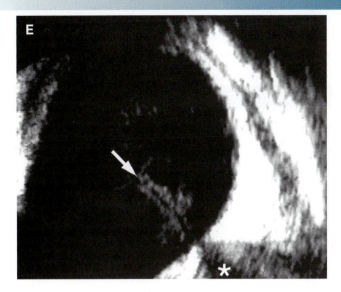

Fig. 19.6E: Saggital kinetic B-scan ultrasound of the optic nerve of the left eye. The location of the optic nerve is seen as a retrobulbar hyporeflective band (white star). An intravitreal tubular hyper reflective structure, consistent with the Cloquet's canal, extending perpendicular from the rim of the optic nerve into the vitreous cavity (white arrow). (From Meyer CH, Rodrigues EB. Optic disc pit maculopathy after blunt ocular trauma. Eur J Ophthalmol. 2004;14:71-73, reprinted with permission.)

The underlying mechanism optic pit maculopathy remains speculative, although many patients develop serous retinal detachments during life. As optic pits are congenital and the corresponding macular detachments develop later during in life, certain unknown events may trigger macular detachments. It is known that most eyes with an optic pit maculopathy have a partial vitreous detachment with firm attachments at the margin of the optic head.[42] We therefore investigated a second 16-year-old boy with a unilateral optic pit, who developed a serous retinal detachment 3 months after a blunt ocular trauma due to a bottle cork.

Funduscopy disclosed a gray oval pit at the temporal margin of the disc. A shallow uniform opaque retinal detachment, about 1.5 disc diameters, extended from the edge of the optic nerve to the macula (Fig. 19.6C). Optical coherence tomography demonstrated an inner layer separation (ISL) with an outer layer detachment (OLD) of the retina. The non-reflective space between them corresponded to a large schisis-like cavity (Fig. 19.6D). B-scan ultrasound revealed a hyper reflective tubular structure at the margin of the optic disc consisted with Cloquet's canal (Fig. 19.6E).

Lincoff and associates[44] hypothesized a two-layered structure in optic pit maculopathy. The serous retinal elevations in optic pits primarily begin at the optic disc with a schisis-like separation of the inner retinal layers. The ILS appears clinically transparent, while the corresponding functional scotoma is mild and central vision may remain intact. When a hole in the outer layer develops, fluid may flow through into the subretinal space creating a secondary OLD.

While the fundus examination demonstrated a serous detachment in the papillomacular area, our OCT-scan confirmed the two-layered structure of the optic pit maculopathy. We hypothesize that the serous retinal detachment was caused by the traumatic event.

- First, the patient reported no visual symptoms prior to the trauma.
- Second, B-scan ultrasound provided additional evidence for a Cloquet's canal terminating at margin of the optic disc. This rare anomalous vitreous attachment may have caused severe traction at the optic nerve during the traumatic event.
- Third, optic pit maculopathies usually occur in older patients (>35 years of age) indicating that an unusually event may have triggered the serous detachment.

Vigorous radial forces transmitted through abnormal vitreous attachment may have therefore exaggerated a schisis-like retinal detachment in our patients with a congenital optic pit.

EPIRETINAL MEMBRANE

The proliferation of epiretinal membranes occur spontaneously or as complication of various diseases on the surface of the retina along the internal limiting membrane. Iwanoff first in 1865 considered epiretinal membrane as the formation of endothelial cells.[45] These cells mainly derive from retinal glial or retinal pigment epithelial cell proliferating along the retinal surface and gain access to the internal limiting membrane by unknown stimuli.[46] The separation or peeling of epiretinal membrane is a rare incidence. It may occur spontaneously without evidence of any intervention by development of a posterior vitreous detachment, Nd:YAG laser or after ocular trauma.

Recently we reported the spontaneous separation of epiretinal membrane and consecutive visual improvement in young patients under 30-years of age.[48] The man noted blurred vision in his left eye. His visual acuity was 0.4 OS. Fundus examination OS demonstrated an epiretinal membrane with a radial folding of the retinal surface from the arcades towards the fovea. We decided to follow with observation as her visual acuity remained stable.

During the follow-up period his vision improved constantly and the epiretinal membrane continued to curl up like a papyrus role. After nine month his visual disturbance disappeared and his VA was 0.8 OS (Figs 7A to C). Similar events may occur in traumatic macular holes, where a spontaneous closure was recently reported.[49]

RETINAL PIGMENT EPITHELIAL TEAR

Retinal pigment epithelial tears occur most commonly in the posterior pole as a complication of age-related macular degeneration (AMD). Retinal pigment epithelial tears associated with blunt ocular trauma have been reported at the posterior pole and periphery.[50,51] Levin and associates[50] suggested that excessive force to the eye transmitting sufficient mechanical stress between the choroid and sclera as well as the retinal pigment epithelium may induce retinal pigment epithelium -tears or choroidal ruptures.

We previously presented three patients with AMD and retinal pigment epithelium -tears in the presence of vitreomacular traction and postulated that shear and abnormal stresses from the vitreoretinal interface may trigger the development of retinal pigment epithelial tears.[52] A 78-year-old white woman, complained of impaired vision. At presentation, her best-corrected VA was 20/70 OD and 20/200 OS. On biomicroscopy there was a V-shaped area of subretinal elevation temporal to the fovea with hyperpigmentation superiorly, consistent with folded retinal pigment epithelium and CNV. Subretinal fluid extended temporally and nasally to the lesion over orange-red, well-demarcated semicircles in the presumed bed of retinal pigment epithelial tears, with focal subretinal hemorrhages at the inferior margin (Fig. 19.8A). On fluorescein angiography there was an area of blocked fluorescence with late leakage, corresponding to the contracted retinal pigment epithelium. Well-demarcated areas of hyperfluorescence were present on either side of the central lesion, corresponding to the bed of the torn retinal pigment epithelium layer (Fig. 19.8B). In the

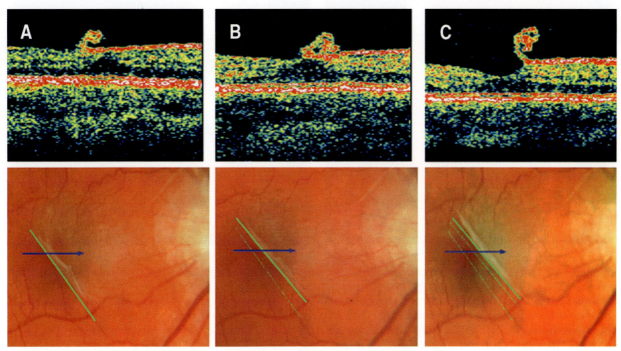

Figs 19.7A to C: A. Fundus picture of the right eye demonstrates the anatomy at the fovea. The blue arrow indicates the location length and direction of the corresponding horizontal OCT scan. The OCT scan demonstrated a hyper reflective band on the retinal surface corresponding to the partially rolled-up membrane. Note the roll is temporal to the fovea and the retinal thickness at the foveola is increased to 243mm. B. Fundus picture of the right eye OS 5 months later. The membrane has continued to peel back towards the optic disc in a roll-up fashion. The old location of the rolled-up membrane is demonstrated by a green dotted line. The current temporal edge of the membrane is marked by a solid green line. The blue arrow indicates the location, length and direction of the corresponding horizontal OCT scan. The OCT scan demonstrates a hyper reflective rolled-up membrane over the fovea. The retinal thickness at the foveola has decreased to 221mm. C. Fundus picture of the right eye 11 months later. The membrane has released the traction on the fovea. The old locations of the rolled-up membrane are demonstrated by two green dotted lines. The new edge of the membrane is marked by a solid green line. The blue arrow indicates the location, length and direction of the corresponding horizontal OCT scan. The OCT scan demonstrates a hyper reflective rolled-up membrane nasal to the fovea. The retinal thickness at the foveola has normalized to 168mm. (obtained from: Graefe's Arch Clin Exp Ophthalmol.: Spontaneous separation of epiretinal membrane in young subjects: personal observations and review of the literature. Meyer CH, Rodrigues EB, Mennel S, Schmidt JC, Kroll P; vol. 242, page 981, Fig. 19.3b-d, year of publication 2004, Springer copyright).

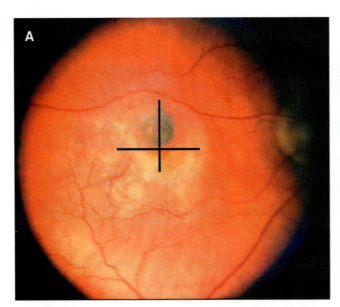

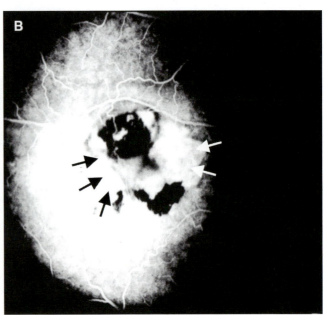

Fig. 19.8A: Fundus picture of the right eye. The fovea appears to be located in an area where the retinal pigment epithelium has been torn away. Subretinal hemorrhage extends to the inferior margin of the V-shaped central hyper pigmented mound of the rolled retracted retinal pigment epithelium. The two adjacent areas are the bed of the presumed retinal pigment epithelial tears. The line indicates the location of the vertical OCT scan.

Fig. 19.8B: Fluorescein angiography of the right eye. During early phase, there is delayed filling with partially blocked fluorescence in the area of folded retinal pigment epithelium. On either side of the central torn retinal pigment epithelium, a well-demarcated crescent shaped area of hyperfluorescence is visible in the bed of the retinal pigment epithelium tear. The arrows indicate the outer borders of the former PED (obtained from: Graefe's Arch Clin Exp Ophthalmol.: Retinal pigment epithelial tear with vitreomacular attachment: a novel pathogenic feature. Meyer CH, Toth CA; vol. 239, page 326, Fig. 19.2A-B, year of publication 2001, Springer copyright).

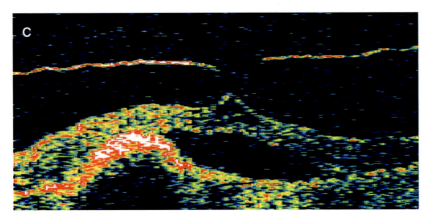

Fig. 19.8C: The vertical OCT scan was obtained from superior to the inferior direction and is plotted from left to right. Superior to the fovea is a highly reflective mass beneath the neurosensory retina, consistent with the dome-shaped reduplicated retinal pigment epithelium–CNV complex. Increased shadowing obscured a view of the underlying structure. Adjacent to the hyper-reflective lesion was a low-reflective region, consistent with subretinal fluid over the area of torn retinal pigment epithelium. Note the increase depth of reflectivity in the choroid in the bed of the retinal pigment epithelial tear consistent with the absence of the retinal pigment epithelium pigment. (obtained from: Graefe's Arch Clin Exp Ophthalmol.: Retinal pigment epithelial tear with vitreomacular attachment: a novel pathogenic feature. Meyer CH, Toth CA; vol. 239, page 328, Fig. 19.4B, year of publication 2001, Springer copyright).

vertical OCT scan of the macula, the neurosensory retina was elevated over a hyper-reflective mass with reduplicated retinal pigment epithelium shadowing the underlying structures. Adjacent to the reflective lesion was a well-demarcated area of low reflectivity in the subretinal space consistent with serous fluid. In the horizontal scan the fovea was tented up by traction and exhibited intraretinal cysts. The partially detached posterior hyaloid could be seen as a highly reflective band with attachments to the center of the fovea (Fig. 19.8C).

REFERENCES

1. Kroll P, Stoll W, Kirchhoff E. Contusion-suction trauma by solid unelastic balls. Klin Monatsbl Augenheilkd. 1983;182:555-559.
2. Berg P, Kroll P, Krause K. Pathogenic mechanism of contusion bulbi. Fortschr Ophthalmol. 1989;86;407-410.
3. Mennel S, Meyer CH, Kroll P. Dislocation of the lenses. N Engl J Med. 2004; 28;351:1913-1914.
4. Williams DF, Mieler WF, Williams GA. Posterior segment manifestations of ocular trauma. Retina. 1990; 10 Suppl 1:S35-44.
5. Delori F, Pomerantzeff O, Cox MS. Deformation of the globe under high-speed impact: Its relation to contusion injuries. Invest Ophthalmol. 1969;8:290-301.
6. Zdenek G, Ryan SJ. Combined posterior contusion and penetrating injury in the pig eye. II. Histological features. Br J Ophthalmol. 1982;66:799-804.
7. Pieramici DJ, Steinberg P, Aaberg TM, et al. The Ocular Trauma classification group: A system of classifying mechanical injuries of the eye (globe). Am J Ophthalmol. 1997;123:820-831.
8. Nettleship E. Peculiar lines in the choroid in a case of post-papillitic atrophy. Trans. Ophthalmol Soc. UK. 1884;4:167.
9. Norton EWD. A characteristic fluorescein angiographic pattern in choroidal folds. Proc R Soc Med. 1969;62:119.
10. Atta HR, Byrne SF. The findings of standardized echography for choroidal folds. Arch Ophthalmol. 1988;106:1234-1241.
11. Cappaert WE, Purnell EW, Frank KE. Use of B-sector scan ultrasound in the diagnosis of benign choroidal folds. Am J Ophthalmol. 1977;84:375-379.
12. Dailey RA, Mills RP, Stimac GK, et al. The natural history and CT appearance of acquired hyperopia with choroidal folds. Ophthalmology. 1986;93:1336-1342.
13. Berlin R. Zur sogenannten commotio retinae. Klin Monatsbl Augenheilkd. 1873;1:42-78.
14. Hesse L, Bodanowitz S, Kroll P. Retinal necrosis after blunt ocular trauma. Klin Monatsbl Augenheilkd. 1996; 209:150-152.
15. Sipperley JO, Quigley HA, Gass DM. Traumatic retinopathy in primates. The explanation of commotio retinae. Arch Ophthalmol. 1978;96:2267-2273.
16. Liem AT, Keunen JE, van Norren D. Reversible cone photoreceptor injury in commotio retinae of the macula. Retina. 1995;15:58-61.
17. Pahor D. Changes in retinal light sensitivity following blunt ocular trauma. Eye. 2000;14:583-589.
18. Miki T, Kitashoji K, Kohno T. Intrachoroidal dye leakage in indocyanine green fundus angiography after experimental commotio retinae. Eur J Ophthalmol. 1992;2:79–82.
19. Kohno T, Miki T, Hayashi K. Choroidopathy after blunt trauma to the eye: a fluorescein and indocyanine green angiographic study. Am J Ophthalmol. 1998; 126:248-260.
20. Dubovy SR, Guyton DL, Green WR. Clinicopathologic correlation of chorioretinitis sclopetaria. Retina. 1997;17:510-520.
21. Mansour AM, Green WR, Hogge C. Histopathology of commotio retinae. Retina. 1992;12:24-28.
22. Ismail R, Tanner V, Williamson TH. Optical coherence tomography imaging of severe commotio retinae and associated macular hole. Br J Ophthalmol. 2002; 86:473-474.
23. Meyer CH, Rodrigues EB, Mennel S. Acute commotio retinae determined by cross-sectional optical coherent tomography. Eur J Ophthalmol. 2003;13:816-818.
24. Von Graefe A. Zwei Fälle von Ruptur der Choroidea. Graefe's Arch Clin Exp Ophthalmol. 1854;1:402.
25. Wagemann A. Zur pathologischen Anatomie der Aderhautruptur und Iridodialyse. Bericht Deutsche Ophthal Ges. 1902;30:278-282.
26. Secretan M, Sickenberg M, Zografos L, Piguet B. Morphometric characteristics of traumatic choroidal ruptures associated with neovascularization. Retina. 1998; 18:62-66.
27. Flower RW, von Kerczek C, Zhu L, et al. Theoretical investigation of the role of choriocapillaris blood flow in treatment of subfoveal choroidal neovascularization associated with age-related macular degeneration. Am J Ophthalmol. 2001; 132:85-93.
28. Mennel S, Hausmann N, Meyer CH, Peter S. Photodynamic therapy and indocyanine green guided feeder vessel photocoagulation of choroidal neovascularization secondary to choroidal rupture after blunt trauma. Graefes Arch Clin Exp Ophthalmol 2004 Aug 4 (epub ahead of print).
29. Aguilar JP, Green WR. Choroidal rupture: A histopathologic study of 47 cases. Retina. 1984;4:269-275.
30. Duane TD. Valsalva retinopathy. Trans Am Ophthalmol Soc. 1972; 70:298-311.
31. Foos RY. Vitreoretinal juncture, topographical variations. Invest Ophthalmology. 1972;11:801-809.
32. Green MA, Lieberman G, Milroy CM, Parsons MA. Ocular and cerebral trauma in non-accidental injury in infancy: underlying mechanisms and implications for paediatric practice. Br J Ophthalmol. 1996;80:282-287.
33. Kroll P, Busse H. Therapy of preretinal macular hemorrhages. Klin Monatsbl Augenheilkd. 1986;188:610-612.
34. Ulbig MW, Mangouritsas G, Rothbacher HH, et al. Long-term results after drainage of premacular subhyaloid hemorrhage into the vitreous with a pulsed Nd:YAG laser. Arch Ophthalmol. 1998;116:1465-1469.
35. Meyer CH, Mennel S, Rodrigues EB, Schmidt JC. Persistent premacular cavity after membranotomy in Valsalva retinopathy on optical coherence tomography. Retina (in press).

36. Schmidt JC, Meyer CH, Rodrigues EB, et al. Staining of the internal limiting membrane in vitreoretinal surgery: A simplified technique. Retina. 2003;23:263-264.
37. Meyer CH, Rodrigues EB, Kroll P. Reduced concentration and incubation of intravitreal Indocyanine green can improve the functional outcome in macular hole surgery. Am J Ophthalmol. 2004;137:386.
38. Garcia-Arumi J, Corcostegui B, Tallada N, Salvador F. Epiretinal membranes in Tersons syndrome. A clinicopathologic study. Retina. 1994;14:351-355.
39. Kranenberg EW. Crater-like holes in the optic disc and central serous retinopathy. Arch Ophthalmol 1960;64:912-924.
40. Sugar HS. Congenital pits in the optic disc with acquired macular pathology. Am J Ophthalmol. 1962;53:307-311.
41. Meyer CH, Rodrigues EB, Schmidt JC. Congenital optic nerve head pit associated with reduced retinal nerve fiber thickness at the papillomacular bundle. Br J Ophthalmol. 2003; 87:1300-1301.
42. Akiba J Kakehasi A, Hikichi T, Trempe CL. Vitreous findings of optic nerve pits and serous macular detachments. Am J Ophthalmol. 1993; 116:38-41.
43. Meyer CH, Rodrigues EB. Optic disc pit maculopathy after blunt ocular trauma. Eur J Ophthalmol. 2004;14:71-73.
44. Lincoff H, Kreissig I. Optic coherence tomography of pneumatic displacement of optic disk pit maculopathy. Br J Ophthalmol. 1998;83:367-372.
45. Iwanoff A. Beiträge zur normalen und pathologischen Anatomie des Auges. Graefes Arch Clin Exp Ophthalmol. 1865;11:135-170.
46. Trese M, Chandler D, Machemer R. Macular pucker. I Prognostic criteria. Graefe's Arch Klin Exp Ophthalmol. 1983;221:12-15.
47. Messner KH. Spontaneous separation of preretinal macular fibrosis. Am J Ophthalmol. 1977;83:9-11.
48. Meyer CH, Rodrigues EB, Mennel S, et al. Spontaneous separation of epiretinal membrane in young subjects: personal observations and review of the literature. Graefe's Arch Clin Exp Ophthalmol. 2004;242:977-985.
49. Yamashita T, Uemara A, Uchino E, et al. Spontaneous closure of traumatic macular hole. Am J Ophthalmol. 2002; 133:230-235.
50. Levin LA, Seddon JM, Topping T. Retinal pigment epithelial tears associated with trauma. Am J Ophthalmol. 1991;112:396–400.
51. Doi M, Osawa S, Sasoh M, Uji Y. Retinal pigment epithelial tear and extensive exudative retinal detachment following blunt trauma. Graefe's Arch Clin Exp Ophthalmol. 2000;238:621-624.
52. Meyer CH, Toth CA. Retinal pigment epithelial tear with vitreomacular attachment: a novel pathogenic feature. Graefe's Arch Clin Exp Ophthalmol. 2001; 239:325-333.

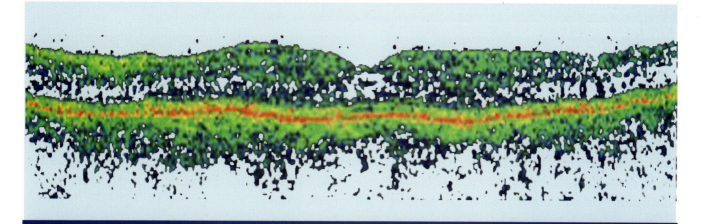

CHAPTER

20

Inflammatory Diseases of Retina and Choroid: An Overview

Andrea Hassenstein, Ulrich Schaudig, Gisbert Richard

INTRODUCTION

Inflammations of the posterior segment can be grouped into two major categories by the most common anatomic features: retinitis and choroiditis. Conditions may present with focal, multifocal or diffuse involvement. A large variety of inflammations of the retina and choroid occurs. It may be the result of an infection (e.g. toxoplasmosis) or of an idiopathic inflammation such as uveitis (Birdshot retinochoroidopathy). Infectious involvement is seen more commonly in the retina and choroid than in the anterior segment. In most cases the blood-retinal barrier is compromised leading to leakage and fluid accumulation, such as detachment of the choroid, retinal pigment epithelium and retina.

Some cases present with typical pathological findings in funduscopy such as toxoplasmosis, but plenty of cases in early stages make a clear diagnosis difficult by funduscopy only.

OPTICAL COHERENCE TOMOGRAPHY

The optical coherence tomography (OCT) is based upon light reflectivity in ocular tissues. Colored B-scans[1-3] are elaborated by the device, and different retinal layers are thus shown in separate colors. The benefit of OCT in inflammatory disease and a possible pathognomonic consideration is demonstrated in this chapter.

The biomicroscopic examination and the fluorescein angiography of the central fundus regions may in some cases not be sufficient to exactly locate lesions, estimate their extent, differentiate lesions of the fovea, see membranes and follow the results of medical or surgical treatment. Fluorescein angiography is two dimensional, perfusion is visualized, however, the nerve fiber layer, pathologic epiretinal structures and the posterior vitreous cannot be observed. A clear cut assignment to retinal layers is often not possible.

Inflammatory diseases of the retina are often accompanied by opaque ocular media due to corneal decompensation, complicated cataracts and vitreous opacities. In those cases the light beam of OCT may not reach the region of interest, particularly the retina and choroid. Therefore a sufficient amount of media clarity is mandatory for an OCT examination.

In inflammatory diseases the OCT detects fluids in or beneath the retina or choroid associated with detachment of the sensory retina, cystoid macular edema, diffuse macular edema and detachment of the retinal pigment epithelium, and allows a precise anatomical localization and quantification. Complications of inflammatory disease of the retina and choroid are persistent macular edema, epiretinal membrane, choroidal neovascularisation and scar formation (e.g. presumed ocular histoplasmosis syndrome, toxoplasmosis). [1-12]

Optical coherence tomography provides additional information in acute and chronic inflammation: Fluid accumulation in different layers is dominating in the former, the incidence of sequelae is predominant in the latter (Figs 20.1 to 20.16)

Acute inflammation
- Cystoid macular edema
- Detachment of sensory retina [10]
- Detachment of retinal pigment epithelium

Chronic inflammation
- Cystoid macular edema
- Epiretinal membrane
- Choroidal neovascularization
- Scar formation

Since the sequelae of the treatment of intraocular inflammations may sometimes be more detrimental than the disease itself, indications for therapy should rely on solid grounds. These features qualify the OCT for use in precisely defined intraocular inflammations when indications are sought for:
- Cytotoxic treatment
- Laser surgery
- Pars plana vitrectomy
- Epiretinal membrane peeling, and
- Excision of subretinal neovascular membrane

INTERESTING CASE EXAMPLES

In our retrospective investigation 117 patients suffered from various inflammatory diseases: choroiditis (n=14), vasculitis (n=4) and serpiginous choroiditis (n=2), toxoplasmosis (n=19), neuroretinitis (n=3), and sarcoidosis (n=75). All patients had a moderately clear visual axis.

Choroiditis

In choroiditis clear media are found due to lacking cellular vitreous infiltration. In acute stages the creamy whitish lesions present in OCT as focal convex thickening of the retinal pigment epithelium and underlying structures with enhanced light transmission into deeper layers in some cases. Only in extensive and acute inflammation a simultaneous sensory detachment is found (Fig. 20.11). Treatment regimens can be changed depending on the amount of subretinal fluid (Figs 20.1 to 20.5)

Serpiginous Choroiditis

In chronic serpiginous choroiditis funduscopy reveals a serpiginous chorioatrophy and hypertrophy of retinal pigment epithelium. In OCT a focal enhancement of backscatter in underlying tissue like in geographic atrophy or laser scars can be seen (Fig. 20.1).

Retinochoroiditis (Toxoplasmosis)

Active lesions in toxoplasmosis can be distinguished from scars by OCT. Vitreous inflammatory cell infiltrates, posterior vitreous detachment, and granulomas at the posterior vitreous layer are visualized.

In acute stage of toxoplasmosis the white retinal infiltration shows a bright reflective inner retinal layer and a thickening of the retina. Due to the backscatter of the nerve fiber layer the underlying outer retinal layers appear optically empty. The predominant infiltration of the nerve fiber layer is consistent with the histological finding of destruction of nerve fibers in retinal infiltration due to toxoplasmosis, therefore called a Retinochoroiditis. The retina is thickened in this area. Depending on the clinical stage, focal or general vitreous infiltration is found (Figs 20.6A, B, and 20.8).

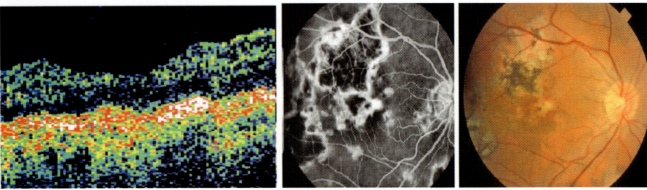

Fig. 20.1: In long-standing serpiginous choroiditis retinal pigment epithelium shows atrophy and scarring. OCT visualizes the enhanced transmission in deeper layers due to lacking backscattering retinal pigment epithelium. The OCT image resembles findings in geographic atrophy. Typical findings in fluorescein angiography and fundus picture, OD.

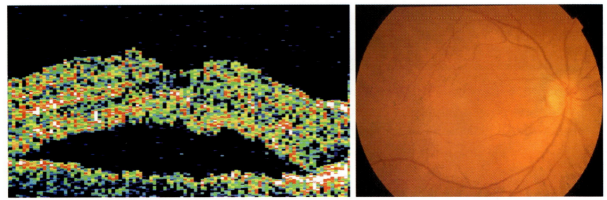

Fig. 20.2: In acute choroiditis OCT reveals a subfoveal accompanying fluid accumulation, deteriorating the vision acuity and only detectable in OCT. Funduscopy is unremarkable, OD.

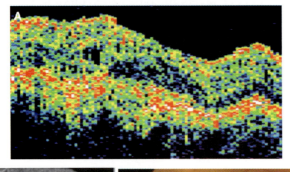

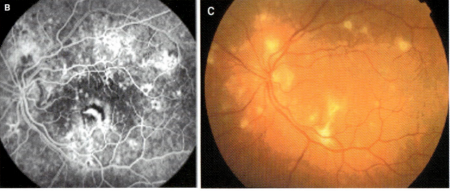

Fig. 20.3: In multifocal choroiditis the high reflective retinal pigment epithelium layer shows a thickening corresponding to infiltration areas. Additionally in fluorescein angiography a subfoveal classic CNV is seen which was not apparent in funduscopy, OS.

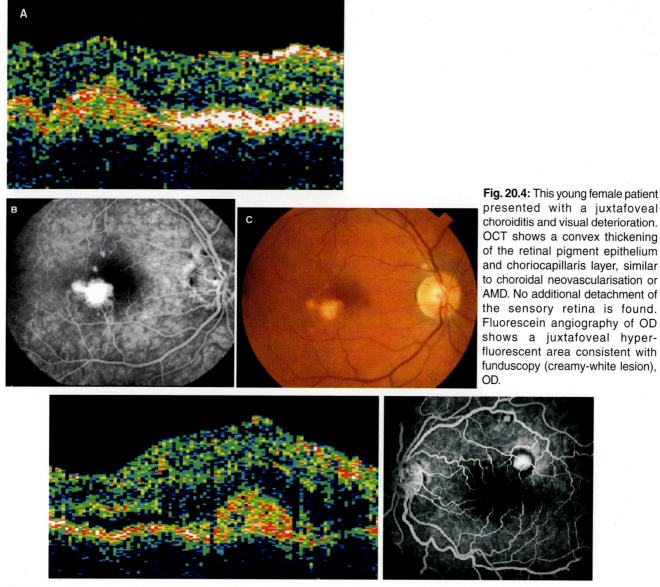

Fig. 20.4: This young female patient presented with a juxtafoveal choroiditis and visual deterioration. OCT shows a convex thickening of the retinal pigment epithelium and choriocapillaris layer, similar to choroidal neovascularisation or AMD. No additional detachment of the sensory retina is found. Fluorescein angiography of OD shows a juxtafoveal hyperfluorescent area consistent with funduscopy (creamy-white lesion), OD.

Fig. 20.5: In long-term follow-up a choroidal neovascularisation (CNV) may present after choroiditis as a sequelae. The fluorescein angiography shows an extrafoveal classic CNV; laser treatment is indicated, OS.

In late scar formation the typical findings of scars are visualized by OCT: focal thinning of the retina, thickening of the retinal pigment epithelium and choriocapillaris and in various degrees an enhanced transmission into deeper layers (Figs 20.7 and 20.12).

The effectiveness of medical treatment (antibiotic drugs and/or high-dose corticosteroids) was obviated by OCT monitoring showing the resolution of vitreous infiltrates and macular edema. [11]

Retinal Vasculitis

Cystoid macular edema (CME) is the prominent pathological findings by OCT. In most cases the CME detected by OCT revealed a far more extensive lesion than biomicroscopy or fluorescein angiography would have suggested (Figs 20.9, 20.10A and B). The medical treatment based on the OCT was more aggressive.

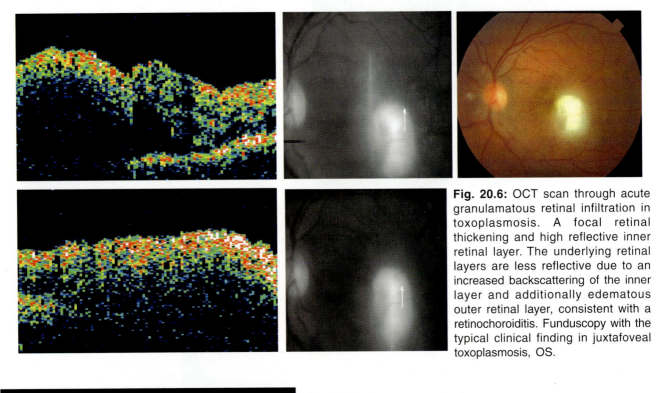

Fig. 20.6: OCT scan through acute granulamatous retinal infiltration in toxoplasmosis. A focal retinal thickening and high reflective inner retinal layer. The underlying retinal layers are less reflective due to an increased backscattering of the inner layer and additionally edematous outer retinal layer, consistent with a retinochoroiditis. Funduscopy with the typical clinical finding in juxtafoveal toxoplasmosis, OS.

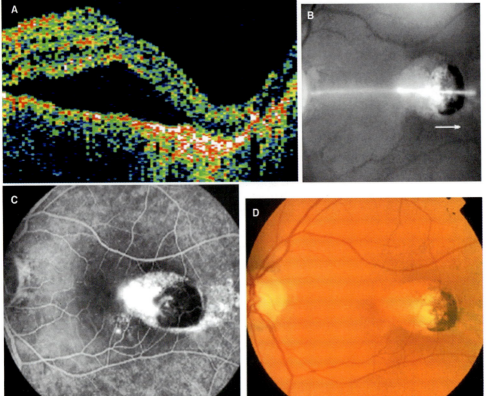

Fig. 20.7: OCT reveals a detachment of the sensory retina in relation to the macular scar not seen in fluorescein angiography. The visual acuity was deteriorated and the recurrence was visualized by OCT. Funduscopy and fluorescein angiography was unremarkable concerning retinal detachment, OS.

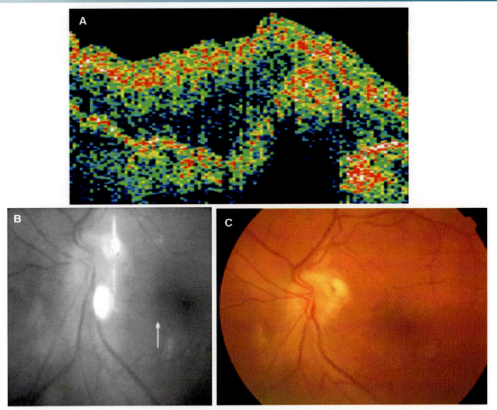

Fig. 20.8: In acute toxoplasmosis Jensen close to the optic nerve head OCT shows a retinal thickening and a reduced light transmission into deeper layers. Funduscopy in peripapillary retinochoroiditis due to toxoplasmosis, OS.

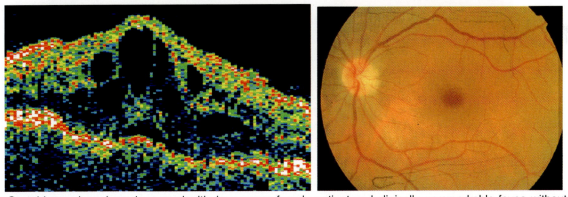

Fig. 20.9: Cystoid macular edema in pars planitis in a young female patient and clinically unremarkable fovea without reflex. OCT shows an extensive cystoid macular edema with large cyst formation, OS.

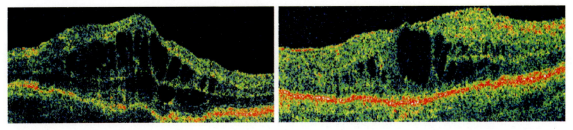

Figs 20.10A and B: Cystoid macular edema in sarcoidosis. This 29-year-old female suffered from sarcoidosis and unilaterally persistent cystoid macular edema with a VA of 20/100. Systemic steroid treatment improved the cystoid macular edema only slightly. She underwent triamcinolone injection into the vitreous and her VA improved to 20/20 in the follow-up, OS.

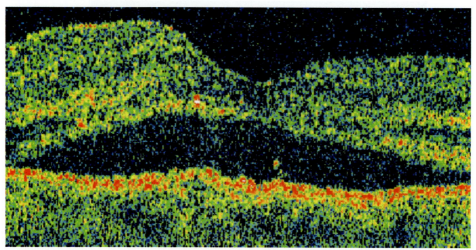

Fig. 20.11: In many inflammatory retinal and choroid diseases an accompanying detachment of the macula is found and is often not detected by funduscopy. The fluid accumulation serves as an activity indicator for treatment decisions, OD.

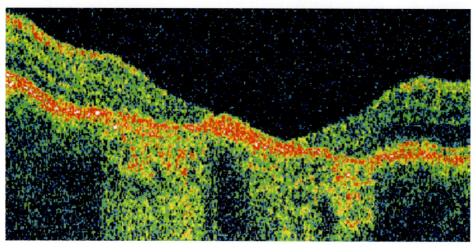

Fig. 20.12: In the follow-up scar formation may occur. In OCT a thinning of the sensory retina and a thickening of the retinal pigment epithelium/choriocapillaris layer are typical findings. In case of retinal pigment epithelium atrophy an enhanced light transmission into deeper areas can be found, OD.

Neuroretinitis

The most common finding in neuroretinitis is a diffuse thickening of the retina. In rare cases a higher backscatter due to hard exudates within the sensory retina may occur.

GENERAL FINDINGS IN INFLAMMATORY DISEASE OF RETINA AND CHOROID IN OPTICAL COHERENCE TOMOGRAPHY

Optical coherence tomography demonstrated 3 different patterns of macular edema in uveitis: detachment of the sensory retina (20%), diffuse macular edema (55%) and cystoid macular edema (25%).

Cystoid fluid accumulation of CME was located predominantly in the outer retinal layer. Patients with CME had significantly greater retinal thickness and worse visual acuity.[4] The sensitivity of OCT for detecting

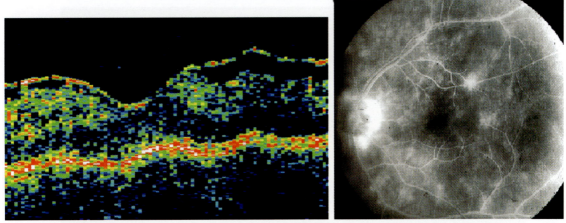

Fig. 20.13: In chronic retinal vasculitis secondary epiretinal membrane may occur. Visual prognosis is good as long as the foveal configuration is concave and no cystoid transformation is present. Typical findings in fluorescein angiography in retinal vasculitis with leakage of retinal vessels, OS.

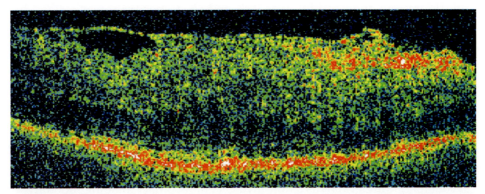

Fig. 20.14: The epiretinal membrane had developed in the course of a prior retinal vasculitis. A diffuse retinal thickening due to tractional forces occurs in secondary epiretinal membrane in chronic inflammatory disease. No cystoid formation is found in the inner retinal layers, OD.

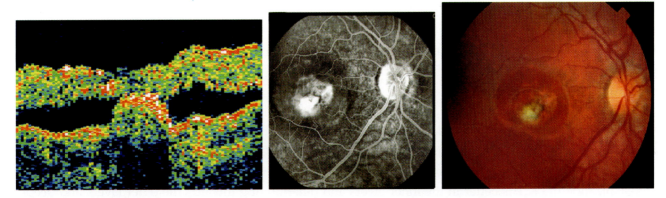

Fig. 20.15: An inflammatory lesion in the fovea of unknown origin presents in OCT as a focal elevation of retinal pigment epithelium/choriocapillaris layer and accompanying detachment of the sensory retina as result of an active process. Fluorescein angiography shows a staining of the macular scar, also funduscopy but no sensory detachment is visible, OD.

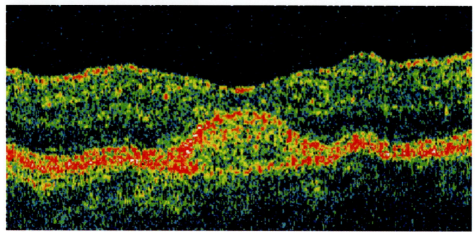

Fig. 20.16: The optical coherence tomography demonstrates a subfoveal dry choroidal neovascularisation without edema beneath the fovea, OS.

CME compared with fluorescein angiography was 96% and OCT specificity was 100%. [5] In 40% of uveitis patients an epiretinal membrane is found in OCT (Figs 20.13 and 20.14). [4]

Choroidal neovascularization (CNV) may follow various inflammatory diseases. The extent and localization to the fovea including fluid accumulation can be visualized by OCT for decision-making strategies. In the OCT, scar formation in presumed ocular histoplasmosis syndrome or toxoplasmosis is similar to a chorioatrophic scar after laser treatment or in geographic atrophy (Fig. 20.12).

Indications for laser or surgical treatment depend primarily on clinical features, and the localization in relation to the macula. Fluorescein angiography shows a mapping of the retinal perfusion with leakage but no relation to retinal layers.

Since the optical coherence tomography is a non-invasive, non-contact imaging modality, which produces high-resolution cross-sectional images of the ocular fundus helping to identify the morphology of intraocular tissue layers, distinct advantages of the OCT compared to fluorescein angiography could be demonstrated. [3]

Our observations suggest applications of OCT evaluation in uveitis with
- Cystoid macular edema, [6]
- Epiretinal membranes, [7]
- Granulomas,
- Detachment of the retinal pigment epithelium or the sensory retina, [5]
- Choroidal neovascularization (Figs 20.15 and 20.16), [8] and
- Subretinal membranes. [8,9]

None of the chorioretinal inflammatory diseases present a typical and unique pathognomonic finding in OCT. Inflammation is due to a breakdown of the blood-retinal barrier and causes fluid accumulation in various layers (retina, retinal pigment epithelium). Therefore OCT will visualize in most cases the fluid accumulation and following structural changes. Due to the light transmission into deeper layers, the clear cut visualization of OCT is better in the inner layers and deteriorating towards the outer layers and deeper structures, such as choroid. Optical coherence tomography helps in indicating treatment and surgical intervention, in visualizing structural changes and relation to the merging structures:
- Direct visualization of inflammation (e.g. toxoplasmosis)

- Visualization of sequelae (e.g. epiretinal membrane)

In conclusion, treatment indications in uveitis patients utilizing the OCT as the main diagnostic tool are membrane peeling, subretinal membrane excision and vitrectomy, laser coagulation and aggressive medical treatment including cytotoxic agents. These observations indicate that the OCT seems to be the most appropriate device to precisely localize secondary CNV and allow decision-making for a surgical strategy (Figs 20.15 and 20.16).

Furthermore, the effectiveness of anti-inflammatory treatment and the surgical outcome can be objectively monitored. This makes the OCT an additional instrument for the visualization of inflammatory processes and sequelae in the central fundus of the eye. Thus, some indications for systemic cytotoxic treatment and laser and intraocular surgery in the patient series presented were exclusively based on the results of this device.[11,12]

Limitations for using this instrument are failure of peripheral fundus imaging due to dense vitreous or media opacities and insufficient patient's fixation or compliance.

REFERENCES

1. Huang D, Swanson EA, Lin CP, et al. Optical coherence tomography. Science. 1991; 254:1178-1181.
2. Hee MR, Izatt JA, Swanson EA, et al. Optical coherence tomography of the human retina. Arch Ophthalmol. 1995; 113:325-332.
3. Toth CA, Narayan DG, Boppart SA, et al. A Comparison of retinal morphology viewed by optical coherence tomography and by light microscopy. Arch Ophthalmol. 1997;115:1425-1428.
4. Markomichelakis NN, Halkiadakis I, Pantelia E, et al. Patterns of macular edema in patients with uveitis: qualitative and quantitative assessment using optical coherence tomography. Ophthalmology. 2004;111:946-953.
5. Antcliff RJ, Stanford MR, Chauhan DS, et al. Comparison between optical coherence tomography and fundus fluorescein angiography for the detection of cystoid macular edema in patients with uveitis. Ophthalmology. 2000;107:593-599.
6. Hee MR, Puliafito CA, Wong C, et al. Quantitative assessment of macular edema with optical coherence tomography. Arch Ophthalmol.1995;113:1019-1029.
7. Wilkins JR, Puliafito CA, Hee MR, et al. Characterization of epiretinal membranes using optical coherence tomography. Ophthalmology. 1996;103:2142-2151.
8. Hee MR, Baumal CR, Puliafito CA, et al. Optical coherence tomography of age-related macular degeneration and choroidal neovascularization. Ophthalmology. 1996;103:1260-1270.
9. Puliafito CA, Hee MR, Lin CP, et al. Imaging of macular diseases with optical coherence tomography. Ophthalmology.1995;102:217-229.
10. Hee MR, Puliafito CA, Wong C, et al. Optical coherence tomography of central serous chorioretinopathy. Am J Ophthalmol. 1995;120:63-74.
11. Hassenstein A, Bialasiewicz AA, Richard G. Optical coherence tomography in uveitis patients. Am J Ophthalmol. 2000;130:669-670.
12. Walter A, Bialasiewicz AA, Hassenstein A, et al. Optical Coherence Tomography Imaging in Ocular Inflammations. In: Süveges I, Follmann P. (eds.): Proc. XIth Congress of the Eur. Soc. Ophthalmology, Bologna, Monduzzi Editore, 1997:1583-1585.

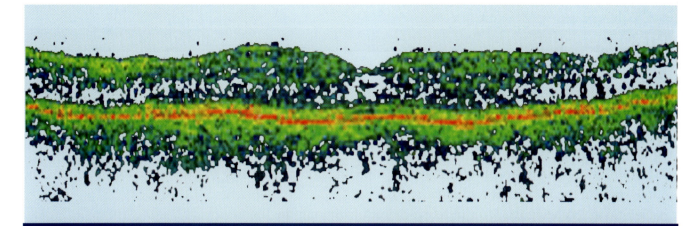

Retinal and Choroidal Inflammation

Jyotirmay Biswas, S Sudharshan

INTRODUCTION

Uveitic conditions are *by nature recurrent*, hence the patients have to be followed up at frequent intervals. Fundus fluorescein angiography and other modalities are also quite sensitive but are invasive and resolution is much lesser when compared to optical coherence tomography (OCT).

Optical coherence tomography thus is helpful in not only in diagnosis but also in follow-up of patients at regular intervals. It is:

- Helpful in the management of intraocular inflammation as it is able to define the extent, depth and thickness of the inflammatory lesion.
- Helpful in localizing the layer of retina-choroid harboring the lesion
- Helpful in not only diagnosing the disease but also in monitoring the response to treatment
- Useful in titrating therapy.

CYSTOID MACULAR EDEMA

Cystoid macular edema (CME) is a classical complication of ocular inflammation. It results from either a breakdown of the inner or outer blood ocular barrier. Clinical CME that is responsible for low visual acuity must be differentiated from CME detected by fluorescein angiography or OCT, which may not be associated with decrease in visual acuity. [1]

Optical coherence tomography can detect precisely even very minimal amounts of fluid in particular layers of retina. Fluid progressively accumulates into the outer plexiform layer of the retina and pools into cystic spaces. However, inflammatory CME must be differentiated from CME resulting from irreversible vascular damage as those found in diabetes or vascular occlusions.

Reinthal and associates [2] have studied the role of OCT in the diagnosis and follow-up of 22 eyes of 18 patients with uveitic macular edema and compared it with fundoscopic and angiographic pictures over a period of 5 months. They found good results even when there was low or medium haze of optical media. There were a few eyes in which OCT detected macular edema, which was not detected by fluorescein angiography. Antcliff and associates [3] compared OCT and fluorescein angiographic detection of CME in patients with uveitis in 121 eyes of 58 patients. Optical coherence tomography and fluorescein angiography had similar results in most of the patients. But in 10 eyes subretinal fluid was detected on OCT but not on angiography. Five of these eyes had CME on angiography but not on OCT. Compared with fluorescein angiography, the OCT sensitivity for detecting CME was 96% and specificity was 100%. Optical coherence tomography is as effective at detecting CME as is fluorescein angiography but is superior in demonstrating axial distribution of fluid. Markomichelakis and associates [4] studied the patterns of uveitic macular edema in 70 consecutive patients with the help of OCT and found macular edema to follow 3 patterns. It can be a diffuse macular edema, cystoid macular edema and serous retinal detachment. Macular edema is mainly located in the outer retinal layers. A serous retinal detachment is noted in the inner retinal layers.

Many workers have studied the advantages of intravitreal triamcinolone in the treatment of refractory cystoid macular edema due to uveitis. It is very effective on short term basis. Intravitreal steroid injections are being used for the treatment of diabetic macular edema, age-related macular degeneration, and other clinical entities. Uveitic macular edema recurs. We have also found that there is need for repeat injections as the macular edema can recur after intravitreal injections. Also is a word of caution in the fact that strict aseptic precautions and monitoring of intraocular pressure is crucial in monitoring this form of therapy. [5-16]

Sourdille and associates [17] have studied the macular thickness changes after uneventful cataract surgery using optical coherence tomography and compared the findings with those of flare and cell measurements of the anterior chamber. They have found that not all eyes with increased macular thickness detected by OCT are due to breakdown of blood aqueous barrier. Most of these changes resolve spontaneously.

OPTICAL COHERENCE TOMOGRAPHY

Interesting Case Examples

Intermediate Uveitis

Intermediate uveitis due to various causes can be recurrent and needs to be followed up at regular intervals. It can vary from severe vitritis, snowball opacities and snow banking to milder forms with minimal vitreous cells. It is commonly idiopathic. Macular edema is an important cause of defective vision.

Case 1: A 33-year old female patient presented with intermediate uveitis associated with cystoid macular edema. Optical coherence tomography examination revealed large cystoid spaces with increase in central macular thickness (Fig. 21.1). Central retinal thickness was measured to be to be 943 microns on retinal map analysis.

Case 2: A 42-year-old male presented with blurred vision in his left eye. On examination he was diagnosed as a case of intermediate uveitis. Fundus examination of the right eye revealed macular edema (Fig. 21.2A). Fluorescein angiography (late phase) showed typical flower petal pattern at the macula suggestive of cystoid macular edema (Fig. 21.2B). Optical coherence tomography revealed multiple cystoid spaces in the macula (Fig. 21.2C). Increased retinal thickness without any obvious cystoid spaces due to retinal edema can cause diminution of vision, which is not generally detected by fundus fluorescein angiography.

Case 3: A 46-year-old male presented with the complaints of defective vision in the left eye of one-week duration. On examination, his vision was 20/40, in his left eye with minimal anterior chamber reaction and vitreous cells 1+. His fundus examination revealed a dull foveal reflex (Figs 3A to C). Optical coherence tomography did not show any obvious cystoid spaces in macula. Central macular thickness was 362 microns. An epiretinal membrane was seen as a highly reflective structure. He regained vision after treatment, with reduction in macular thickness and restoration of the foveal contour.

Case 4: A 53-year-old female presented with complaints of defective vision in the left eye. On examination, she was found to have pars planitis. Her fundus examination revealed cystoid macular edema. The vision in the left eye was 20/80 (Fig. 21.4A). Optical coherence tomography showed loss of foveal contour with retinal thickness measuring 371 microns and presence of cystoid spaces. She was treated conventionally with topical steroids and posterior sub tenon's injection of triamcinolone acetonide in her left eye. On her 4-week follow up, her vision improved to 20/20, in both the eyes and her OCT revealed complete resolution of macular edema and restoration of the foveal contour (Fig. 21.4B).

Case 5: A 22-year-old female, a known case of pars planitis underwent phacoemulsification and intraocular lens implantation in her left eye, which was uneventful. Four months post operatively she presented with the complaints of floaters and blurred vision in her left eye. On examination her vision in the left eye was

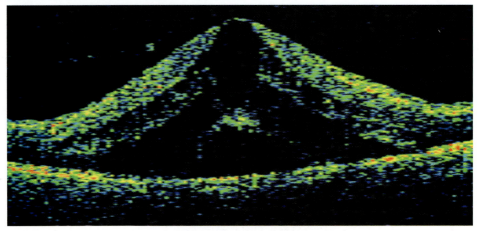

Fig. 21.1: OCT scan through the fovea showing multiple cystoid spaces. Central macular thickness is 943 microns

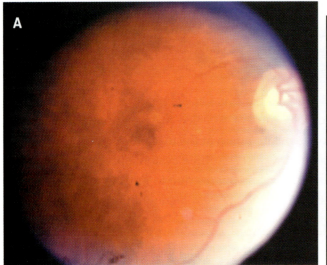

Fig. 21.2A: Fundus photograph revealing macular edema

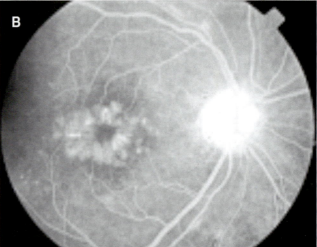

Fig. 21.2B: Fluorescein angiography – late phase revealing typical flower petal pattern suggestive of cystoid macular edema

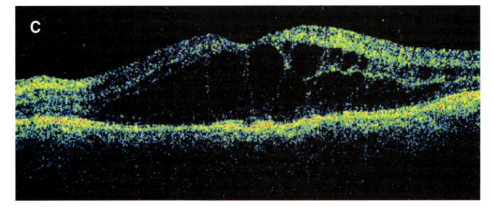

Fig. 21.2C: OCT revealing cystoid macular edema

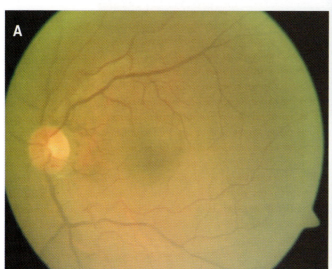

Fig. 21.3A: Fundus photograph of the left eye showing a dull foveal reflex

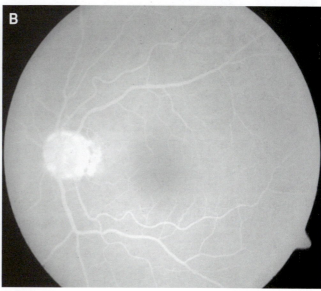

Fig. 21.3B: Fluorescein angiography of the left eye of the same patient showing no evidence of macular edema even in the late phase

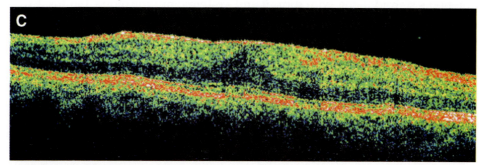

Fig. 21.3C: OCT of the left eye revealing an increase in retinal thickness (382 microns) suggestive of diffuse macular edema. There is a high reflective structure (arrow) suggestive of epiretinal membrane

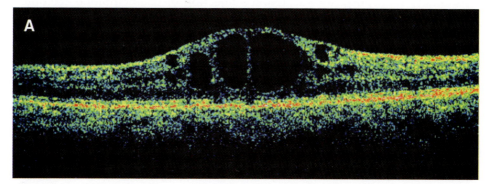

Fig. 21.4A: OCT of the left eye revealing cystoid macular edema with a central macular thickness of 371 microns with multiple cystoid spaces

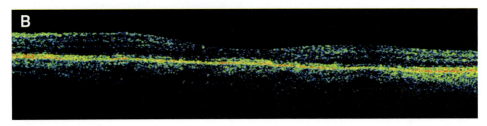

Fig. 21.4B: OCT revealing complete resolution of macular edema and restoration of the foveal contour

20/100 (Fig. 21. 5A). Central macular thickness was 506 microns. She was treated with periocular and systemic steroids. and After 6 weeks of treatment, her vision was 20/30 (Fig. 21.5B). Optical coherence tomography revealed central macular thickness of 154 microns, few small cystic spaces and normal foveal contour.

Case 6: A 43-year-old male, a known patient of suspected multiple sclerosis that was being treated for intermediate uveitis presented with recurrence. Magnetic resonance imaging showed a well-defined lesion at the medial longitudinal fasciculus. His vision in the right eye was 20/80 (Fig. 21.6A). Optical coherence tomography revealed multiple cystoid spaces. Central macular thickness was 442 microns. He was treated with posterior subtenon's steroid along with topical and systemic prednisolone. On his 4-week follow up he still complained of defective vision though he felt it was better than his earlier visit. His vision in the right eye showed slight improvement at 20/60 (Fig. 21.6B). Repeat OCT showed cystoid spaces still present in the macula, however, macular thickness had reduced only by about 50 microns when compared to the previous visit. Macular thickness was 390 microns. Patient was treated with 4 mg intravitreal injection of triamcinolone acetonide injection (Fig. 21.6C). Optical coherence tomography revealed almost complete disappearance of the cysts and his vision had improved to 20/30 (Fig. 21.6D).

Case 7: A 55-year-old female, on treatment for intermediate uveitis, presented with the complaints of defective vision in her left eye. The vision in her left eye was 20/80. On her initial presentation, left eye showed evidence of CME. Optical coherence tomography showed large cystoid spaces in the macula, which was treated conventionally with posterior sub-tenon's injection of triamcinolone acetonide and systemic steroids (Fig. 21.7A). But at 2-month follow up, the patient complained of further loss of vision, and OCT was repeated. Optical coherence tomography revealed increase in the number and size of the cystoid spaces in the macula and macular thickness was 419 microns. Foveal thickness was 855 microns (Fig. 21.7B). Intravitreal triamcinolone was given and 1 month later, her vision had improved considerably to 20/100. Optical coherence tomography revealed complete resolution of macular edema with the disappearance of cysts and restoration of foveal contour. Macular thickness was 192 microns (Fig. 21.7C).

Case 8: A 43-year-old female, a known patient of intermediate uveitis with persistent CME presented with counting finger vision in both eyes. She was a known diabetic. Her fundus examination revealed a dull foveal reflex. Her left eye showed cystoid macular edema. She was treated with intravitreal triamcinolone. On 2 month follow-up her vision improved to 20/80, in the left eye and 4 months later her left eye vision had improved to 20/60 (Figs 21.8A and B).Optical coherence tomography revealed increased macular thickness and few high reflective dot like structures just beneath the retinal nerve fiber layer (Fig. 21.8C).

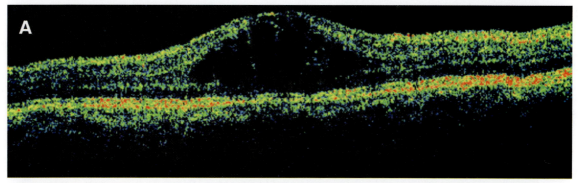

Fig. 21.5A: OCT of the left macula revealing cystoid macular edema with the central macular thickness being 506 microns

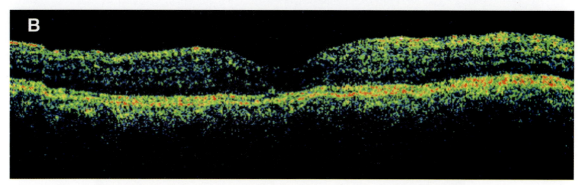

Fig. 21.5B: OCT revealing central macular thickness of 154 microns, few small cystic spaces and normal foveal contour

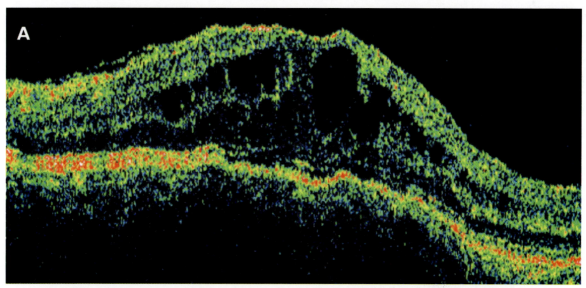

Fig. 21.6A: OCT revealing multiple cystoid spaces in the macular edema. Central macular thickness measured by retinal map analysis showed 442 microns thickness

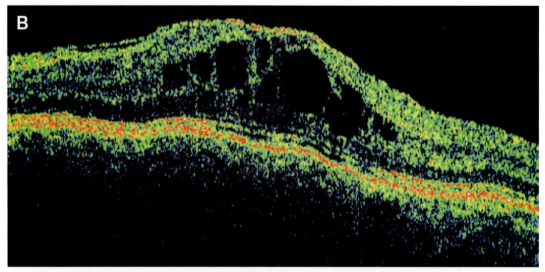

Fig. 21.6B: OCT scan passing through the fovea showing the persistence of multiple of cystoid spaces in the macula and retinal map analysis showing the average macular thickness of 390 microns

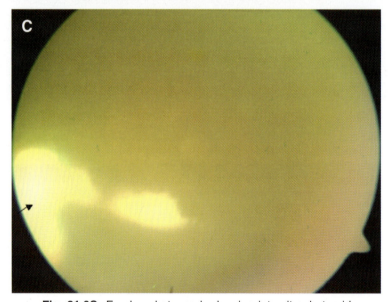

Fig. 21.6C: Fundus photograph showing intravitreal steroid

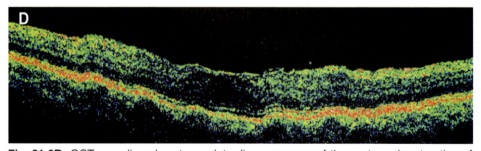

Fig. 21.6D: OCT revealing almost complete disappearance of the cysts and restoration of the foveal contour

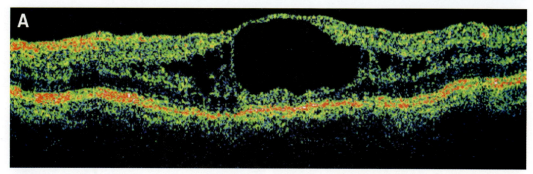

Fig. 21.7A: OCT showing large cystoid spaces in the macula. The retinal thickness being 340 microns

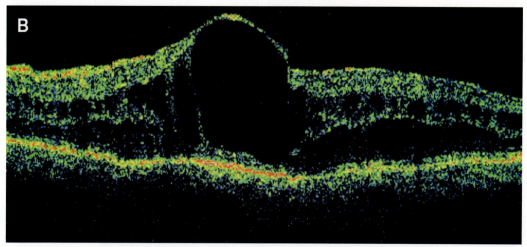

Fig. 21.7B: OCT revealing increase in the number and size of the cystoid spaces in the macula. Macular thickness is 419 microns and foveal thickness 855 microns

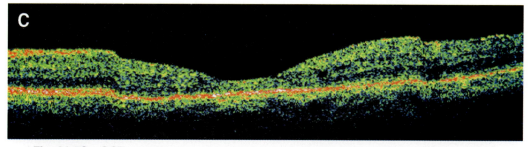

Fig. 21.7C: OCT revealing complete resolution of macular edema. The cysts have totally disappeared and foveal contour has been restored. Macular thickness is192 microns

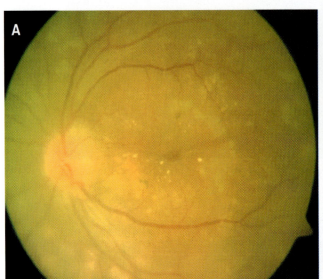

Fig. 21.8A: Fundus photograph showing cystoid macular edema

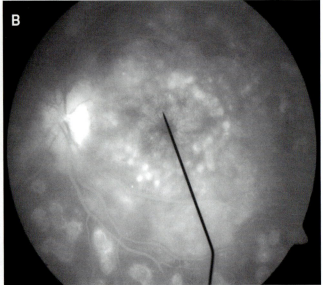

Fig. 21.8B: Fluorescein angiography of the left eye revealing cystoid macular edema with a typical flower petal pattern on late phase. A few scattered hard exudate are also seen at the posterior pole

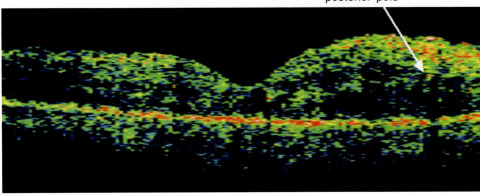

Fig. 21.8C: OCT revealing increased macular thickness and few high reflective dot like structures just beneath the retinal nerve fibre layer showing the exudates

Case 9: A 39-year old patient was diagnosed with intermediate uveitis. His vision in the left eye was 20/100. On examination he had CME in his left eye. Fundus examination of the left eye revealed cystoid macular edema and a typical flower petal pattern on late phase fluorescein angiography. There was no obvious pooling of dye suggestive of neurosensory detachment (Figs 21.9A and B). Optical coherence tomography not only confirmed the presence of cystoid macular edema but also detected a subtle neurosensory detachment in the left eye (Fig. 21.9C)

Case 10: A 55-year old male presented with history of blurred vision of 6 months duration. He was being treated with topical steroids. On examination, he had intermediate uveitis and fundus examination revealed a dull foveal reflex with suspicion of cystoid macular edema (Figs 21.10A and B). Optical coherence tomography revealed thin epiretinal membrane in the temporal quadrant juxtafoveally. Central macular thickness was 513 microns. He was found to have a high reflective structure. This is was probably a retinal pigment epithelial tear. This highly reflective structure was seen at a level in the retina. He was treated conventionally with topical and periocular steroids.

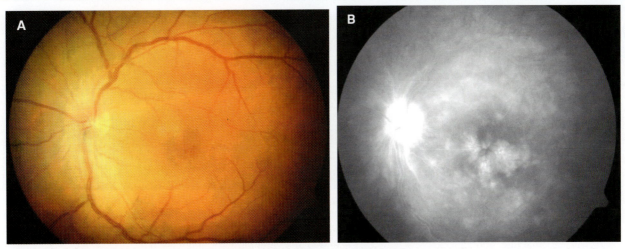

Fig. 21.9A and B: Fundus photograph and fluorescein angiography of the left eye revealing cystoid macular edema and a typical flower petal pattern on late phase angiogram. There is no obvious pooling of dye suggestive of neurosensory detachment

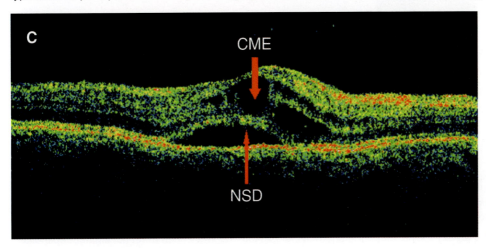

Fig. 21.9C: But OCT not only confirming the presence of cystoid macular edema, it also detecting a subtle neurosensory detachment in the left eye

Hypotonic Maculopathy

Ciliary body shut down is an important cause of severe hypotony in long standing uveitic patients. Other causes include choroidal detachment and retinal detachment.

Case 11: A 42-year-old patient, a known patient of recurrent anterior uveitis, underwent phacoemulsification and intraocular lens implantation in both the eyes. On his 6-week post operative visit, he complained of blurred vision and distorted images in his right eye. On examination, he had vitreous haze and his intraocular pressure was low. He was diagnosed to have hypotonic maculopathy and had a dull foveal reflex (Fig. 21.11A). His OCT examination revealed macular edema with choroidal folds suggestive of hypotonic maculopathy and macular edema (Fig. 21.11B). He was treated with intravitreal and systemic steroids. He had an improvement in vision of about 2 lines only, at 6 month follow-up.

Pigment Epithelial Detachment

Case 12: Optical coherence tomography was performed on a 40-year patient with suspicion of cystoid macular edema which revealed retinal pigment epithelial detachment (Fig. 21.12). Retinal pigment epithelial detachments and small neurosensory detachments at the fovea are sometime difficult to recognize clinically.

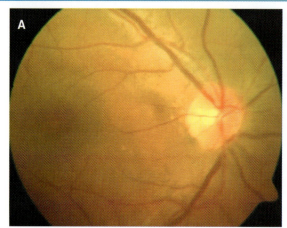

Fig. 21.10A: Fundus photograph revealing cystoid macular edema

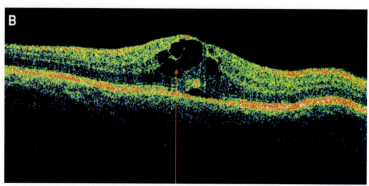

Fig. 21.10B: OCT scan through the fovea revealing a thin epiretinal membrane seen at temporal quadrant juxtafoveally. Central macular thickness is 513 microns. Note the high reflective structure, which is probably a retinal pigment epithelial tear

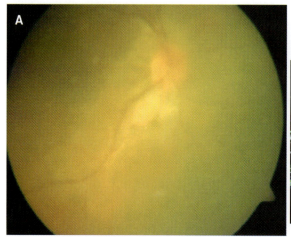

Fig. 21.11A: Fundus picture showing hazy media with choroidal folds, not seen clearly, and a dull foveal reflex

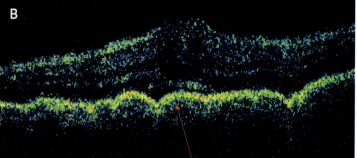

Fig. 21.11B: OCT scan revealing cystoid macular edema along with the choroidal folds. Note the wavy lines of retinal pigment epithelium suggestive of choroidal folds and hypotony

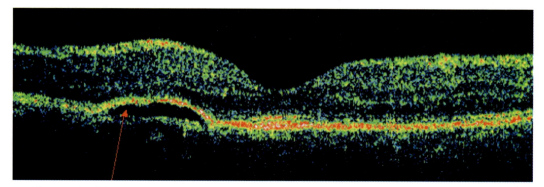

Fig. 21.12: OCT showing hyporeflective, empty space beneath the retinal pigment epithelium (arrow) suggestive of a retinal pigment epithelial detachment

Epiretinal Membrane and Vitreomacular Traction

Epiretinal membrane comprises of thin translucent membranes that are seen in the inner retinal surface in the macular area (Fig. 21.13). Diagnosis of an epiretinal membrane through a visually significant cataract can be difficult but knowledge of its existence has a tremendous impact on counseling for postoperative expectations. Optical coherence tomography allows an accurate diagnosis of vitreomacular traction and allows monitoring of progression. Spontaneous resolution with normalization of retinal contour or persistent traction with progressive edema is easily documented. It is very useful in determining the need for and timing of surgical intervention. The postoperative anatomic response can be correlated with visual recovery.

Case 13: A 59-year-old female patient with intermediate uveitis of 10 years duration presented with recent deterioration of vision in both the eyes. Her vision was 20/100 in the right eye and count fingers at 2 meters in the left eye. Her fundus picture is shown in Fig. 21.14A.

Optical coherence tomography of the left eye showed an epiretinal membrane and macular edema (Fig. 21.14B). After treatment for 3 months, her vision was 20/100 in both eyes. Optical coherence tomography of the right eye revealed CME and an epiretinal membrane but foveal thickness had reduced to 491 microns (Fig. 21.14C). Optical coherence tomography of the left eye showed cystic changes and an epiretinal membrane (Fig. 21.14D). She was treated conservatively and was followed up regularly. Six months later, OCT of the left eye was the same as her previous visit (Fig. 21.14E). It was decided to observe the patient for increase in traction or loss of vision.

Case 14: A 57-year old female, with pan uveitis and retinal vasculitis both eyes, was under follow-up. During one of her review visits, her left eye fundus examination showed a suspicious tractional retinal detachment at the macula and a thickened posterior hyaloid face. There was the presence of an epiretinal membrane with patches of choroiditis (Fig. 21.15A). Her OCT showed vitreomacular traction, epiretinal membrane and cystoid macular edema (Fig. 21.15B). Right eye underwent vitrectomy and belt buckle for vitreous hemorrhage whereas the left eye was treated conservatively.

Case 15: A 58-year old female with complaints of defective vision in the left eye of 3 months duration was examined. Her right eye showed early nuclear sclerosis whereas the left eye showed cystic changes in the macula. Optical coherence tomography of the left eye revealed epiretinal membrane and early macular hole (Fig. 21.16). Since her vision was 20/30 in that eye, it was decided to observe and she was treated medically.

Macular Hole

Macular hole is the end result of a chronic macular edema in various uveitic conditions especially intermediate uveitis, retinal vasculitis and traction due to any cause.

Case 16: A 31-year old female presented with complaints of pain and redness in her right eye. She was diagnosed to have scleritis in the right eye. Visual acuity in her right eye was 20/80. Fundus examination suggested a full thickness macular hole incidentally. Investigations for her scleritis revealed c-ANCA positive. Optical coherence tomography revealed a near full thickness macular hole. (Fig. 21.17A).Vitreoretinal intervention was deferred and the patient was treated for scleritis. Full thickness macular holes show a breach in all the layers of retina while lamellar hole shows only partial loss of tissue with steep foveal contour (Fig. 21.17B).

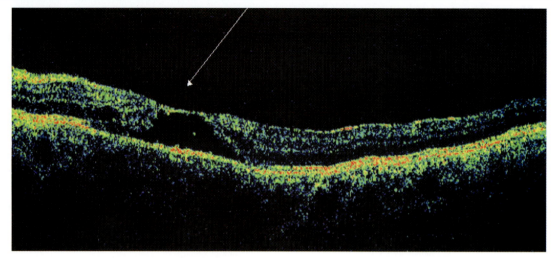

Fig. 21.13: Epiretinal membrane bridging an inner macular hole

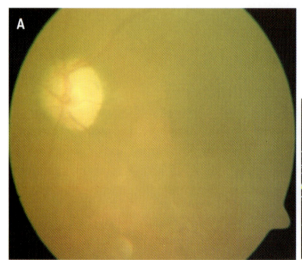

Fig. 21.14A: Fundus photograph of the right eye showing dull foveal reflex

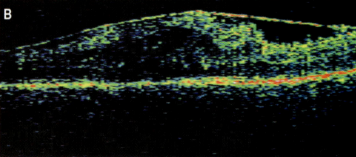

Fig. 21.14B: OCT of the right eye revealing epiretinal membrane and macular edema with the foveal thickness being 522 microns

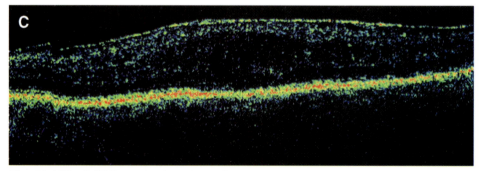

Fig. 21.14C: OCT line scan through the fovea showing the presence of a hyper reflective membrane extending from optic disc both nasally and temporally.

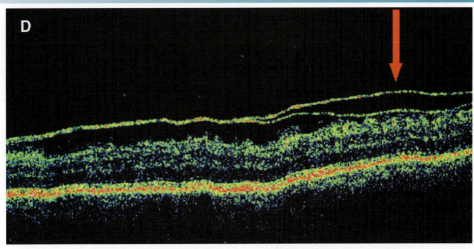

Fig. 21.14D: OCT scan of left eye revealing tenting of fovea with vitreomacular traction with CME

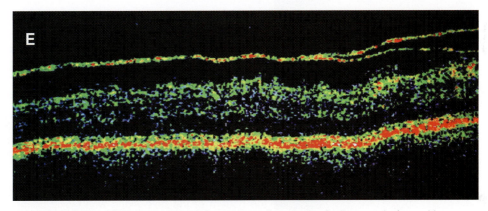

Fig. 21.14E: OCT scan of the left eye revealing similar findings as before with no increase in vitreomacular traction

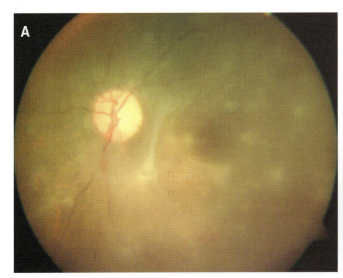

Fig. 21.15A: Fundus photograph showing showing an epiretinal membrane with patches of choroiditis

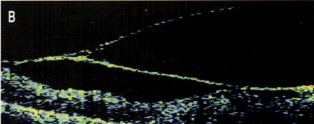

Fig. 21.15B: OCT showing vitreomacular traction, epiretinal membrane and cystoid macular edema

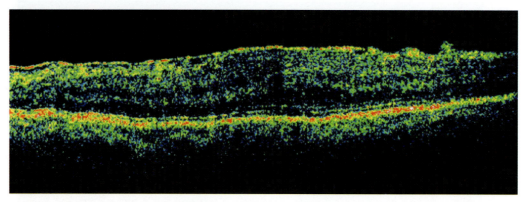

Fig. 21.16: OCT examination of the left eye revealing an epiretinal membrane with early macular hole

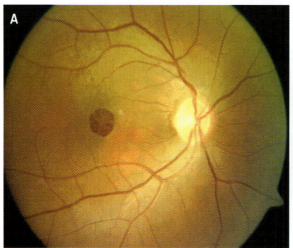

Fig. 21.17A: Fundus photograph showing a macular hole

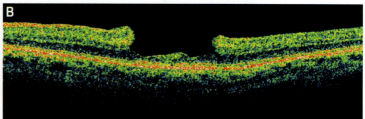

Fig. 21.17B: OCT scan through fovea showing retinal dehiscence. Surrounding retina showing thickening measuring 385 microns from the bottom of the hole along with cystic changes characterized by hyporeflective spaces in the neuro sensory retina. The diameter of the hole is 360 microns

Lamellar Macular Hole

Case 17: A 48-year old known patient of intermediate uveitis, presented with the complaints of blurred vision in his right eye of 2 months duration. On examination, his vision was 20/30 in his right eye. He had anterior vitreous cells. Fundus examination revealed retinal pigment epithelial changes at the macula suggestive of old resolved CME (Fig. 21.18A). Optical coherence tomography of the right eye showed outer lamellar macular hole (Figs 21.18B and C).

Serous Retinal Detachment

Optical coherence is most useful in assessing the presence of sub retinal fluid and monitoring their changes after treatment. Minimal subretinal space appears as a non reflective space between the retinal pigment epithelium and neurosensory retina while retinal edema is visualized as increase in retinal thickness and diffuse decrease in retinal reflectivity. Serous detachment of the retinal pigment epithelium is characterized by the elevation of the hyper reflective layer corresponding to the retinal pigment epithelium.

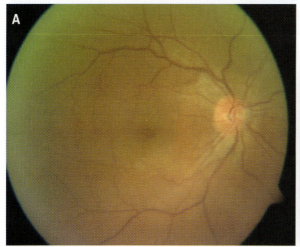

Fig. 21.18A: Fundus examination revealing retinal pigment epithelial changes at the macula suggestive of old resolved CME.

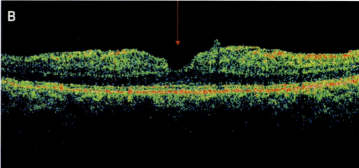

Fig. 21.18B: OCT examination of his right eye revealing a lamellar macular hole

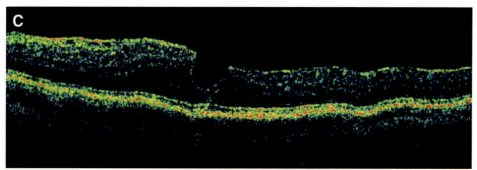

Fig. 21.18C: Inner lamellar hole

Sympathetic Ophthalmia

Sympathetic ophthalmia is a bilateral granulomatous panuveitis that occurs after either surgery or penetrating trauma to one eye. The traumatized eye is called the exciting eye and the non injured eye is called the sympathizing eye. It is not so common, but still feared because of its potentially blinding effects in both eyes. Optical coherence tomography is extremely sensitive in identifying neurosensory retinal elevation because of the distinct difference in optical reflectivity between photoreceptors and underlying retinal pigment epithelium/choriocapillaris.[18] In patients with retinal detachment, OCT can detect the presence of shallow subretinal fluid or CME that may be difficult to identify by other methods, confirming a macula-involving retinal detachment. In the acute phase, the fluorescein angiogram typically demonstrates multiple hyperfluorescent sites of leakage at the level of the retinal pigment epithelium which persist during the venous phase. In severe cases, these foci may coalesce with pooling of dye beneath areas of exudative retinal detachment. The sites of early blocked fluorescence generally correspond to the clinically observed Dalen Fuchs nodules.

Case 18: A 26 year old male with history of blunt trauma in right eye of 2 weeks duration presented with complaints of pain, redness and diminution vision in the left eye. Vision in the right eye was light perception and count finger 3 meters in the left eye. Primary wound repair was done in the right eye and appeared not salvageable. Left eye showed exudative retinal detachment and a hyperemic disc (Figs 21.19 A to F). He was treated with intravenous methylprednisolone. Post treatment, the vision in the left eye was 20/100 (Figs 21.20 A and B).The patient was administered immunosuppressive therapy. On examination his vision in the left eye was 20/30 and his only complaint was some amount of metamorphopsia. Fundus examination did not reveal any exudative retinal detachment and B-scan appeared normal (Fig. 21.20C). His 2nd and 3rd monthly visits were normal (Fig. 21.20D), his vision in the left eye being 20/20.

Vogt Koyanagi Harada's Syndrome

Vogt-Koyanagi-Harada (VKH) syndrome is a rare systemic disease involving various melanocyte-containing organs. Bilateral uveitis associated with cutaneous, neurologic, and auditory abnormalities characterizes this syndrome. As first described by Vogt in 1906 and Koyanagi in 1929, predominantly anterior uveitis associated with poliosis, vitiligo, and auditory disturbances characterizes Vogt-Koyanagi syndrome. In 1926, Harada reported a patient with idiopathic uveitis affecting the posterior segment with retinal detachment and meningeal irritation. At present, these 2 disorders are considered variations of a single entity referred to as Vogt-Koyanagi-Harada syndrome or uveoencephalitis. The findings associated with posterior uveitis, serous retinal detachment and CSF pleocytosis in the absence of extra ocular manifestations are often termed Harada's form of this syndrome. A single or multifocal serous retinal detachment within the posterior fundus is the major ocular complication in the acute phase. Optical coherence tomography can detect axial distribution of fluid better than fluorescein angiography.

Two patterns of serous retinal detachments can occur in VKH, namely, a true serous detachment and a cystic space with intraretinal fluid accumulation in the outer retina. Maruyama et al[19] have studied the tomography features of serous retinal detachment in VKH in 42 consecutive eyes of 21 patients. In their series they found a true serous retinal detachment in 69% patients and 40% had intra retinal fluid accumulation with no associated serous retinal detachment. Four eyes had both features in the same fundus. A true detachment has a lenticular optical empty space in the subretinal space. The outer surface being clearly demarcated forms a sharp angle with the retinal pigment epithelium. The subretinal space does not contain reflective dots or reflective tissue on the retinal pigment epithelium. Intraretinal fluid accumulation has cystoid spaces generally delineated by surrounding retinal tissue and has a thin reflective layer on the retinal pigment epithelium. The intraretinal cystoid space has highly reflective dots.

The classic course of VKH syndrome consists of the following 3 phases: meningoencephalitis phase, ophthalmic-auditory phase and convalescent phase. The convalescent phase is characterized by cutaneous signs developing after uveitis and begins to subside usually within 3 months from the onset of the disease. During this phase, depigmentation of the fundus gives rise to the classical sunset glow fundus. It is more common in Asian patients. Retinal pigment epithelium migration and Dalen Fuchs nodules are very obvious at this stage. Okamoto and associates[20] have studied the physiological characteristics of the macula in patients with VKH during the convalescent stage with specific reference to kinetics of foveal cone photopigment regeneration. They studied 6 eyes of three patients at the convalescent stage. The regeneration kinetics of foveal cone photopigment improved in three of six eyes whereas the other three remained delayed. Optical coherence tomography was normal in all the eyes suggesting that a disorder of foveal cone photopigment regeneration and its recovery requires a significantly longer time than that of other macular functions in some patients with VKH.

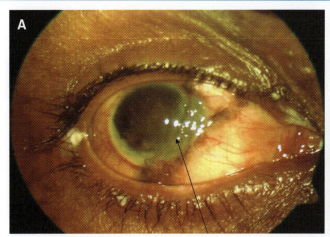

Fig. 21.19A: Clinical picture of the right eye, with history of penetrating trauma, showing corneal scleral tear which has undergone primary repair

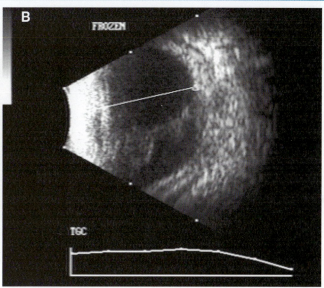

Fig. 21.19B: B-scan of the right eye showing grossly shrunken globe, with an axial length of 16 mm. Total retinal detachment with retinal incarceration is seen. Choroidal thickening of 3mm

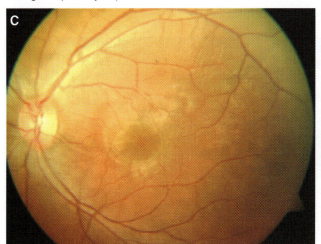

Fig. 21.19C: Fundus photograph of the left eye showing multiple pockets of fluid at the posterior pole

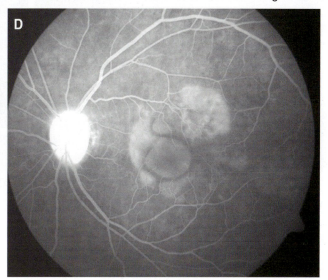

Fig. 21.19D: Fluorescein angiogram of the left eye showing pooling of the dye

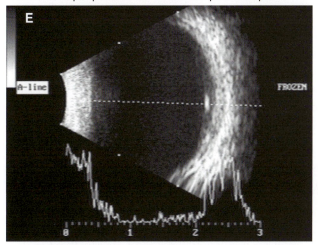

Fig. 21.19E: B-scan of the left eye showing a shallow retinal elevation and choroidal thickness was 1.5 mm

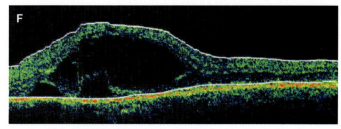

Fig. 21.19F: OCT scan of the left showing multiple neurosensory detachments at the macula

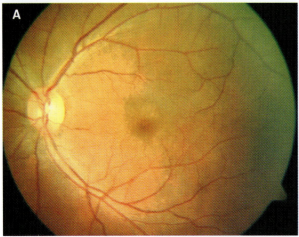

Fig. 21.20A: Fundus photograph of the left eye appearing normal

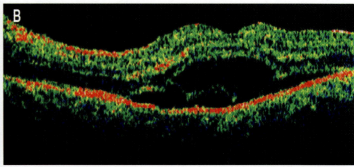

Fig. 21.20B: OCT scan of the left eye showing neurosensory detachment, though the height and the numbers have reduced compared to previous pictures

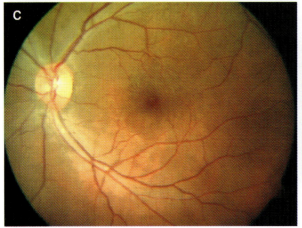

Fig. 21.20C: Fundus photograph of the left eye – normal

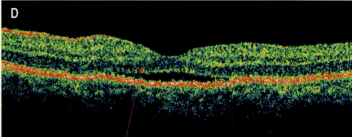

Fig. 21.20D: OCT line scan passing through the center of macula showing a small hypo reflective area just above the retinal pigment epithelium suggestive of a shallow neurosensory detachment at the fovea

Acute Vogt Koyanagi Harada Syndrome

Case 19: A 40-year old female, presented with diminished vision in both the eyes. Her vision was 20/100 OU. Fundus, fluorescein angiography and B-scan of the right eye are shown in Figs 21.21 A to F. Optical coherence tomography of the right eye showed multiple neurosensory detachments and fluid in the outer retinal space. There are areas with hyporeflective clumps of echoes suggestive retinal pigment epithelium clumps or localized retinal pigment epithelium detachment (Fig. 21.21G). Optical coherence tomography scan of the left macula showed area of pigment epithelial detachment and neurosensory detachment. There is hypertrophy of the retinal pigment epithelium (Fig. 21.21 H). After initial course of intravenous methylprednisolone, immunosuppressive therapy was started. Her vision had improved to 20/60 in both the eyes (Figs 21.22 A to D)

Case 20: A 41-year old male patient presented with the complaints of pain, redness and photophobia in both the eyes of 2 weeks duration. His vision was 20/200 OU. Fundus examination revealed disc hyperemia and bullous exudative retinal detachments in both the eyes (Figs 21.23 A to F and 21.24 A to D). He was

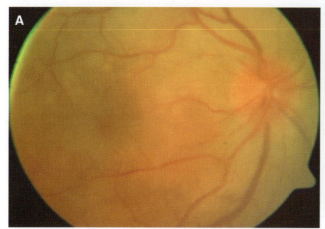

Fig. 21.21A: Fundus picture of the right eye showing disc hyperemia and multiple areas of serous elevation and pigment epithelial detachments

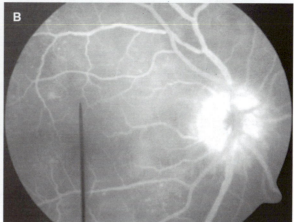

Fig. 21.21B: Fluorescein angiography showing staining of the disc

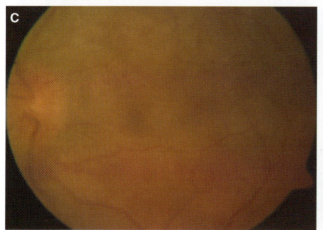

Fig. 21.21C: Fundus photograph of the left eye showing disc hyperemia and multiple pockets of fluid

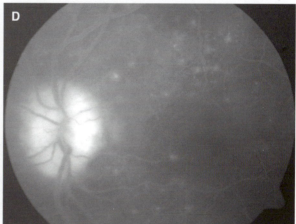

Fig. 21.21D: Fluorescein angiogram of the left eye showing disc staining and pin point leaks

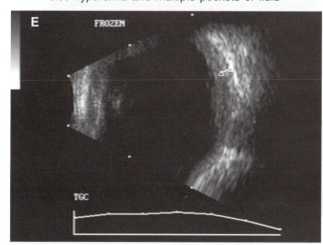

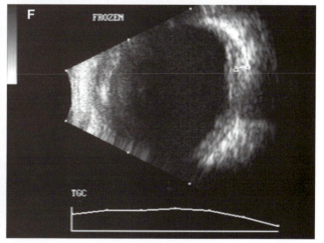

Figs 21.21E and F: B-scan of the right eye showing retinal detachment with shifting fluid suggestive of exudative retinal detachment. Choroidal thickness is 1.6 mm. B-scan of the left eye showing retinal detachment with shifting fluid suggestive of exudative retinal detachment. Choroidal thickness is 1.7 mm

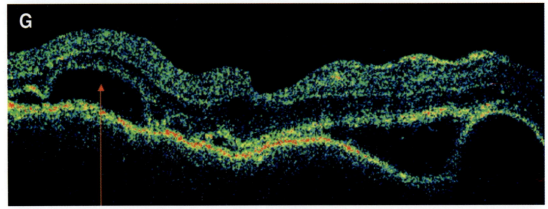

Fig. 21.21G: OCT picture of the right eye showing multiple neuro sensory detachments and fluid in the outer retinal space. There are areas with hyporeflective clumps of echoes suggestive retinal pigment epithelium clumps or localized retinal pigment epithelial detachment

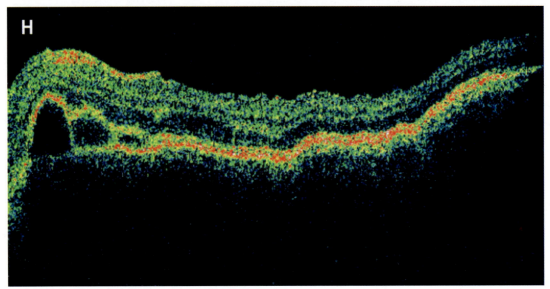

Fig. 21.21H: OCT scan of the left macula showing area of pigment epithelial detachment and neurosensory detachment.

diagnosed to have Harada's disease and was treated with intravenous methylprednisolone. After 3 days of intravenous methylprednisolone, his vision had improved to 20/100 and 20/80 in right and left eyes respectively (Figs 21.25 A to F).

Case 21: A 54-year old female presented with diminution of vision in both eyes. One examination, she was found to have granulomatous anterior uveitis. Her fundus examination appeared to be normal in both the eyes (Figs 21.26 A to C). B-scan of the right eye revealed a shallow retinal detachment at the posterior pole and OCT confirmed the same (Figs 21.26D to H). Pre and post treatment OCT pictures are shown in Figs 21.27 A to D.

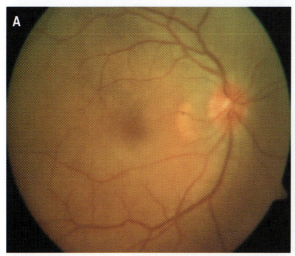

Fig. 21.22A: Fundus picture of the right eye showing settled retinal detachment with few areas of pigment epithelial detachment

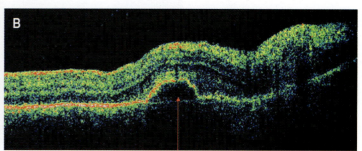

Fig. 21.22B: OCT scan revealing pigment epithelial detachment

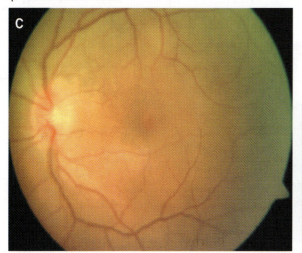

Fig. 21.22C: Fundus picture of the left eye showing normal posterior pole

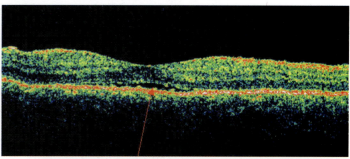

Fig. 21.22D: OCT scan of the left eye picking up a subtle neurosensory detachment at the fovea

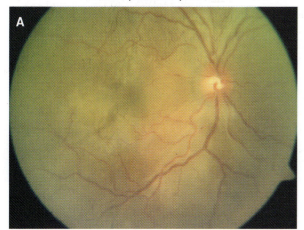

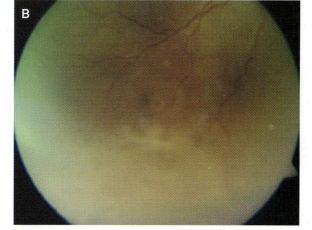

Figs 21.23A and B: Fundus photograph of the right eye. Fundus examination revealing disc hyperemia and bullous exudative retinal detachments in both the eyes.

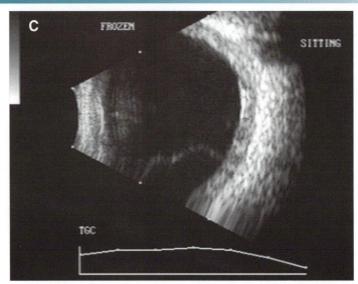

Fig. 21.23C: B-scan of the right eye revealing retinal detachment with shifting fluid suggestive of exudative detachment with increased choroidal thickness

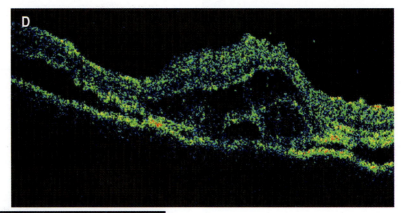

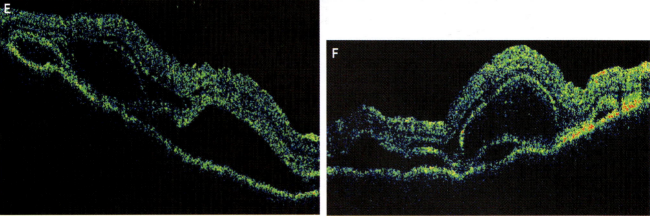

Figs 21.23D to F: OCT scans at different points in the fundus showing retinal detachment and multiple hyporeflective areas just above the retinal pigment epithelium suggestive of exudative retinal detachment (neurosensory detachment)

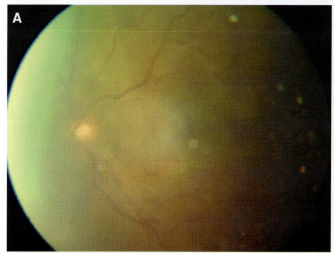

Fig. 21.24A: Fundus picture of the left eye showing exudative retinal detachment

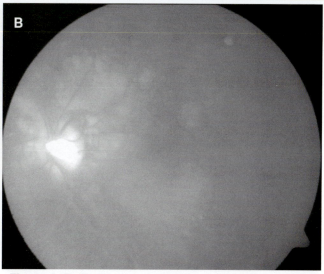

Fig. 21.24B: Fluorescein angiography of the left eye – late phase – showing pooling of the dye

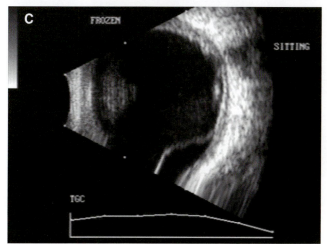

Fig. 21.24C: B- scan of the left eye showing retinal detachment

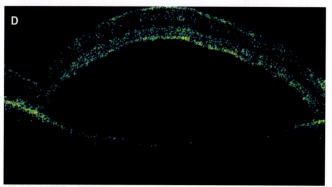

Fig. 21.24D: OCT scan showing large bullous neurosensory detachment

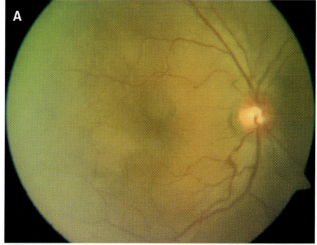

Fig. 21.25A: Post intravenous methylprednisolone fundus photograph appearing normal

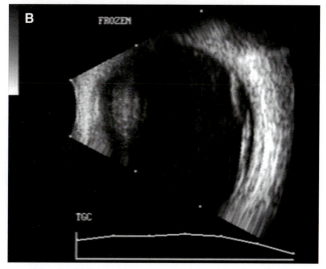

Fig. 21.25B: B-scan showing retinal detachment

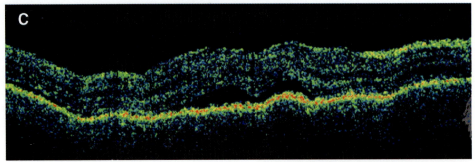

Fig. 21.25C: OCT showing choroidal folds and neurosensory detachment

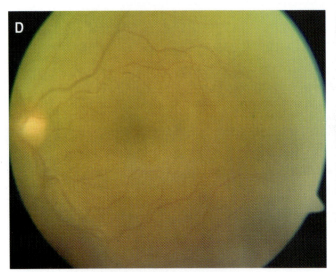

Fig. 21.25D: Fundus photograph of the left eye appearing normal

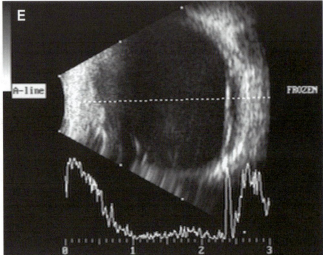

Fig. 21.25E: B-scan of the left eye showing retinal detachment

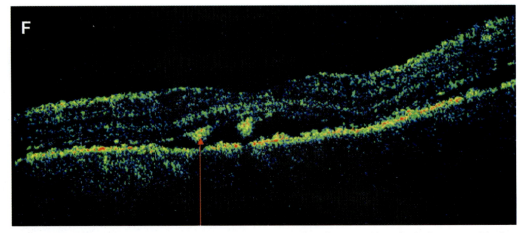

Fig. 21.25F: OCT of the left eye showing neuro sensory detachment with retinal pigment epithelium clumps suggestive of retinal pigment epithelial tear/rip. The gaps in the retinal pigment epithelium can be noted which are suggestive. Also note that high reflective exudates can also block echoes and can be seen as gaps beneath the high reflective structures

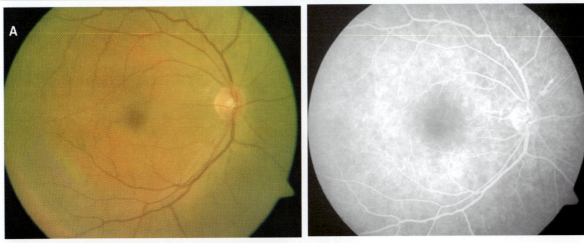

Fig. 21.26A and B: Fundus and fluorescein angiography of the right eye appearing normal

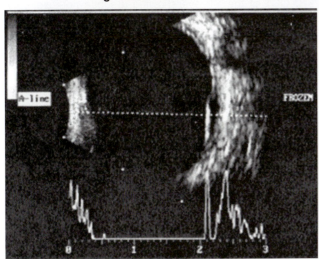

Fig. 21.26C: B-scan of the right eye picked up a subtle retinal detachment at the posterior pole

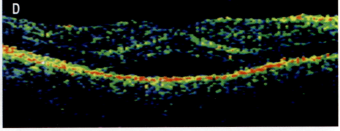

Fig. 21.26D: OCT macular scan of the right eye passing through the fovea picked up a neurosensory detachment thus confirming the ultrasound findings

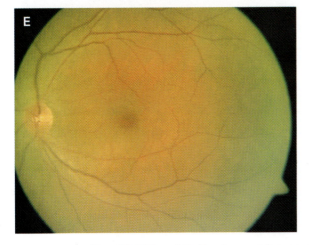

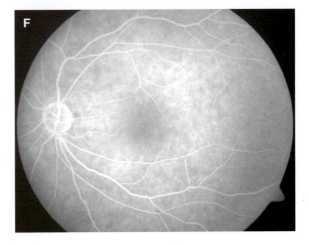

Figs 21.26E and F: Fundus and fluorescein angiography of the left eye appearing normal

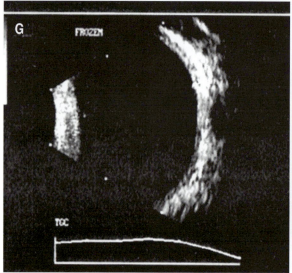

Fig. 21.26G: B-scan of the left eye is normal

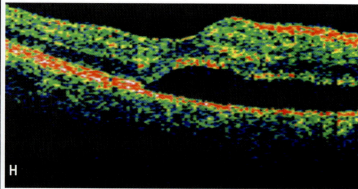

Fig. 21.26H: OCT of the left eye showing a subtle neurosensory detachment. Clinical photograph of the same patient showing the vitiligo patch which appeared later in the course of the disease

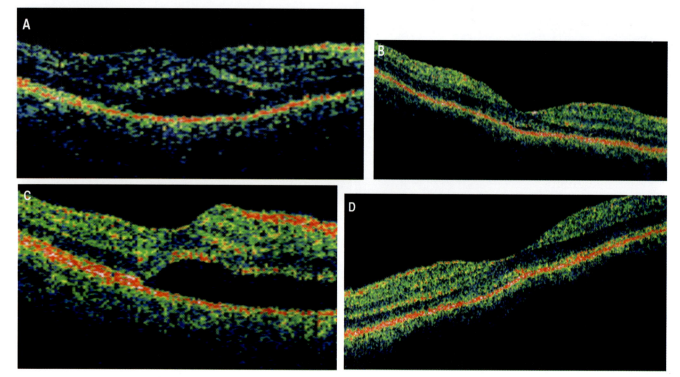

Fig. 21.27A to D: OCT pictures showing pre and post treatment scans

Convalescent Stage of Vogt Koyanagi Harada's Syndrome

Case 22: A 28-year old patient in convalescent stage of Vogt Koyanagi Harada's disease presented on her follow-up with 20/20 vision in both eyes. Fundus of the right eye showed typical sunset glow fundus with areas of depigmentation. Dalen Fuchs spots could be seen in the mid periphery along with pigment clumps at the posterior pole (Fig. 21.28A). Optical coherence tomography scans at different areas in the fundus showed areas of hyper reflectivity and acoustic shadowing beneath the hypertrophied retinal pigment epithelium (Figs 21.28B and C). Line scan passing through the center of macula through the pigment clumps showed hyper reflective dots at the retinal pigmentary epithelial layer with acoustic shadowing beneath them (Fig. 21.28D). Fundus of the left eye showed typical sunset glow fundus with pigmentary clumping at the posterior pole and Dalen Fuchs nodules (Fig. 21.28E). OCT scan showed hyper reflectivity and acoustic shadowing beneath the hypertrophied retinal pigment epithelium. Optical coherence tomography line scans passing through the Dalen Fuchs nodule showed a high reflective clump like structure beneath the retinal pigment epithelium (Figs 21.28 F to I)

Posterior Scleritis

Posterior scleritis presents with protean manifestations. It can rarely be confused with central serous retinopathy, VKH, and tumor. Ultrasound and fluorescein angiography play an important role in the diagnosis of posterior scleritis.

Case 23: A 40-year old female patient presented with gradual decrease in vision of 1 month duration in her right eye. On examination she was found to have fundus lesions suggestive of posterior scleritis. Her vision in the right eye was 20/100. Fundus examination revealed pockets of fluid and choroidal folds (Fig. 21.29A). Fluorescein angiography showed multi hyperfluorescent spots and pooling of dye (Figs 21.29 B and C). Optical coherence tomography showed a subtle neurosensory detachment along with cystoid macular edema (Fig. 21.29D). After 6 weeks of treatment, her vision had improved to 20/30 in her right eye. Optical coherence tomography scan showed reduction in neurosensory detachment as well as macular edema (Fig. 21.29E)

Focal Choroiditis

Focal choroiditis can result from many causes. Toxoplasmosis is one of the common causes, especially in younger age groups.

Case 24: A 45-year old female presented with complaints of diminished vision in left eye for 1 month. Her vision was 20/20 in the right eye and 20/40 in the left eye. Fundus examination revealed focal choroiditis (Fig. 21.30A). Laboratory investigations revealed low IgG positivity for toxoplasma. OCT line scan passing through the lesion showed lesions beneath the retinal pigment epithelium with few areas of moderate back scatter (Fig. 21.30B). OCT line scan passing through center of the fovea appeared normal (Fig. 21.30C).

Healed Toxoplasmosis

Case 25: A 13-year old girl complained of defective vision in her left eye since 1 month. On questioning she was found to have contact with pets. Her vision in the right eye was 20/20 and in the left eye was 20/400. Her fundus examination showed old choroiditis scar with epiretinal membrane (Fig. 21.31A). Fluorescein angiography also showed staining of these lesions (Fig. 21.31B). Macular hole was suspected and OCT was done. Focal choroiditis can be due many causes. It is commonly due to infection and toxoplasma is one of the common causes of unifocal choroiditis especially in younger age groups showed scarring with hyper reflective echoes, retinal thinning and epiretinal membrane and cystoid macular edema temporal to the fovea (Fig. 21.31C). ELISA test revealed high titers for toxoplasmosis. The patient was treated with anti toxoplasma medication.

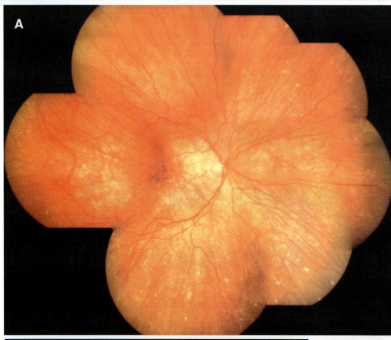

Fig. 21.28A: Fundus picture showing the typical sunset glow fundus with lots of areas of depigmentation. Dalen Fuchs spots can be seen in the mid periphery. Also pigmentary clumping is seen at the posterior pole

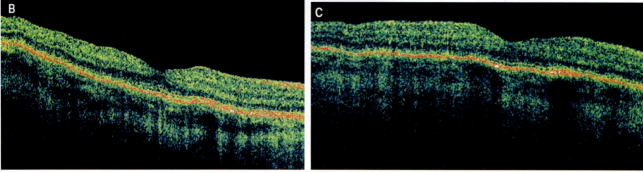

Figs 21.28B and C: OCT scans at different areas in the fundus showing areas of hyper reflectivity and acoustic shadowing beneath the hypertrophied retinal pigment epithelium

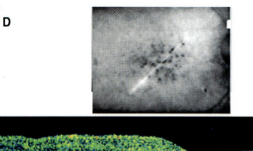

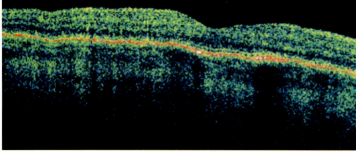

Fig. 21.28D: OCT line scan passing through the center of macula through the pigmentary clumping at the posterior pole showing hyper reflective dots at the retinal pigmentary epithelial layer with acoustic shadowing beneath them

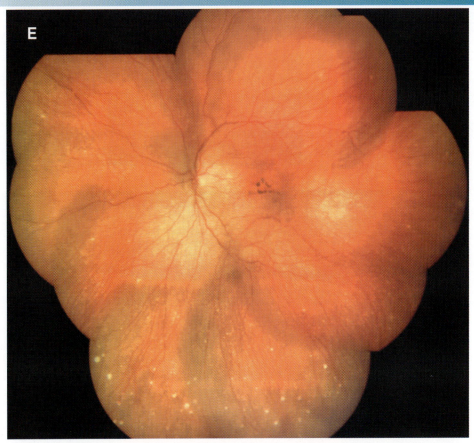

Fig. 21.28E: Fundus picture of the left eye showing typical sun set glow fundus with pigmentary clumping at the posterior pole and Dalen Fuchs nodules

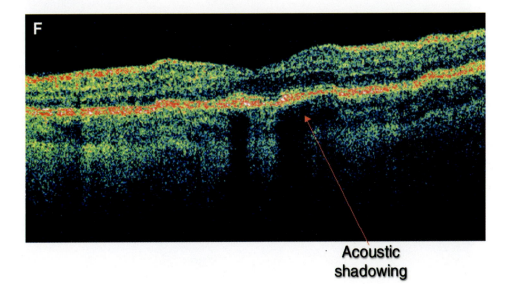

Acoustic
shadowing

Fig. 21.28F: OCT scan showing hyper reflectivity and acoustic shadowing beneath the hypertrophied retinal pigment epithelium

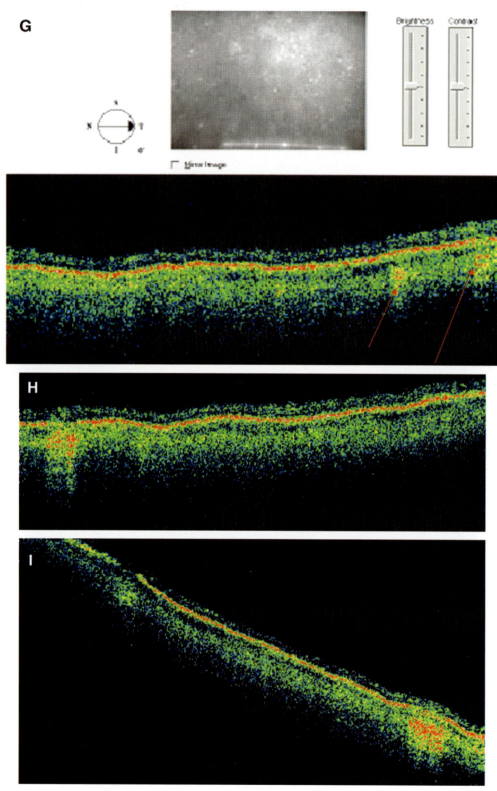

Figs 21.28G to I: OCT line scans passing through the Dalen Fuchs nodule showing a high reflective clump like structure beneath the retinal pigment epithelium

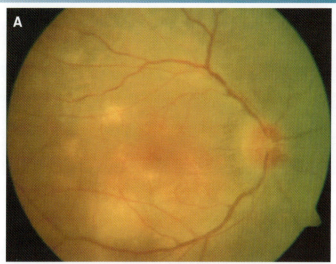

Fig. 21.29A: Fundus lesions suggestive of pockets of fluid and choroidal folds

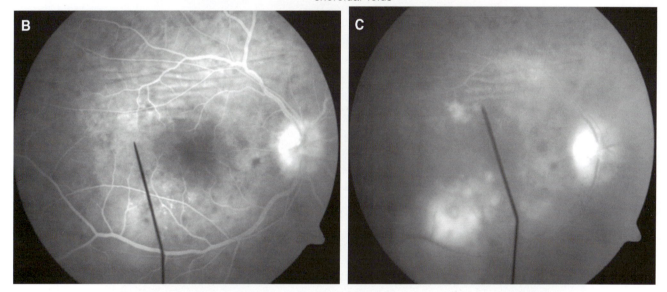

Figs 21.29B and C: Fluorescein angiography showing multi hyperfluorescent spots and a vague pooling of dye

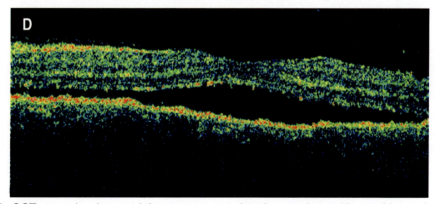

Fig. 21.29D: OCT scan showing a subtle neurosensory detachment along with cystoid macular edema

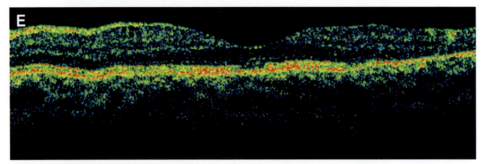

Fig. 21.29E: OCT scan post treatment showing reduction neuro sensory detachment as well as macular edema

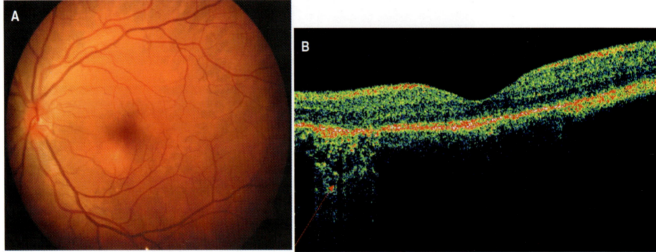

Fig. 21.30A: Fundus photograph showing a focal choroiditis lesion

Fig. 21.30B: OCT line scan passing through the lesion showed lesions beneath the retinal pigment epithelium with few areas of moderate back scatter

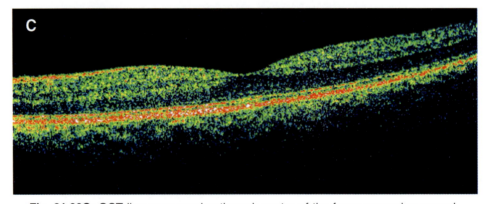

Fig. 21.30C: OCT line scan passing through center of the fovea appearing normal

Tuberculous Choroiditis

Case 26: A patient with systemic history of tuberculosis was diagnosed to have tuberculous choroiditis in the right eye. Fundus showed healed tuberculous choroiditis lesions (Fig. 21.32A). Optical coherence tomography line scans passing through different lesions showed scars and neurosensory detachment (Figs 21.32B to E).

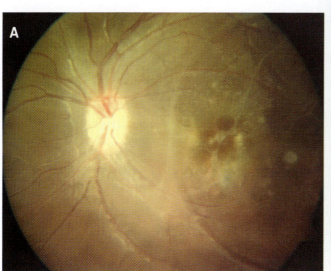

Fig. 21.31A: Fundus photograph showing healed chorioretinal scars with full thickness defects

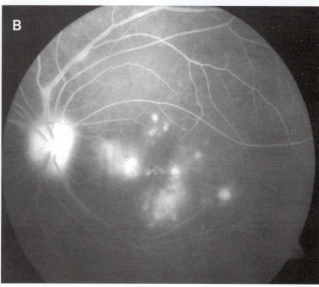

Fig. 21.31B: Fluorescein angiography showing staining of the healed scars

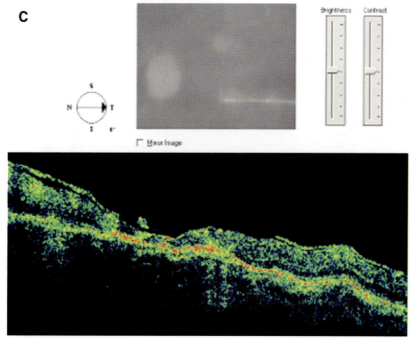

Fig. 21.31C: OCT scan through the inferior margin of the scar showing hyper reflectivity from the underlying retinal pigment epithelium and choroid with loss of neuro sensory retina

Multifocal Choroiditis

Recurrent multifocal choroiditis is usually seen in the 2nd to 4th decade of life and is characterized by the presence of multiple, discrete lesions at the level of choriocapillaris and retinal pigment epithelium. Visual loss is commonly due to macular scarring, choroidal neovascularization or sub retinal fibrosis.

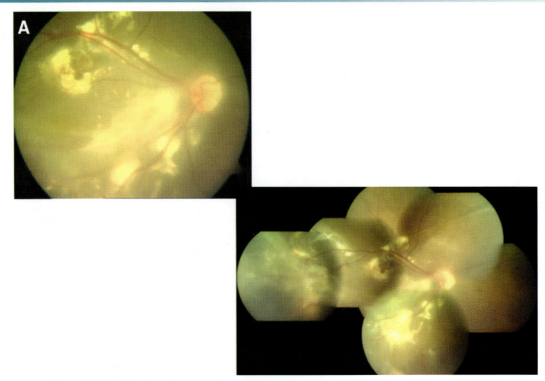

Fig. 21.32A: Fundus photograph showing healed tuberculous choroiditis

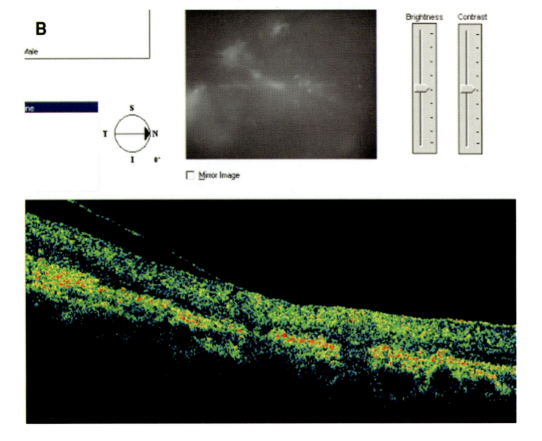

Fig. 21.32B

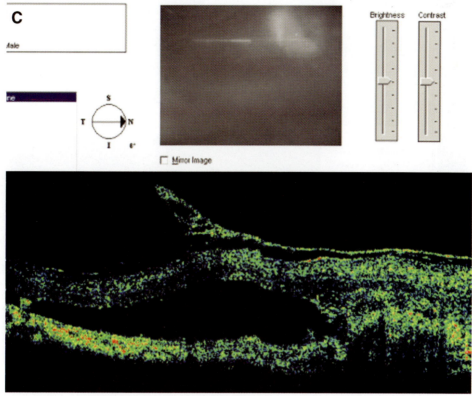

Figs 21.32B and C: OCT line scans passing through different lesions showing scars and neurosensory detachment

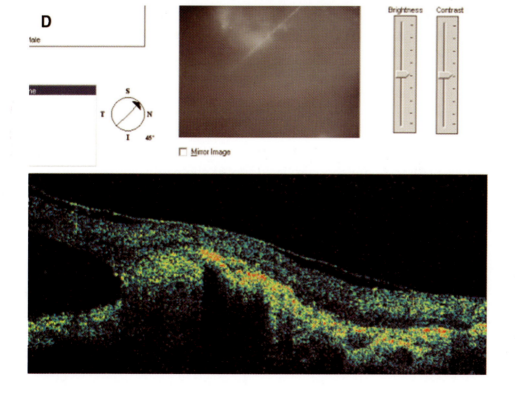

Fig. 21.32D

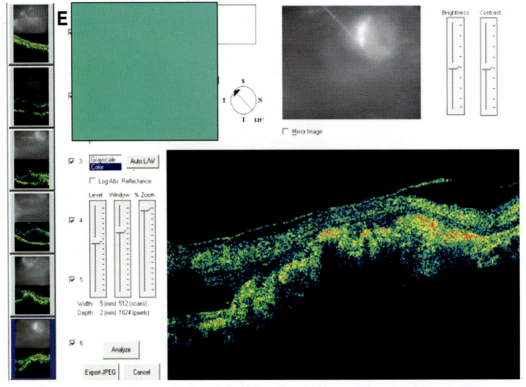

Fig. 21.32D and E: OCT line scans passing through the inferior margin of the disc

Case 27: A 23-year-old female was referred to us with complaints of sudden onset of pain associated with loss of vision in her left eye of 12 days duration. She had no systemic complaints. Her vision was 20/20 in the right eye and counting fingers close to face in the left eye. Her fundus examination revealed multifocal choroiditis and a large choroidal granuloma at the posterior pole (Fig. 21.33A). B-scan of the left eye revealed a mass like lesion abutting optic nerve head temporally measuring antero-posterior 10 mm, transverse 12.3 mm, and height 4.3 mm, with overlying shallow retinal detachment. Choroid was thickened irregularly with evidence of echolucent zone in the suprachoroidal space (Fig. 21.33B). Laboratory investigations to rule out granulomatous conditions were normal. She was treated with intravenous methylprednisolone for 3 days and then with systemic azathioprine and prednisolone for 3 months. After 3 months, her vision had improved to 20/60 in the left eye. Fundus examination showed healed choroiditis with subretinal scarring and gliosis (Fig. 21.34A). B-scan also showed resolution of lesion. Optical coherence tomography scan passing through the scar showed retinal pigment epithelial hypertrophy with intra retinal cyst and fibrovascular complex and disrupted retinal pigment epithelium at few points (Figs 21.34C and D).

Healed Multifocal Choroiditis

Case 28: A middle aged male presented with complaints of hazy vision in both the eyes for 1 week. His vision was 20/30 and 20/60 in right and left eyes respectively. Fundus examination revealed healed multifocal choroiditis in both the eyes (Fig. 21.35A). Fluorescein angiography showed resolved lesions and window defects (Fig. 21.35B). Optical coherence tomography line scan passing through the lesions and the scar

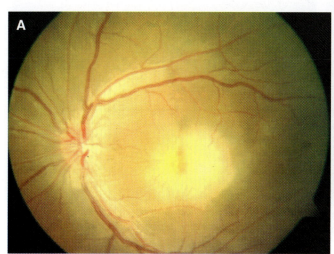

Fig. 21.33A: Fundus examination revealing multifocal choroiditis and a large choroidal granuloma at the posterior pole.

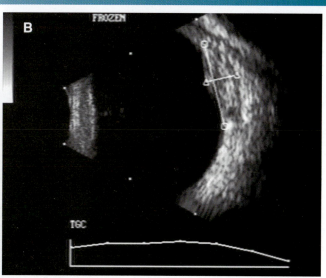

Fig. 21.33B: B-scan of the left eye revealing a mass like lesion abutting optic nerve head temporally measuring Anteroposterior 10 mm, transverse 12.3 mm, and height 4.3 mm with overlying shallow retinal detachment. Choroid was thickened irregularly with evidence of echolucent zone in the suprachoroidal space

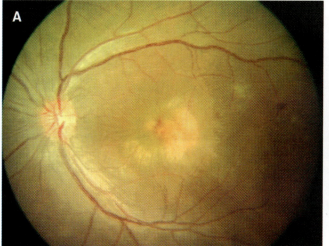

Fig. 21.34A: Fundus photograph showing healed choroiditis with sub retinal scarring and gliosis

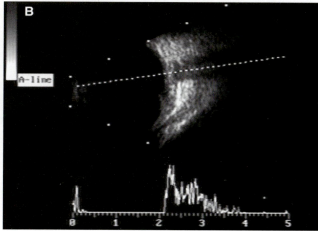

Fig. 21.34B: B-scan showing resolution of lesion

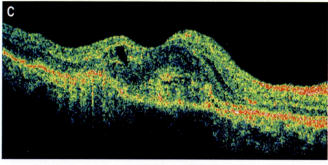

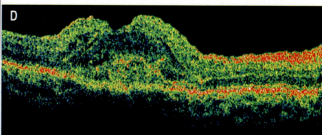

Figs 21.34C and D: OCT scan passing through the scar showing retinal pigment epithelium hypertrophy with intra retinal cyst and fibrovascular complex and disrupted retinal pigment epithelium at few points

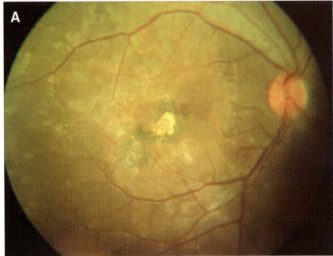

Fig. 21.35A: Fundus picture of the right eye showing healed choroiditis lesions with sub retinal gliosis and scarring at the posterior pole

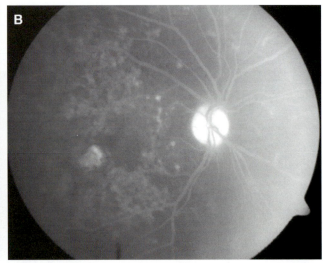

Fig. 21.35B: Fluorescein angiography showing resolved lesions and staining due to window defects

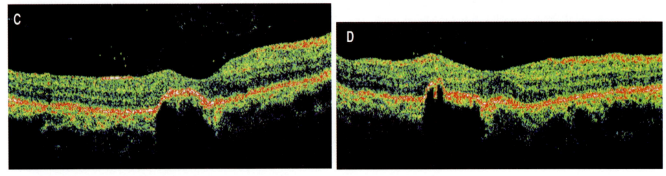

Figs 21.35C and D: OCT line scan passing through the lesions and the scar showing hypertrophied and irregular retinal pigment epithelium layer and overall thinning of the retina. Also seen are scars beneath the retinal pigment epithelium

showed hypertrophied and irregular retinal pigment epithelium layer and overall thinning of the retina (Figs 21.35C and D).

Choroidal Neovascular Membrane in Multifocal Choroiditis

Case 29: A 25-year old male patient was being treated for multifocal choroiditis in both the eyes for 3 years. He presented with history of slight diminution of vision in the right eye for 10 days. His vision was 20/100 in the right eye and 20/20 in the left eye. Fundus picture of the right eye showed choroidal neovascular membrane (Fig. 21.36A). Fluorescein angiography revealed a classic choroidal neovascular membrane in the right eye (Figs 21.36B and C). Optical coherence tomography revealed choroidal neovascular membrane in the right eye along with neuro sensory separation (Figs 21.36 D to G).

Macular Choroiditis with Choroidal Neovascular Membrane

Case 30: A 42-year old female patient was referred with history of having been treated for choroiditis with systemic steroids in the past. Fundus examination showed choroidal neovascularization (Fig. 21.37A). Fluorescein angiogram showed leakage (Figs 21.37 B and C).

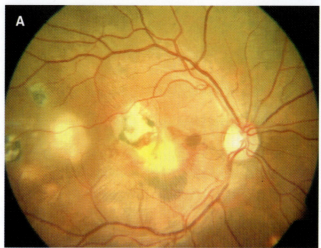

Fig. 21.36A: Fundus photograph of the right eye showing choroidal neovascular membrane

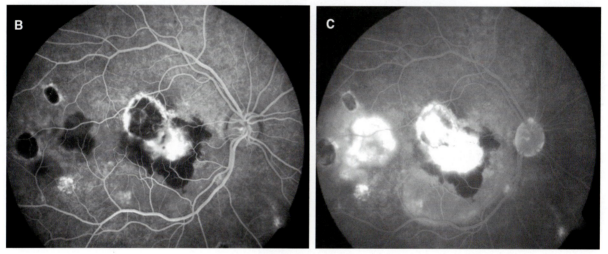

Figs 21.36B and C: Fluorescein angiography revealing a classic choroidal neovascular membrane in the right eye (early and late phase)

Optical coherence tomography scan passing through the different specified points in the scar and the hemorrhage are seen. It shows disrupted retinal pigment epithelium with fibrovascular complex and scar and pigment epithelium detachment (Figs 21.37D and E). She was treated with photodynamic therapy. Optical coherence tomography revealed normal foveal contour with no edema or any neuro sensory separation. Patient was treated with systemic steroids and after 1 month, patient's vision had improved to 20/20.

Retinal Vasculitis

It is a sight threatening inflammatory eye disease involving the retinal blood vessels. Most frequently retinal veins are involved and the term retinal periphlebitis is used to describe this condition. It can occur as primary idiopathic retinal vasculitis or as a manifestation of systemic disease including sarcoidosis, collagen

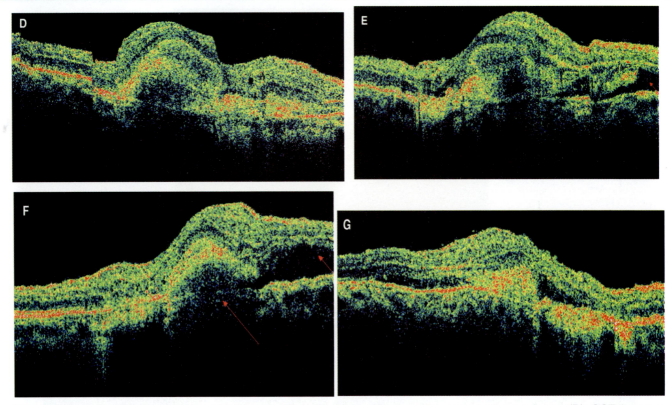

Figs 21.36D to G: OCT line scans passing through different points on the choroidal neovascular membrane (D). OCT line scan showing areas of disrupted retinal pigment epithelium with increases hyper reflectivity from the outer retinal layers with adjacent hypo reflective areas suggesting of the presence of intra retinal fluid (E). These findings were consistent with classic choroidal neovascular membrane (F). There are areas of pigment epithelial detachment with underlying choroidal scars and areas of neuro sensory detachment (G).

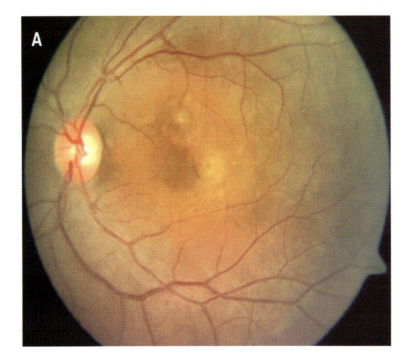

Fig. 21.37A: Fundus photograph showing choroidal neovascular membrane

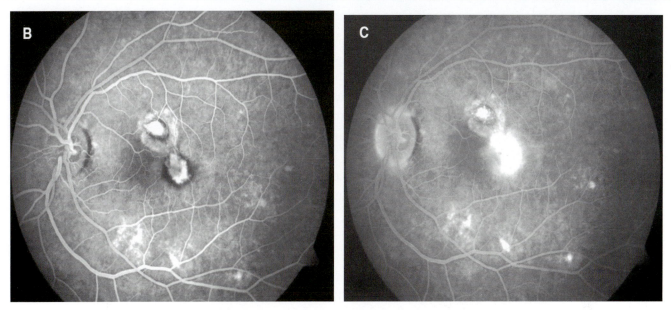

Figs 21.37B and C: Fluorescein angiography showing leakage

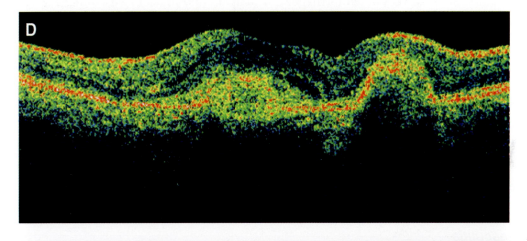

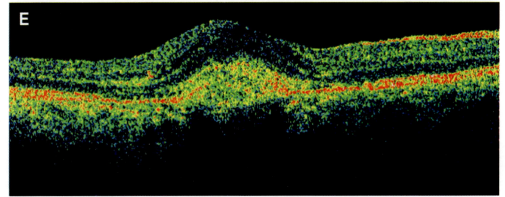

Figs 21.37D and E: OCT scan passing through the different specified points in the scar and the hemorrhage are seen. It shows disrupted retinal pigment epithelium with fibrovascular complex and scar. Note the pigment epithelium detachment.

vascular diseases, malignancy, neurologic conditions and systemic infections. It occurs in other ocular inflammatory diseases like pars planitis etc. Fundus flourescein angiography is the gold standard in the investigation of vasculitis. It is important to note the active vasculitic patches, useful in the follow-up and in the detection of neovascularization which indicates the need for laser therapy. Diffuse capillary leakage is a common finding in patients with idiopathic retinal vasculitis. Macular ischemia is most readily identified on fluorescein angiography and it is important to recognize particularly in patients whose visual acuity fails to improve despite aggressive medial therapy and inflammatory control. Late staining of vessels occurs in 2/3rd of patients and it affects arteries veins or both. Vision loss in vasculitic lesions can be either due to macular edema or macular ischemia. Optical coherence tomography is helpful in diagnosis and quantification of macular edema in vasculitis. It helps in identifying cystoid macular edema and is a great non invasive tool in monitoring response to an intervention.

Central Eales' Disease

Case 31: A 35-year old male came to us with diminished vision in his right eye. On examination he had central sub hyaloid hemorrhages and retinal vasculitis and was diagnosed as Central Eales' disease in the right eye. His fundus appeared to have macular edema, but due to the hemorrhage, it could not be confirmed. Fundus examination showed retinal hemorrhage, macular fan and areas of vasculitis (Fig. 21.38A). Optical coherence tomography line scan of the right macula shows hyper reflective areas suggestive of hard exudates (Fig. 21.38B).

Tubercular Retinal Vasculitis

Case 32: A 17-year old female with history of tuberculous colitis came to us with diminished vision in both eyes. She was found to have vasculitis and was treated accordingly with anti tubercular therapy and systemic steroids. After her treatment, she had macular scar in both the eyes. Her vision remained stable at 20/100 in both the eyes. Fundus examination showed healed scar (Fig. 21.39A). Optical coherence tomography line scan passing through the scar showed thinned retina. The retinal thickness was only 81 microns (Fig. 21.39B)

Idiopathic Vasculitis

Case 33: A 46-year old male presented to us with diminished vision in left eye of 2 months duration. On examination his vision was 20/20, in the right eye and left eye was 20/100. Fundus examination revealed pars planitis in both eyes and vasculitis in the left eye. His vasculitis workup did not yield anything and he was treated with posterior subtenons injection and was started on systemic steroids. On his 3 month follow up, his vision was 20/20 in the right eye and in the left eye it had improved to 20/40. Fundus examination revealed a dull foveal reflex. Fundus examination revealed a dull foveal reflex and the presence of a macular star (Fig. 21.40A). Fluorescein angiography showed macular star and doubtful macular edema (Fig. 21.40B). Optical coherence tomography lines scan passing through the scar in the center revealed cystoid spaces suggestive of cystoid macular edema and few high reflective echoes suggestive of hard exudates. Also a thin hyper reflective structure was seen suggestive of epiretinal membrane and increased retinal thickness (Fig. 21.40C). Patient was maintained on systemic steroids and reviewed 1 month later when his vision had returned to normal.

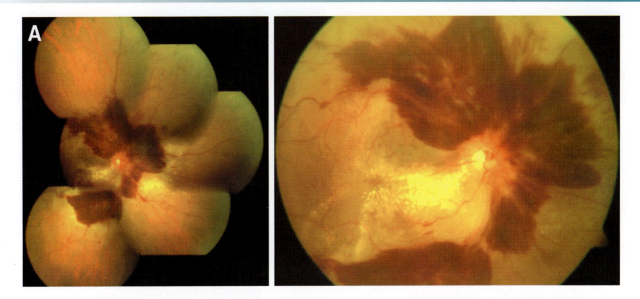

Fig. 21.38A: Fundus photograph showing hemorrhages, macular fan and areas of vasculitis

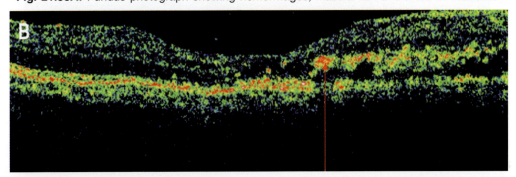

Fig. 21.38B: OCT line scan of the right macula shows hyper reflective areas suggestive of hard exudates. Retinal thickness is 298 microns. Foveal thickness is 191 microns

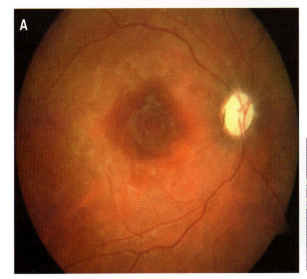

Fig. 21.39A: Fundus photograph showing a healed scar

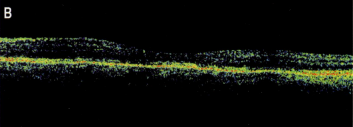

Fig. 21.39B: OCT line scan passing through the scar showing thinned retina. The retinal thickness here was only 81 microns

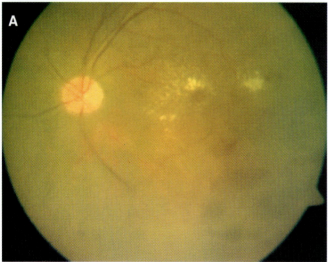

Fig. 21.40A: Fundus examination revealing a dull foveal reflex and the presence of a macular star

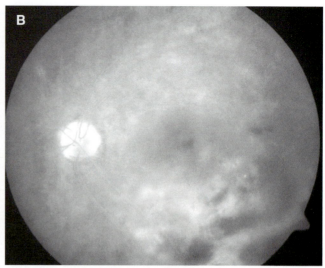

Fig. 21.40B: Fluorescein angiography showing macular star and doubtful macular edema

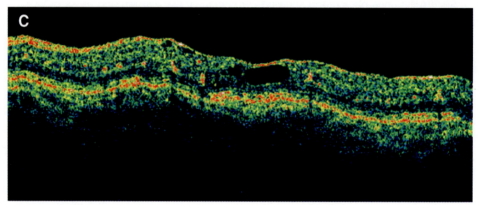

Fig. 21.40C: OCT lines scan passing through the scar in the center revealing cystoid spaces suggestive of cystoid macular edema and few high reflective echoes suggestive of hard exudates. Also a thin hyper reflective structure is suggestive of epiretinal membrane and increased retinal thickness

Healed Viral Retinitis

Case 34: A 26-year old patient with history of viral retinitis treated was examined during one of his follow up visits. Fundus picture showed central macular scar (Fig. 21.41A). Fluorescein angiography showed staining of the lesions (Figs 21.41 B and C).OCT picture line scan passing through the scar in the center of macula showing thinned retina and hypertrophied retinal pigment epithelium (Fig. 21.41D).

Intraocular Lens Induced Uveitis

Intraocular lens induced uveitis can be a reaction against haptics, manufacturing impurities, certain methods of sterilization, and degradation of lens haptics.

Causes:

- release of prostaglandins and cytokines

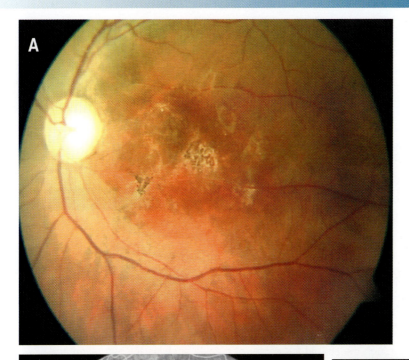

Fig. 21.41A: Fundus photograph showing central macular scar

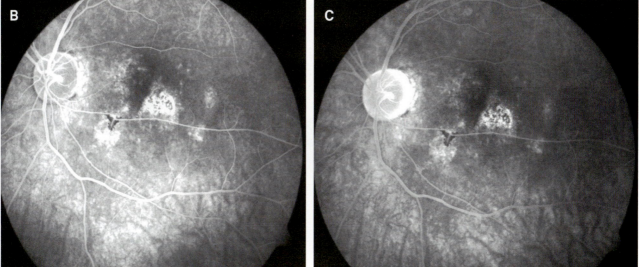

Figs 21.41B and C: Fluorescein angiography showing staining of the lesions

- recruitment of lymphocytes and other inflammatory cells
- secondary immune mediated inflammation more toxic than the initial toxic reaction

Case 35: A 61-year old patient came with history of gradual decrease in vision in his right (pseudophakic) eye which was operated 3 yrs ago. His vision was 20/400 in his right eye. On examination he was found to have anterior chamber reaction and partly decentered intraocular lens with a dull foveal reflex. Clinical photograph of intraocular lens induced uveitis is shown in Fig. 21.42A. Optical coherence tomography revealed large cystoid spaces in the macula with macular thickness being 271 microns and foveal thickness being 456 microns (Fig. 21.42B). He was started on topical steroids and sub tenon's triamcinolone injection.

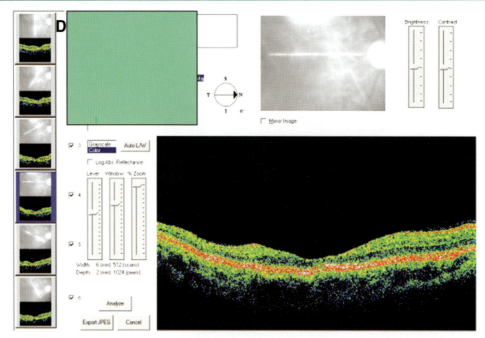

Fig. 21.41D: OCT picture line scan passing through the scar in the center of macula showing thinned retina and hypertrophied retinal pigment epithelium

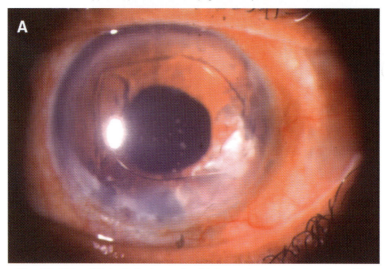

Fig. 21.42A: Clinical photograph of intraocular lens induced uveitis

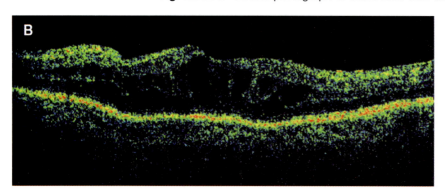

Fig. 21.42B: OCT showing cystoid macular edema

On his 1 month review his vision had improved to 20/60 in the right eye with reduction in cystoid macular edema. His repeat OCT revealed very few cystoid spaces with decrease in foveal thickness.

REFERENCES

1. Guex-Crosier Y. The pathogenesis and clinical presentation of macular edema in inflammatory diseases. Doc Ophthalmol 1999;97:297-309.
2. Reinthal EK, Volker M, Freudenthaler N, et al. Optical coherence tomography in the diagnosis and follow up of patients with uveitic macular edema – Ophthalmologe – 2004 May 20.
3. Antcliff RJ, Stanford MR, Chauhan DS, et al. Comparison between optical coherence tomography and fundus fluorescein angiography for the detection of cystoid macular edema in patients with uveitis. Ophthalmology. 2000; 107:593-599.
4. Markomichelakis NN, Halkiadakis I, Pantelia E, et al. Patterns of macular edema in patients with uveitis: qualitative and quantitative assessment using optical coherence tomography.: Ophthalmology. 2004;111:946-953.
5. Chen SD, Mohammed Q, Bowling B, Patel CK. Vitreous wick syndrome—a potential cause of endophthalmitis after intravitreal injection of triamcinolone through the pars plana. Am J Ophthalmol. 2004;137:1159-1160.
6. Massin P, Andren F, Haouchine B, et al. Intravitreal triamcinolone acetonide for diffuse macular edema. Ophthalmology 2004; 111: 218-225.
7. Young S, Larkin G, Branley M, Lightman S. Safety and efficacy of intravitreal triamcinolone for cystoid macular edema in uveitis. Clin Experiment Ophthalmol. 2001;29:2-6.
8. Castillo BD, Sanchez JM, Garcia Sanchez J. [Intravitreal injection of triamcinolone acetonide in non infectious uveitis] Arch Soc Esp Oftalmol. 2001;76:661-664.
9. Sonoda KH, Enaida H, Ueno A, et al. Pars plana vitrectomy assisted by triamcinolone acetonide for refractory uveitis: a case series study. Br J Ophthalmol. 2003;87:1010-1014.
10. Nelson ML, Tennant MT, Sivalingam A, et al. Infectious and presumed non-infectious endophthalmitis after intravitreal triamcinolone acetonide injection. Retina. 2003;23:686-691.
11. Roth DB, Chieh J, Spirn MJ, et al. Noninfectious endophthalmitis associated with intravitreal triamcinolone injection. Arch Ophthalmol. 2003;121:1279-1282.
12. Sutter FK, Gillies MC. Pseudo-endophthalmitis after intravitreal injection of triamcinolone. Br J Ophthalmol. 2003;87:972-974.
13. Jonas JB, Kreissig I, Degenring R. Intraocular pressure after intravitreal injection of triamcinolone acetonide. Br J Ophthalmol. 2003;87:24-27.
14. Beer PM, Bakri SJ, Singh RJ, Liu W, Peters GB 3rd, Miller M. Intraocular concentration and pharmacokinetics of triamcinolone acetonide after a single intravitreal injection. Ophthalmology. 2003;110:681-686.
15. Jonas JB, Kreissig I, Degenring RF. Endophthalmitis after intravitreal injection of triamcinolone acetonide. Arch Ophthalmol. 2003;121:1663-1664.
16. Sourdille P, Santiago PY. Optical coherence tomography of macular thickness after cataract surgery. J Cataract Refract Surg. 1999;25:256-261.
17. Voo I, Mavrofrides EC, Puliafito CA. Clinical applications of optical coherence tomography for the diagnosis and management of macular diseases. Ophthalmol Clin N Am 2004;17:21-31.
18. Maruyama Y, Kishi S. Tomographic features of serous retinal detachment in Vogt-Koyanagi Harada syndrome. Ophthalmic Surg Lasers Imaging. 2004;35: 239-242.
19. Okamoto Y, Miyake Y, Horio N, et al. Delayed regeneration of foveal cone photopigments in VKH at the convalescent stage. Invest Ophthalmol Vis Sci. 2004; 45:318-322.

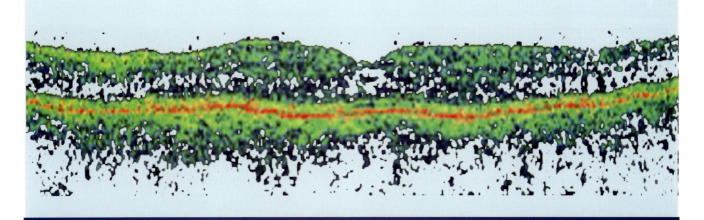

CHAPTER
22

Optic Disc Pit
Maculopathy

*Borja F Corcostegui, Max Motta,
Jose Garcia-Arumi, Carlos Mateo,
A Boixadera*

INTRODUCTION

Optic disc pits are a congenital depression oval or round within the nerve head. They are seen in association with other abnormalities of the optic nerve as well as of the retina around the disc. They are believed to develop secondary to a defect in the development of the primitive papilla, but some optic disc pits have been associated with colobomata lesions of optic nerve head and inferonasal retinal coloboma. They occur in less than 1/11000 patients[1] and are bilateral in 10-15% of cases, and men and women are equally affected.[2] Optic disc pits are normally sporadic, but rarely have they been seen to be related in an autosomal dominant pattern.[3]

About one third of optic disc pits are located centrally and two third eccentrically on the disc, but the majority are located on the temporal side. Pits have been observed to vary in depth and color. Around 60% are grey, 30% are yellow and 10% are black.[4] Their size can range from small to large occupying most of the facade of the optic disc. Some visual field defects have been described associated with optic disc pits. Arcuate scotoma is the most frequently one seen due of the absence of the wedge of nerve fibers displaced by the optic disc pit. Larger pits can be associated with sector defects extending from the disc or even altitudinal visual field defects. Nasal and temporal steps are often detectable. Less frequently seen are the paracentral scotomata and generalized constriction of the visual field.[2] Other visual field defect is that associated with the serous detachment of the macula.

Serous detachment of the macula is now known as a common complication of optic disc pits. Between 40% and 50% of patients with optic disc pits have either an associated nonrhegmatogenous serous retinal detachment or retinal changes suggestive of previous detachment.[2,5] The majority of the detachments are located in the macular region. Centrally located pits are normally not associated with detachment and appear more commonly when pits are located in the temporal region of the optic disc or in larger pits.[2] Serous detachments occurs most commonly in the second and third decades of life. Although spontaneous reattachment has been reported, most eyes with optic disc pits associated macular detachment have poor visual prognosis if left to the natural course.[6]

The origin of the fluid associated with optic disc pits remains unclear; several theories of the pathophysiology were reported. Leaked fluid occurs from the blood vessels around the pit, which then enters in the subretinal space.[5] Others have speculated that there may be a direct source of fluid from the choroid that penetrates through Bruch's membrane under subretinal space.[7] Others investigators have suggested that cerebrospinal fluid may leak from the optic nerve subarchanoid space into the optic pit, and from there into the subretinal space.[8,9] But currently, the most accepted explanation is that the fluid from the vitreous leaks through the optic pit to fill the subretinal space.[10,11] Regardless of the origin, however, it has been accepted, since Lincoff's report,[12] that the fluid initially enter in the retinal stroma, forming a schisis, and then reaches the subretinal space, creating a less extensive circumscribed detachment of the outer layer (Fig. 22.1).Optical coherence tomography (OCT) studies of this entity have confirmed the bilaminar structure of the macular detachment. OCT studies also help assess the anatomical results after the surgical treatment.

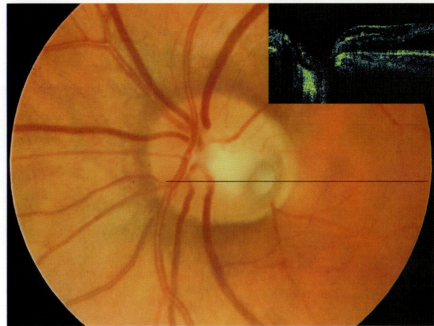

Fig. 22.1: Optical coherence tomography shows the optic pit as a deep and wide excavation within the optic nerve head. Cystoid changes and schisis cavity formation are seen in the inferior peripapillary retina affecting more than one retinal layer.

OPTICAL COHERENCE TOMOGRAPHY

Anatomical Findings

The OCT findings support the concept introduced by Lincoff [12] of a bilaminar structure. Probably a schisis-like cavity starts in the outer retina adjacent to the optic disc pit and extends to the fovea (Fig. 22.2). The schisis-like cavity mimics a true schisis cavity in some cases, although vertical retinal elements can be detected on the OCT in the inner retina. A degree of cystoid edema can be present in the inner retina. These findings are very similar to those shown histopathologically.[13] Initially, the schisis cavity has cystoid changes. They appear in the peripapillary retina adjacent to the pit and progress. Nerve fibers bridging the schisis allow synaptic transmission and permit a functional retina. Eventually schisis involves the macula and an inner macular transparent layer becomes persistent.

In retinal detachment, fluid may enter from the retinal stroma and not directly into the subretinal space. There is variability in the extension of the neurosensory macular retinal detachment and the cystoid changes. Some cases have small area of schisis-like cavity with a extensive retinal detachment (Fig. 22.3). In other cases schisis is prominent with a small detachment of neurosensory retina. Another feature seen is the presence of subretinal precipitates. They appear as small yellow foci of varying size located on the outer surface of the elevated retina. Optical coherence tomography shows a hyper reflectivity of these deposits which probably correspond to pigment-laden macrophages (Fig. 22.4).[8] In most of the cases we found no evidence of outer wall breaks in eyes with macular detachment. There are possibilities that the breaks are minute and the resolution of OCT cannot detect these breaks. In other eyes a lamellar hole has been detected in the outer retina (Fig. 22.5). The pseudohole is covered by a thin inner foveal tissue. Variability in the thickening of the central macula depends on the schisis-like extension in the fovea and the neurosensory

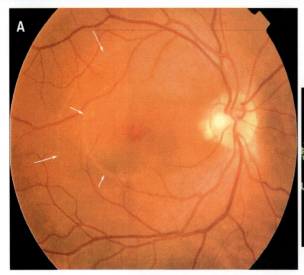

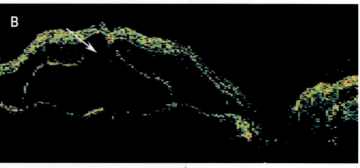

Fig. 22.2A: Limits of schisis lesion (long arrows) and retinal detachment (short arrows), in a case of optic pit maculopathy. An irregular laminar macular hole is present.

Fig. 22.2B: Optical coherence tomography shows clearly the neurosensory retinal detachment with a discontinuity (arrow), corresponding to an outer layer hole. A large schisis-like separation in the overlying and surrounding retina is present

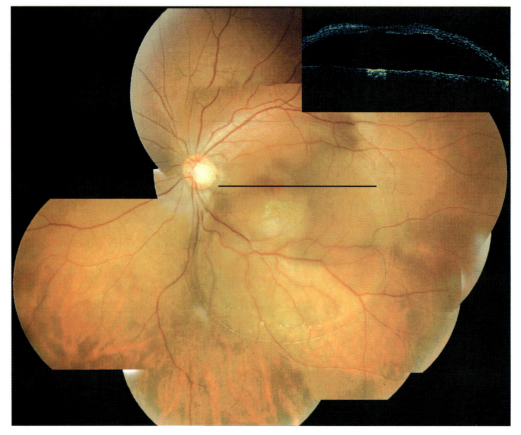

Fig. 22.3: Large retinal detachment in an optic disc pit. The OCT shows a large retinal detachment.

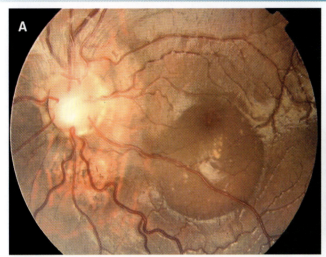

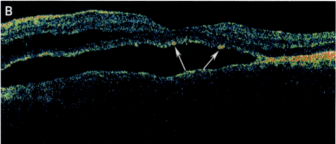

Fig. 22.4A: Retinal detachment in a patient with large optic pit or small coloboma of the optic nerve.

Fig. 22.4B: Optical coherence tomography show an inner layer separation, and an outer layer detachment. Hyper reflectivity dots are corresponding to the subretinal exudates (arrows).

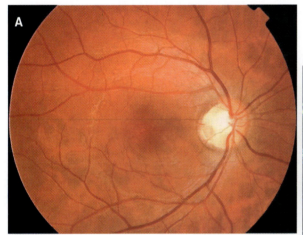

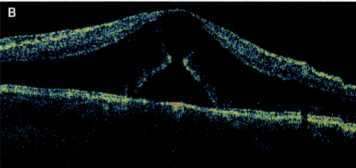

Fig. 22.5A: A dome-shaped retinal elevation is present in the macula. Fluid is in connection with an optic pit at the temporal side of the optic nerve head. A lamellar hole is present centrally with a small surrounding retinal detachment.

Fig. 22.5B: Vertical OCT scan through the fovea shows a neurosensory retinal detachment with overlying and surrounding outer edema.

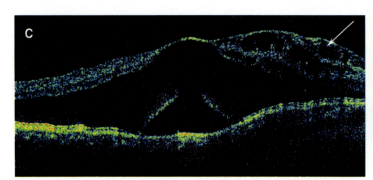

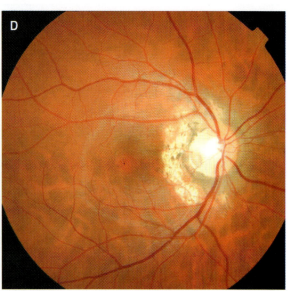

Fig. 22.5C: Horizontal OCT scan through the macula. The neurosensory retinal detachment shows a central discontinuity corresponding to an outer retinal layer hole. A large, schisis-like separation is present in the overlying and surrounding retina. Inner cystic appearances are present in the temporal retina close to the pit (arrow).

Fig. 22.5D: Three months postoperatively, the macula appears flat and the lamellar hole cannot be demarcated.

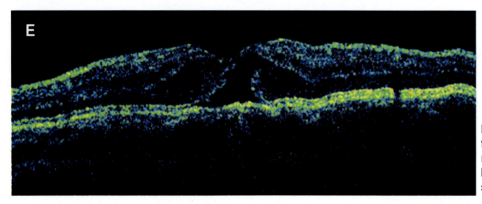

Fig. 22.5E: Horizontal OCT scan through the macula shows that the retinal elevation has diminished, but still persisting is the schisis and small outer-layer separation.

elevation from the retinal pigment epithelium. This thickening may range between 300 to 840 microns or more. Thickening can change with the evolution of morphology of the disease.

SURGICAL TREATMENT

Optical coherence tomography is a useful tool for monitoring the therapeutic effect for retinal detachment associated with optic disc pits. The visual prognosis in untreated cases is poor.[6] Various authors have reported the results of treatment with laser photocoagulation,[14,15] intravitreal gas injection [14,16,17] posterior scleral buckling,[18] and vitrectomy combined with laser and gas injection. [14,15,19-21] The best functional results seem to be achieved with vitrectomy, although some cases still persist or recur. Several reports have appeared on vitrectomy for treatment of optic pit maculopathy [14,15,19-21] with referred reattachment rates of around 80% and recurrence in 20% cases. The goal of the surgical technique used in these series was to release vitreous

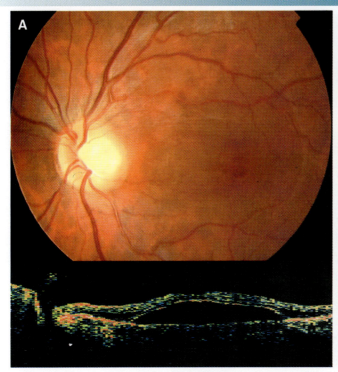

Fig. 22.6A: An optic pit disc and retinal detachment with a bilaminar appearance.

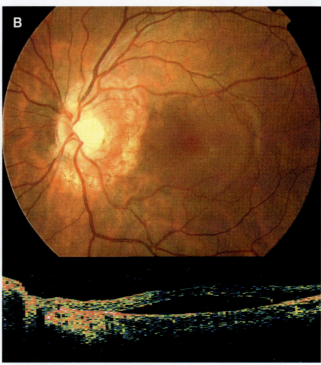

Fig. 22.6B: Some weeks after treatment subretinal fluid is persistent.

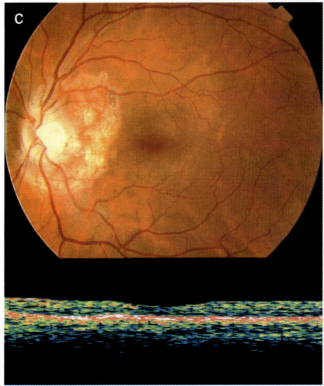

Fig. 22.6C: One year after surgical treatment the retina is totally reattached.

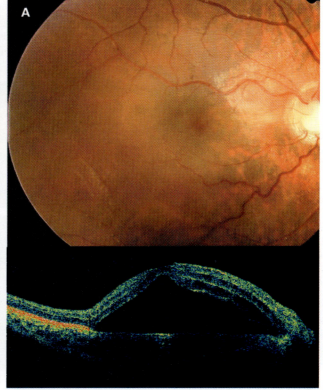

Fig. 22.7A: Large serous retinal detachment in a case of optic pit. Optical coherence tomography shows a retinal schisis and serous detachment.

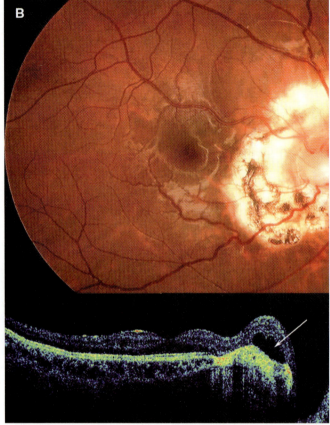

Fig. 22.7B: After surgery a scar is present avoiding the fluid pass to the subretinal space. Fluid is in the edge of the optic disc (arrow).

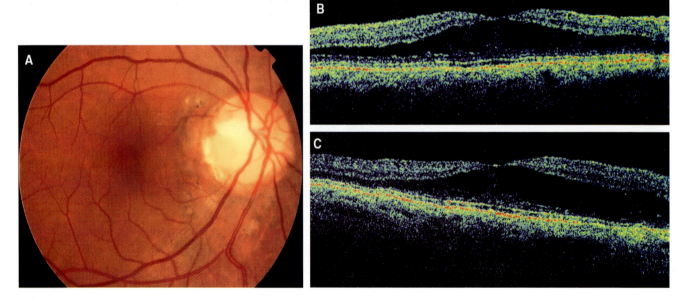

Figs 22.8A to C: A. Radiating retinal folds are seen in the inner retina after surgical treatment of optic disc pit. B. Vertical OCT shows diffuse thickness of the neurosensory retina. C. Horizontal OCT shows schisis separation present in connection with the optic pit disc, without serous retinal detachment. Visual acuity has been stable at 20/25 during the past three years.

traction and seal the communication between the pit and the adjacent inner retinal layers by compressing the retinal layers, using laser and gas tamponade creating an intraretinal scar, after laser photocoagulation around the disc. In most of the cases some subretinal fluid persists for a variable period of time after surgery. Optical coherence tomography can help in monitoring the macular elevation that resolves gradually (Figs 22.6 and 22.7). Increase in visual acuity coincides with the reabsortion of subretinal fluid [21] and the macula can regain its normal thickness. In some cases laser applications are unlikely to close the intraretinal cysts and fluid keeps on passing under the macula (Fig. 22.8), or to the subretinal space, and the visual acuity keeps on decreasing. A new treatment may be repeated with laser and gas compression, to create an adhesive barrier for fluid from the pit.

In some cases recurrence appears months or years after surgery. Optical coherence tomography has revealed a recurrence of a shallow neuroretinal elevation at the macular area and schisis cavities in the intraretinal space adjacent to the pit. Normally these findings are coincident with a diminished visual acuity. A new treatment with laser and gas normally closes the fluid pass. Using OCT, the cross-sectional structure of the affected retina can be viewed easily the actual retinal thickness can be measured objectively. Optical coherence tomography is a useful tool for monitoring the therapeutic effect of surgery.

REFERENCES

1. Kranenburg EW. Crater-like holes in the optic disc and central serous retinopathy. Arch Ophthalmol. 1960; 64:912-928.
2. Brown GC, Shields JA, Goldberg RE. Congenital pits of the optic nerve head. II. Clinical studies in humans. Ophthalmology. 1980; 87:51-65.
3. Slusher MM, Weaber RG, Greven CM, et al. The spectrum of cavitary optic disc anomalies in a family. Ophthalmology. 1989; 96:342-347.
4. Brown GC, Tasman WS. Congenital Anomalies of the Optic Disc, New York, Grune & Stratton 1983;97-127.
5. Gordon R, Chatfield RK. Pits in the optic disc associated with macular degeneration. Br J Ophthalmol. 1969;53:481-489.
6. Sobol WM, Blodi CF, Folk JC, Weingeist TA. Long-term visual outcome in patients with optic nerve pit disc and serous retinal detachment of the macula. Ophthalmology. 1990;97:1539-1542.
7. Wise G, Dollery C, Henkind P. The retinal circulation. New York, Harper & Row Publishers. 1971:471.
8. Gass JDM. Serous detachment of the macular secondary to congenital pit of the optic nerve head. Am J Ophthalmol.1969;67:821-841.
9. Irvine AR, Crawford JB, Sullivan JH. The pathogenesis of retinal detachment with morning glory disk and optic pit. Retina. 1986;6:146-150.
10. Sugar HS. Congenital pits in the optic disc with acquired macular pathology. Am J Ophthalmol. 1962;53:307-311.
11. Brockhurst RJ. Optic pits and posterior retinal detachment. Trans Am Ophthalmol Soc. 1975;73:264-291.
12. Lincoff H, Schiff W, Kreissig , et al. Retinoschisis associated with optic nerve pits. Arch Ophthalmol.1988;106:61-67.
13. Ferry AP. Macular detachment associated with congenital pit of the optic nerve head. Pathologic findings in two cases simulating malignant melanoma of the optic nerve head. Arch Ophthalmol. 1963;70:346-357.
14. Cox MS, Witherspoon CD, Morris RE, Flynn HW. Evolving techniques in the treatment of macular detachment caused by optic nerve pits. Ophthalmology. 1998;95:889-896.
15. Schatz H, McDonald HR. Treatment of sensory retinal detachment associated with optic nerve pit or coloboma. Ophthalmology. 1988; 95:178-186.
16. Lincoff H, Kreissig I. Optical coherence tomography of pneumatic displacement of optic disc pit maculopathy Br J Ophthalmol. 1998;82:367-372.
17. Lincoff H, Schiff W, Krivoy D, Ritch R. Optic coherence tomography of optic disk pit maculopathy. Am J Ophthalmol.1996;122:264-266.
18. Theodossiadis GP, Theodossiadis PG. Optical coherence tomography in optic disc maculopathy treated by macular buckling procedure. Am J Ophthalmol. 2001;132:184-190.
19. Snead MP, James N, Jacobs PM. Vitrectomy, argon laser, and gas tamponade for serous retinal detachment associated with an optic disc pit: a case report. Br J Ophthalmol. 1991;75:381-382.
20. Taiel-Sartral M, Mimoun G, Glacet-Bernard A, et al. Vitrectomy-laser-gas for treating optic disk pits complicated by serous macular detachment. J Fr Ophthalmol. 1996;19:603-609.
21. Garcia-Arumi J,Corcostegui B, Boixadera A, et al. Optical coherence tomography in optic pit maculopathy managed with vitrectomy-laser-gas. Graefe´s Arch Clin Exp Ophthalmol. 2004; 242:819-826.

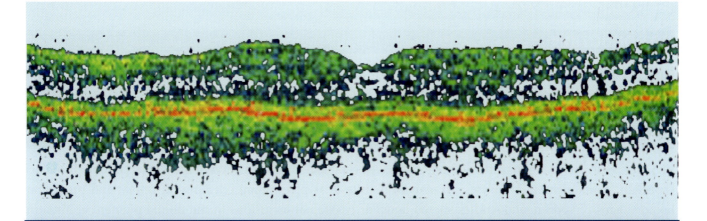

CHAPTER
23

Miscellaneous
Retinal Disorders

**Pradeep Venkatesh,
Parul Sony, Satpal Garg**

INTRODUCTION

Optical coherence tomography (OCT) is a useful diagnostic tool in the evaluation of a variety of retinal disorders.[1] This chapter discusses application of OCT in certain other clinical situations.

MACULAR INFARCTION

Retinal toxicity in form of macular infarction is a well established complication of intravitreal aminoglycosides especially gentamicin and amikacin. It usually manifests as pale retinal edema with retinal and pre-retinal hemorrhages. Experimental studies shown lamellar lysosomal inclusions in the retinal pigment epithelium as the earliest finding in such cases.[2] A sub-epithelial accumulation of amorphous and granular material, consistent with the morphologic features of hard drusen, and staining positively with periodic acid-Schiff, has also been reported.[2]

Optical Coherence Tomography

Ischemic retina has been shown exhibit hyper reflectivity on OCT.[3] In addition to this; fresh infarction may also show macular edema, with elevation of neurosensory retina, and accumulation of hyper-reflective material under the neurosensory retina.

Interesting Case Example

A fifty-one-year-old man presented with severe visual loss in the right eye. He had received intravitreal injection of 1000 μg vancomycin, 400 μg of amikacin and 400 μg of dexamethasone for post-cataract extraction endophthalmitis. He regained some peripheral field of vision but the central vision remained poor. At the time of presentation he had a BCVA of finger counting close to face in the right eye. The anterior chamber and the pupillary reactions were normal. There was no vitreous haze. Macular area had a pale edema, a cherry red spot, retinal hemorrhages and cotton wool spots along inferior vascular arcade (Fig. 23.1A). Peripheral retina was normal. OCT showed an increased macular thickness in the right eye (central foveal thickness 352 microns OD and 204 microns OS). There was hyper-reflectivity of the inner retinal layers, corresponding to the area of retinal pallor and edema. Neurosensory retina was elevated with accumulation of hyper-reflective material under the neurosensory retina. Loss of normal alternate layers of hyper-reflectivity that represent different layers of retina was also seen (Fig. 23.1B). At three month the BCVA improved to 20/200. Fundus showed resolution of macular edema and hemorrhages (Fig. 23.1C). Optical coherence tomography revealed persisting hyper-reflectivity in area of ischemic retina, with resolution of sub-neurosensory deposits (Fig. 23.1D).

SOLAR RETINOPATHY

Solar retinopathy is characterized by visual distortion in patients with history of sungazing or exposure to solar eclipse. Viewing of sun results in damage to the outer retinal layers. Fundus examination usually reveals a central yellow spot in early period after injury. Later this yellow spot is replaced by small sharply red lesion or a hypopigmented lesion with irregular margins. Fundus fluorescein angiography is usually unremarkable; but occasionally it may show window defect in the area of the lesion.

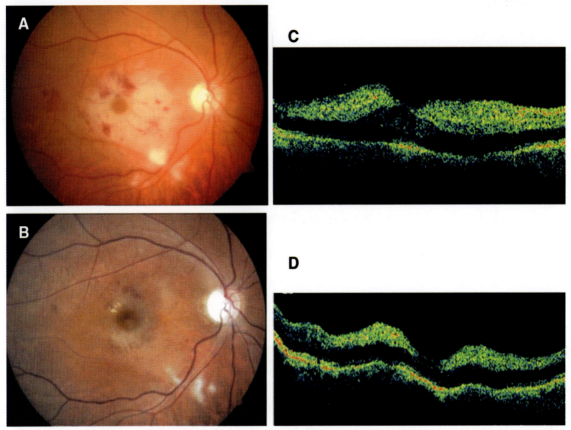

Figs 23.1A to D: A. Fundus photograph (Day 1) of right eye showing macular edema, and retinal hemorrhages. B. Fundus photograph (month 3) of right eye showing resolved macular edema, retinal hemorrhages and few cotton wool spots. C. OCT macular thickness map scan (Day 1) showing macular edema, with elevation of neurosensory retina, and accumulation of hyper-reflective material under the neurosensory retina. D. OCT macular thickness map scan (Month 3) showing partial resolution of macular edema, hyper-reflective ischemic retina and loss of normal alternate layers of hyper reflectivity.

Optical Coherence Tomography

Optical coherence tomography is helpful in delineating the exact site of injury *in vivo* in these eyes. Both early and late damage can be picked up with OCT.

- *Early changes*: OCT demonstrates hyper-reflectivity in all the foveal layers 48 hours after watching the solar eclipse. These changes generally disappear with-in a period of one week to one month.[4]
- *Late changes*: OCT in eyes with chronic solar retinopathy demonstrates selective retinal pigment epithelium and photoreceptor damage. OCT findings correlate well with the histological studies in solar retinopathy eyes. [5-7] OCT shows a normal and preserved foveal contour. A small hyporeflective/optically clear space is seen in the foveal region in the area corresponding to the outer photoreceptors and retinal pigment epithelium. [5-7] The remaining Retinal pigment epithelium is usually normal. A small area of hyper-reflectivity immediately adjacent to the clear area has also been described.[7] These findings represent the damaged photoreceptors and retinal pigment epithelium and may account for the visual complaints.

Interesting Case Examples

Case 1

A-40-years-old-male presented with bilateral diminution of vision for past 6 months. He had history of prolonged sun gazing. The best-corrected visual acuity was 20/40 OU. Fundus showed small hypopigmented foveal lesions OU (Fig. 23.2A and B). OCT revealed focal optically clear area in the outer hyper reflective layers corresponding to RPE-choriocapillaris complex and outer segments of photo receptors (Fig. 23.2C and D).

Case 2

A-16-year-old female presented with distorted vision in her left eye. She watched the solar eclipse with her left eye 6 months back. Fundus showed a small hypopigmented lesion in her left eye (Fig. 23.3A). Right eye was normal.

A small central optically clear area was seen on OCT, in the outer hyper reflective layers corresponding to RPE-choriocapillaries complex and outer segments of photo receptors. The area just adjacent to this showed mild hyper-reflectivity (Fig. 23.3B).

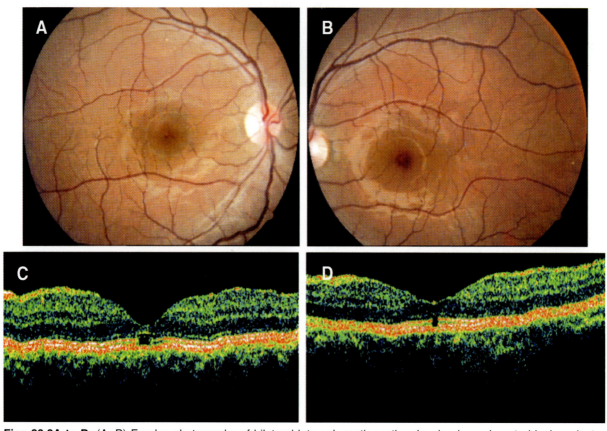

Figs 23.2A to D: (A, B) Fundus photographs of bilateral late solar retinopathy showing hypopigmeted lesions (outer lamellar macular hole) in both eyes. (C, D) OCT line scan showing optically clear area in the macular area corresponding to focal defect in retinal pigment epithelium and outer segment of retinal photoreceptors.

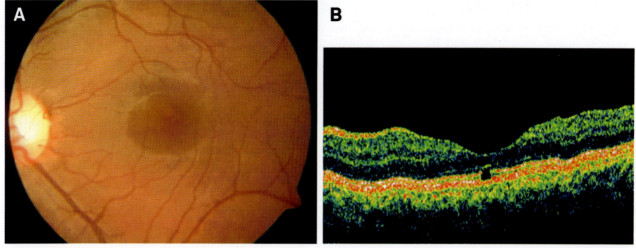

Figs 23.3A and B: A. Photographs of unilateral solar retinopathy showing a small hypopigmented lesion. B. OCT line scan showing optically clear area in the macular area corresponding to focal defect in Retinal pigment epithelium and outer segment of retinal photoreceptors.

BERLIN'S EDEMA

Commotio retina is characterized by acute retinal opacification and whitening following blunt trauma. A mild commotio retina present with transient visual loss and usually settles spontaneously with minimal sequelae. More severe cases may be associated with permanent visual loss.

In acute stage there is disruption of the outer segments of photoreceptors. This is followed by its phagocytosis by retinal pigment epithelium. Retinal pigment epithelium cells migrate onto retina by next 48 hours to reach the inner plexiform layer or the ganglion cell layer. Thus Retinal pigment epithelium may present as multilayered, disorganized structure on the Bruch's membrane with atrophy of outer segment seen as overlying neurosensory atrophy.

Optical Coherence Tomography

OCT is an effective tool in identifying post-traumatic retinal edema with definitive objectivity. Apart from the increase in the thickness of the involved area OCT shows other retinal alterations like changes in the reflectivity and contour of various retinal layers. OCT findings depend on the severity and the duration of commotio retinae.[8,9] Severe cases with extensive photoreceptor disruption show optically clear spaces in the area corresponding to the photoreceptors.[8] The major site of retinal trauma on OCT appears to be at the level of the photoreceptor outer segment/Retinal pigment epithelium interface. These changes generally disappear within few weeks. Delayed observation with OCT in these cases may demonstrate moderate increase in the reflectivity in the area corresponding to the photoreceptors probably representing the migrated Retinal pigment epithelium cells with disorganized overlying neuro-sensory retina.[20-21] Studies have shown that the OCT images are consistent with histological changes in commotio retinae which include fragmentation of photoreceptor outer segments and damaged cell bodies.[8,9]

Interesting Case Examples

Case 1

A-12-year-old-boy presented with acute vision loss in right eye following blunt trauma 1 week back. The BCVA was 20/200. Anterior segment was normal. Fundus showed severe commotio retinae with pale retina (Fig. 23.4A). He had superonasal retinal dialysis with vitreous base avulsion. Optical coherence tomography showed altered reflectivity in the area of photoreceptor outer segment. There was increased reflectivity in the inner layer of the retina as well probably representing the migrated Retinal pigment epithelium cells with disorganized overlying neurosensory retina. There were few small clear areas denoting extensive photoreceptor disruption (Fig. 23.4B). Foveal thickness was marginally increased when compared to the fellow normal eye.

Case 2

A-9-year-old-boy presented with poor vision in right eye following blunt trauma 1 year back. The BCVA was 10/200. Anterior segment was normal. Fundus showed pale disc with marked scarring and pigmentary changes at macula (Fig. 23.5A). Optical coherence tomography showed marked neurosensory atrophy with extensive RPE changes, (Fig. 23.5B). Foveal thickness was markedly decreased when compared to the fellow normal eye.

RETAINED INTRAOCULAR FOREIGN BODY

Optical coherence tomography may serve as a helpful tool in assessing the concurrent macular damage in a case of retained intraocular foreign body.[10] Metallic retained intraocular foreign body (RIOFB) is seen as

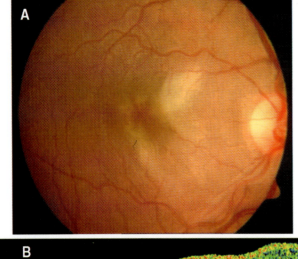

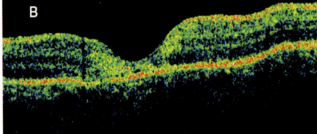

Fig. 23.4A and B: A. Fundus photograph showing pale retinal opacification with macular edema; B. OCT scan showing altered reflectivity in the area of photoreceptor outer segment with increased reflectivity in inner retina representing the migrated RPE cells.

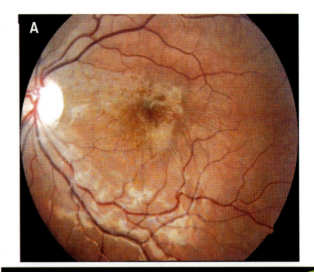

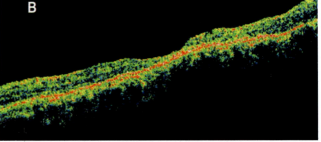

Fig. 23.5A and B: A. Fundus photograph showing old macular scar; B. OCT scan showing increased reflectivity with marked neurosensory atrophy.

area of hyper reflectivity with marked posterior shadowing. Occasionally attachment of posterior hyaloid (when thickened) or membranous tract may also be seen.

Optical Coherence Tomography

Postoperatively OCT helps in prognosticating the visual outcome by providing the structural details of macula and also the foreign body impaction site. The site of impaction is generally seen as intense and hyper reflective area following surgery; with complete loss of definition of various retinal layers on OCT scan.

In our series of ten eyes with retained intraocular foreign body (all the eyes had metallic RIOFB impacted in the posterior pole with a clear media) OCT revealed marked hyper reflectivity with posterior shadowing in the region of RIOFB.

Interesting Case Example

A 13-year-old boy presented with history of penetrating trauma to his right eye while working with chisel and hammer. His BCVA was 20/160. Fundus examination showed a metallic foreign body impacted superotemporal to the optic disc. There was mild dispersed vitreous hemorrhage (Fig. 23.6A). Optical coherence tomography showed intense reflectivity in the area of foreign body with marked posterior shadowing. Attachment of posterior hyaloid was visible at the edges of the foreign body (Fig. 23.6B). Adjacent retina showed mild edema. There were a few dot like hyper reflectivity signals in the vitreous

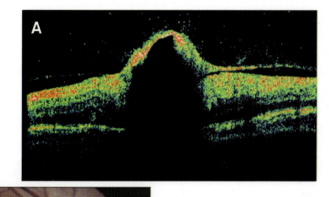

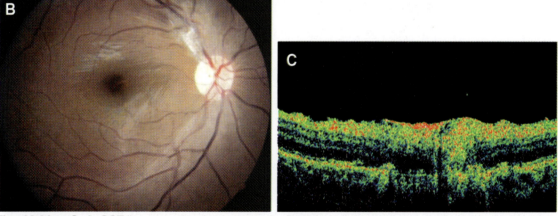

Figs 23.6A to C: A. OCT line scan showing increased reflectivity in the area corresponding to the foreign body with marked posterior shadowing. B Post-operative photograph showing scarring the area of foreign body, with epiretinal membrane formation; C. OCT showing increased reflectivity in the scar area.

cavity corresponding to mild dispersed vitreous bleed. Patient underwent pars plana vitrectomy with removal of foreign body. Follow-up OCT revealed a small epiretinal membrane with underlying scar of increased reflectivity (Fig. 23.6C).

SUBHYALOID HEMORRHAGE

Vitreous hemorrhage is not infrequently encountered after ocular trauma. Occasional subhyaloid hemorrhage may also occur. Hemorrhage results in high reflectivity with shadowing of the underlying layers in the Optical coherence tomography image. The shadowing is more severe with subhyaloid hemorrhage which is thick and dense. The OCT may be useful in differentiating subhyaloid hemorrhage from sub-Internal Limiting membrane hemorrhage.

Interesting Case Examples

Case1

A 11-year-old boy presented with diminution of vision in his right eye following a blunt trauma. Anterior segment was normal. Fundus examination a showed boat shaped subhyaloid hemorrhage (Fig. 23.7A). OCT demonstrated a dome shaped elevation of increased reflectivity. There was marked posterior shadowing. Attachment of thin membrane was seen at one edge suggesting the sub-internal limiting membrane location of the blood rather then a retrohyaloid bleed (Fig. 23.7B).

Case 2

A-41-year-old man presented poor vision for past three months in his right eye following a blunt trauma. Anterior segment was normal. Fundus examination showed an old pale subhyaloid hemorrhage in the right eye (Fig. 23.8A). Optical coherence tomography demonstrated a dome shaped elevation of increased reflectivity with marked posterior shadowing (Fig. 23.8B).

TRAUMATIC MACULAR HOLE

Optical Coherence Tomography

Optical coherence tomography demonstrates the detailed topography of traumatic macular hole. Various characteristics like elevation of the hole edges, cystoid changes at the margins, hole size, and changes at the base of the hole and associated retinal pigment epithelium changes can be better evaluated with OCT. Depending on the duration of trauma, the hole may exhibit elevated edges with cystoid changes in recent trauma. Optical coherence tomography of old macular holes usually demonstrate flat edges with associated neurosensory atrophy.

Interesting Case Example

A 29-year-old man presented with sudden diminution of vision in his left eye following a blunt trauma. The BCVA was 10/200. Anterior segment was normal. Fundus examination of the left eye revealed a full-thickness macular hole (Fig. 23.9A). Optical coherence tomography demonstrated a full thickness macular hole with cystoid changes at the edges of the hole (Fig. 23.9B). The patient underwent pars-plana vitrectomy

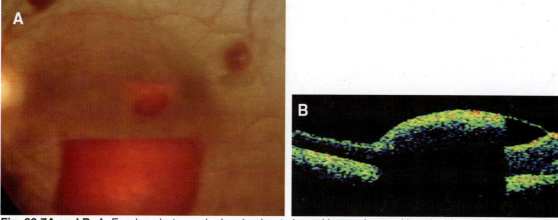

Fig. 23.7A and B: A. Fundus photograph showing boat shaped hemorrhage with retinal hemorrhages; B. OCT scan showing a sub-internal limiting membrane collection of blood seen as increased reflectivity and posterior shadowing.

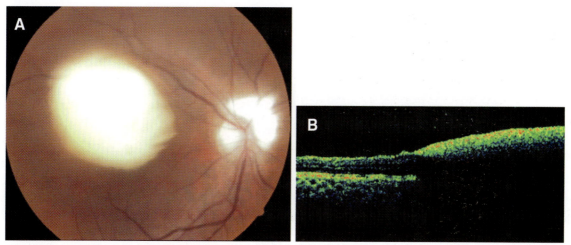

Fig. 23.8 A and B: A.Fundus photograph showing old pale colored round subhyaloid hemorrhage; B. OCT scan showing a sub-hyaloid collection of blood seen as increased reflectivity and posterior shadowing.

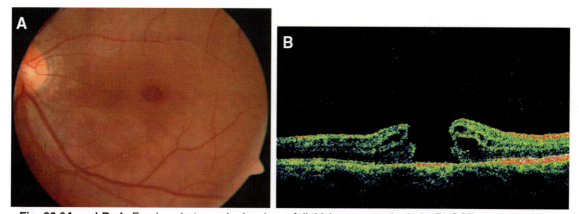

Fig. 23.9A and B: A. Fundus photograph showing a full thickness macular hole; B. OCT scan showing full thickness macular hole with cystoid changes at the edge.

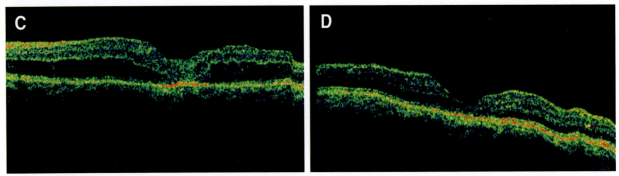

Fig. 23.9C and D: C. OCT scan showing closed macular hole with intraretinal edema (2 weeks) following pars plana vitrectomy and ILM peeling; D. OCT scan showing closed hole with resolution of macular edema (6 weeks post-operative)

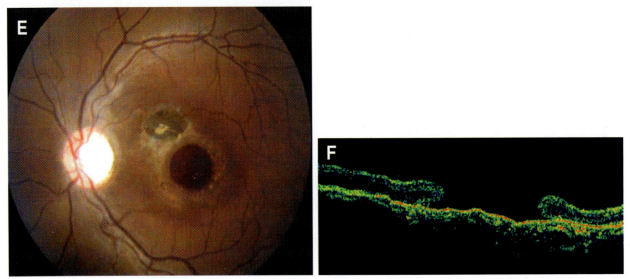

Fig. 23.9E and F: E. Fundus photograph showing an old full thickness macular hole; F. OCT scan showing a full thickness macular hole with flat edges with marked neurosensory atrophy.

with ILM peeling. At 2 weeks post-surgery the visual acuity was 20/200 and fundus examination demonstrated clinical closure of macular hole.

Optical coherence tomography confirmed closure of the hole however marked intraretinal edema was seen (Fig. 23.9C). At 6 weeks follow-up the visual acuity improved to 20/100 with resolution of intraretinal edema on OCT (Fig. 23.9D).

ELECTRIC BURNS

Trauma to ocular tissue following high voltage electric current injury is well documented. Current traveling through retinal pigment epithelium is converted into heat and destroys the overlying retina. Macular manifestations include macular edema, macular cyst, and full thickness macular hole.

Optical Coherence Tomography

Optical coherence tomography imaging is valuable in such cases and may clearly depict the retinal involvement in form of cystoid macular edema, macular hole or a macular cyst. Macular cysts may simulate a full thickness macular hole clinically and the OCT can easily differentiate intra-retinal macular cysts from full thickness macular hole. It has been suggested that these cysts may undergo spontaneous resolution with improvement in visual acuity. Therefore, OCT helps in providing an initial conclusive diagnosis in these cases and may obviate the need of early surgical intervention.

Interesting Case Example

A 28-year-old-man presented with bilateral acute loss of vision 3 months back following a high voltage injury. Visual acuity was 20/200 right eye and 20/120 in the left eye. Anterior segment was normal. On Watzke-Allen testing he described narrowing of light beam bilaterally. Fundus of the right eye had a well-defined round lesion resembling a full thickness macular hole, with yellowish deposits at the center. Left eye had yellow deposits in the macular area (Fig. 23.10A and B).

Optical coherence tomography showed bilateral macular cysts larger in the right eye, without any surrounding edema. The outer and inner retinal layers were intact. Six months later the patient had BCVA of 20/200 OD and 20/40 OS. Fundus picture was similar to the initial presentation. OCT showed a persistent macular cyst in the OD. Left eye showed a spontaneous resolution of the macular cyst (Figs 23.10 C to F).

MEDULLATED RETINAL NERVE FIBERS

Optical Coherence Tomography

Medullated nerve fibers are seen as area of increased reflectivity with posterior shadowing on peripapillary retinal nerve fiber layer scan. Retinal nerve fiber layer thickness analysis shows increased values in the corresponding area. We performed OCT in seven patients with medullated retinal nerve fiber layer. All the eyes showed marked increase in the thickness and reflectivity signal in the retinal nerve layer of OCT scan along with posterior shadowing, in the area corresponding to the area of involvement.

Interesting Case Example

A 35-year-old female reported to the outpatient department. Her unaided visual acuity was 20/63 OU. With refraction she improved to 20/20 OU. Dilated fundus examination of the right eye revealed myelinated nerve fibers around the optic nerve head (Figs 23.11A and B). A fast retinal nerve fiber layer scan centered on to the optic nerve head showed an area of increased reflectivity at the level of the nerve fiber layer, in the region correlating with the myelinated fibers. There was marked shadowing below the area of hyper-reflectivity (Figs 23.11C and D).

PSEUDOPHAKIC MACULAR EDEMA

Incidence of postoperative cystoid macular edema (CME) has gone down with advent of phacoemulsification and better medical care. However it may still be encountered following an intraocular surgery, and cataract extraction still remains the most common cause for postoperative CME. The diagnosis of CME is based on fundus examination and confirmed by fluorescein angiography.

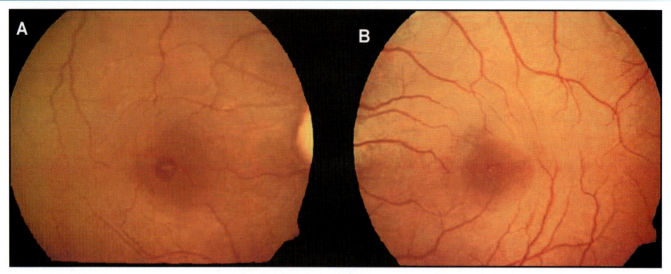

Fig. 23.10A and B: Fundus photographs (a) showing macular lesion simulating full thickness macular hole in the right eye and (b) yellow macular deposits in the left eye.

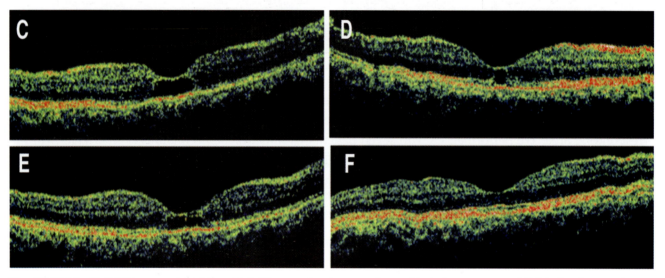

Figs 23.10C to F: OCT images right (c) and left (d) eyes showing macular cyst in both eyes; repeat OCT showing persistence of macular cyst in the right eye (e) and spontaneous resolution of macular cyst in the left eye (f).

Optical Coherence Tomography

Optical coherence tomography has a very important application in evaluation and management of patients with CME of varied origin.[11,12] Optical coherence tomography is a very effective modality for confirmation of CME with distinct advantages of being a noninvasive and a quick technique.

Cystoid macular edema is seen as intraretinal cystic cavities which are optically clear or possess very low reflectivity and associated increased macular thickness. An OCT enables exact quantitative assessment of macular edema in terms of increased macular thickness and volume parameters. These parameters can be used to decide the mode of treatment and also to monitor the effect of intervention with good precision. [11,12]

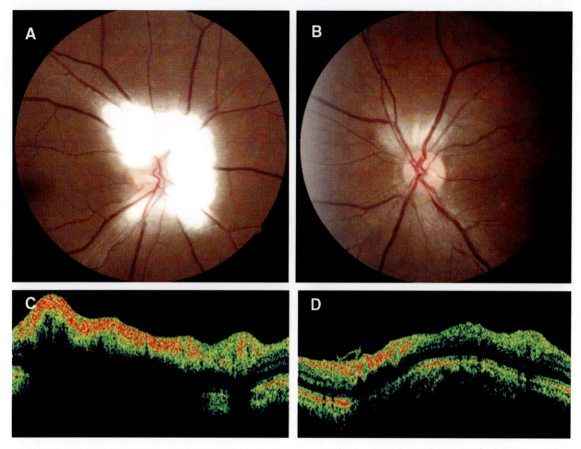

Figs 23.11A to D: (A, B) Fundus photograph showing bilateral medullated retinal nerve fibers more extensive in the right eye. (C,D) Peripapillary retinal nerve fiber layer scan showing marked increase in reflectivity with posterior shadowing in the area corresponding to the medullated nerve fibers.

Interesting Case Examples

Case 1

A 45-year-old presented with complaints of poor visual recovery following an uncomplicated phacoemulsification 2 weeks back. Her visual acuity was 20/100 in the right eye. Fundus examination showed a cystoid macular edema (Fig. 23.12A). An OCT scan revealed increased retinal thickness in the right eye compared to the fellow eye with large optically clear cystoid spaces (Fig. 23.12B). The patient received a subtenon injection of 20 mg triamcinolone following which the visual acuity improved to 20/50 with no evidence of macular edema clinically or on OCT (Fig. 23.12C).

Case 2

A 55-year-old presented with poor visual recovery following an uncomplicated phacoemulsification 1week back. The BCVA was visual acuity was 20/240 in the right eye. Fundus examination showed a cystoid macular edema. OCT imaging revealed increased retinal thickness in the right eye with large optically clear cystoid spaces, subretinal fluid collection with a thin strip of bridging tissue (Fig. 23.13A). Following a subtenon injection of triamcinolone the visual acuity improved to 20/160, however the OCT imaging showed mild decrease in the cystoid spaces with conversion to a full thickness defect (Fig. 23.13B).

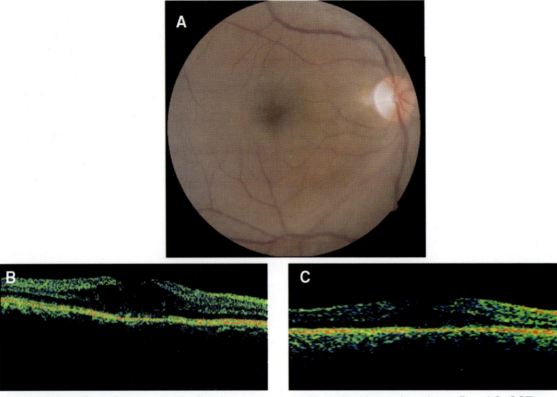

Figs 23.12A to C: A. Fundus photograph showing postoperative cystoid macular edema. B and C. OCT scan showing increased macular thickness with cystoid cavities; c) marked resolution of cystoid space with decrease in macular thickness following subtenon tricort injection.

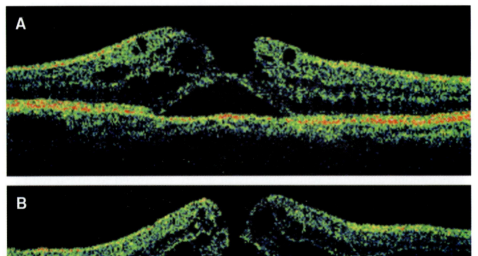

Figs 23.13A and B: A. OCT scan showing increased macular thickness with cystoid cavities with thin bridging tissue with small area of subretinal fluid collection; B. OCT scan showing conversion to full thickness defect with persistence of cystoid spaces following subtenon tricort injection.

REFERENCES

1. Puliafito CA, Hee MR, Lin CP, et al. Imaging of macular diseases with optical coherence tomography. Ophthalmology 1995;102:217-229.
2. Tabatabay CA, D'Amico DJ, Hanninen LA, Kenyon KR. Experimental drusen formation induced by intravitreal aminoglycoside injection. Arch Ophthalmol. 1987;105:826-830.
3. Gupta V, Gupta A, Dogra MR. Retinal vascular occlusions. In: Gupta V, Gupta A, Dogra MR eds. Atlas. Optical coherence tomography of macular disorders. Jaypee New Delhi. First edition 2004 p103-105.
4. Bechmann M, Ehrt O, Thiel MJ et al. Optical coherence tomography findings in early solar retinopathy. Am J Ophthalmol. 2000;84:546-547.
5. Jorge R, Costa RA, Quirino L S et al. Optical coherence tomography in patients with late solar retinopathy. Am J Ophthalmol. 2004:137:1139-1142.
6. Garg S, Martidis A, Nelson ML, Sivalingam A. Optical coherence tomography of chronic solar retinopathy. Am J Ophthalmol. 2004;137:351-354.
7. Kaushik S, Gupta V, Gupta A. Optical coherence tomography findings in solar retinopathy. Ophthalmic Surg Lasers Imaging. 2004;35:52-55.
8. Ismail R, Tanner V, Wiliamson S. Optical coherence tomography imaging of severe commotio retinae and associated macular hole. Br J Ophthalmol. 2002;86:473-474.
9. Meyer CH, Rodrigues EB, Mennel S. Acute commotion retinae determination by cross-sectional Optical coherence tomography. Eur J Ophthalmol. 2003;13: 816-818.
10. Pal N, Azad RV, Sony P, Chandra P. Localization of retained intraocular foreign body with optical coherence tomography. Eye. 2004;3.
11. Hee MR, Puliafito CA, Wong C, et al. Quantitative assessment of macular edema with optical coherence tomography. Arch Ophthalmol 1995;113:1019-1029.
12. Nelson ML, Martidis A. Managing cystoid macular edema after cataract surgery. Curr Opin Ophthalmol. 2003;14:39-43.

INDEX